Emergency Ambulance Driving

Bradford J. Childs & Donald J. Ptacnik

Library of Congress Cataloging in Publication Data

Childs, Bradford J.
Emergency ambulance driving.

Includes index.
1. Ambulance driving. I. Ptacnik, Donald J.
II. Title. [DNLM: 1. Allied Health Personnel.
2. Ambulances. 3. Automobile Driving. 4. Emergency
Medical Services. WX 215 C537e]
TL152.5.C48 1986 629.28'3234 85-5710
ISBN 0-89303-427-4

Production Editor/Text Designer: Leonard Blasso
Production Manager: Paula Huber
Art Director: Bernard Vervin
Manufacturing Director: John Komsa

Printed in the United States of America

1 2 3 4 5 6 7 8 9 10

ISBN 0-89303-427-4

Prentice-Hall of Australia, Pty., Ltd., Sydney
Prentice-Hall Canada, Inc., Scarborough, Ontario
Prentice-Hall Hispanoamericana, S.A., Mexico
Prentice-Hall of India Private Limited, New Delhi
Prentice-Hall International (UK) Limited, London
Prentice-Hall of Japan, Inc., Tokyo
Prentice-Hall of Southeast Asia Pte. Ltd., Singapore
Editora Prentice-Hall Do Brasil LTDA., Rio de Janeiro
Whitehall Books, Limited, Petone, New Zealand

Contents

About the Authors

Brad Childs, an Oregon-certified EMT III, has been involved in EMS since 1971, when he became an EMT and took a position with Medical Services, Inc. the ambulance provider in Eugene, Oregon at that time. Mr. Childs's involvement with emergency ambulance driving instruction has continued since 1973, when he was appointed driver trainer. In 1974, he was placed in charge of all training for the company, a position he held until 1981. Mr. Childs attended the Center for Driver Education and Safety at St. Cloud State University in St. Cloud, Minnesota, in 1979 where he became certified as an Advanced Driving Techniques Instructor. He has taught extensively on many subjects concerning EMS and has spoken at various conferences. In July of 1982, he became nationally recognized for his expertise in the field of emergency ambulance driving with the introduction of his regular column, *Rules of the Road,* which appeared for two years in *jems* (Journal of Emergency Medical Services).

Mr. Childs makes his home near Eugene, Oregon, where he divides his time between working actively on an ambulance for Medic-4 in Roseburg, as a consultant and instructor with Don Ptacnik's EMS Consulting, and as Lieutenant in charge of EMS with the Pleasant Hill Volunteer Fire Department. He is married and has two children.

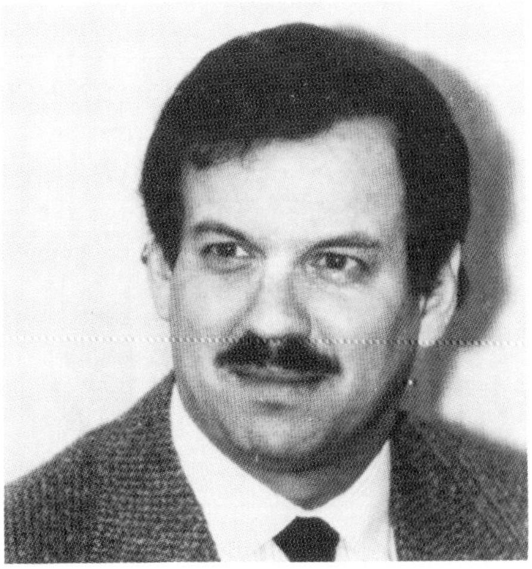

Involved in pre-hospital care since 1972, Don Ptacnik has acted as an emergency medical technician, an EMS instructor and an EMS educational consultant for the Oregon State Health Division. Since 1975 he has been a part-time instructor at the Central Oregon Community College where he provides students with a knowledge of the functions of the emergency medical care team and public safety agencies. An Oregon State-Certified EMT instructor, Mt. Ptacnik is a member of the National EMT Instructor Coordinator's Society, the National Society of EMS Administrators, and is the Communications Officer of the Paramedics Society of the National Association of EMTs. He has been a lecturer at many state and national EMS education conferences.

Don Ptacnik has two other EMS books to his credit and is a regular columnist for the National Association of EMTs' Quarterly Newsletter. He was officially recognized for his services in 1981 when the Oregon State EMT Association presented him with the EMS Service Award, the highest EMS award given in Oregon. Currently a nationally registered EMT and an Oregon-certified EMT II, Mr. Ptacnik is owner of EMS Consulting, a nationally based consulting firm offering services in EMS system development, public and industrial safety, education, and management.

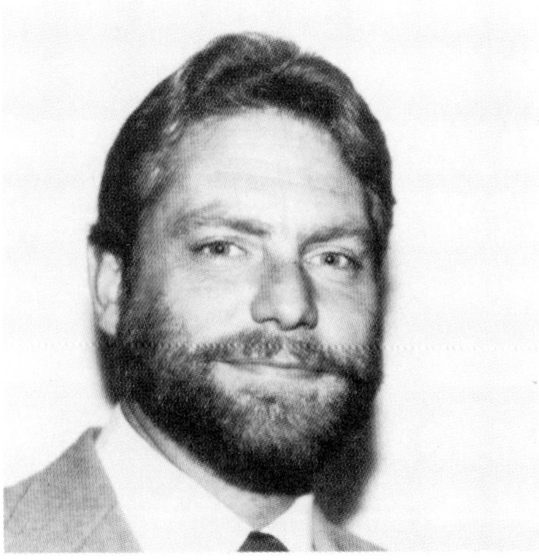

Acknowledgments

Writing a book, especially a technical one, cannot be done by one or two people. What doesn't show up on the title page is a large support team hiding somewhere behind the authors. Their involvement must, however, be acknowledged. In the case of this book there were several people who were a tremendous help to both Don and myself. Some were an asset to the development of the book in general, others showed their support to us as individuals. To include each, we decided each of us would provide our own thanks.

For my part a special thanks is deserved by Jim Huckstep, longtime ambulance fleet mechanic and, on occasion, builder of specialized units. Jim was always available to educate us, field questions, and proofread copy with an expert's eye for accuracy. Truly invaluable help.

Jon Jenkins too must receive special thanks. It was he who first taught me to drive an ambulance and through the years has provided me with a wealth of insight and knowledge. Jon originally compiled much of the material presented in this book for use in an in-house training manual. Later he turned the project over to me.

Dave Schultz of the St. Cloud State University Center for Drivers Education and Safety also deserves special attention. He was the instructor to the instructor and always available to answer technical questions and guide us over very technical material.

The book also could not have made it if not for the help and understanding of those fellow employees at Medic/4 who were so understanding while the book was being written. They filled in on occasion washing dishes and the ambulance without me so the manuscript could go forward. They were my sounding board for ideas and frustration. Many became involved from time to time but three must be singled out for service above and beyond the call of duty. They were, at various times throughout the long process, my regular partners; Patrice Coate, Mike Winkler, and J.D. Berlingeri.

The fire departments of Springfield, Eugene and Bend, Oregon, were gracious enough to allow us to ride along, photographing their equipment and personnel.

I have saved the one most valuable to me for last; my wife and greatest champion Debbie Childs. Forced to put up with endless hours of discussion about driving, her support and encouragement never wavered.

There were many other friends too, patient enough to listen, offering support and taking an interest in the project. Although they are too numerous to mention, each had a vital part in the final outcome.

Brad Childs
Springfield, Oregon

Acknowledgments

When an author sits down to write what is called the "front matter" of a book, he or she is faced with a very emotional, personal task. You want to include everyone possible . . . but you never can quite get everybody's name who really helped in the book. I'll try by starting with the folks that talked me into co-authoring this text. Chuck Mondin, Claire Merrick, and Rick Weimer—all of the Brady company. Once they succeeded, Joanne Haworth, Paula Huber and Len Blasso of Brady ably kept Brad and me apprised of every step . . . up and sometimes down.

My secretaries, Barbara Finley and Joyce Brewer, dealt with the incredible mess Brad and I called a manuscript. Your professionalism, patience, and friendships are truly appreciated.

The City of Bend, Oregon, its Fire Department, Firemedics, and Officers—all were extremely cooperative, giving up both city time and some laid-back Sunday shifts for photo sessions. Thanks, guys. Oh, I think I just heard three bells! Drive safely.

Vern Bartley, Bend Firemedic and a professional photographer, earned a special thanks. He helped me, a neophyte photographer, compose many of the shots seen in this text.

Leonard C. Parker, J.D., legal counsel and close friend—thanks for your assistance with Chapter 2. Kathy West, R.N., B.S.N., was kind enough to contribute to our text's appendix. Len Swanzy, along with Jim Huckstep, also gave mechanical advice for Chapter 1.

A special thanks is given to some really close friends that, once again, chose to pull the load with me. Tom Burton; Margaret McMicken, M.S.; Chuck Peterson; T. J. Ward, J.D.; and my daughter, Rose—don't know what I'd do without your support. Guess I'd just be a madman in a pickup truck trying to get it on paper and then trying to make some sense of it all. That seems to be the big key . . . and then chapters would turn into books.

Thanks, Jimmy B.

Don Ptacnik
Bend, Oregon

Preface

The term "ambulance driver," commonly used by society until recently, fortunately has fallen into general disuse. Because it oversimplifies the task of the EMT and EMT-Paramedic, the term is generally viewed by EMS personnel as degrading. After all, EMTs now render highly technical medical care. However, in their haste to rid themselves of such a limiting label, EMTs and EMT-Paramedics may have forgotten one of the primary functions of the job—transportation of the sick and injured.

The act of driving the ambulance is more than just an activity which gets the patient from the scene to the hospital. Proper ambulance driving is, in fact, an extremely important component of the actual care of the patient. Driving can get the patient to the hospital safely, quickly, and with a minimum of discomfort while allowing medical care to continue. On the other hand, it can also be done in a treacherous, unsafe manner which causes the patient greater discomfort, perhaps even further injury, and leaves the crewperson attending the patient holding on for dear life instead of continuing patient care.

After observing ambulance driving for the past several years, we have become concerned that the training required of many EMS personnel—before they are placed behind the wheel of an ambulance—is not on a par with the rest of their training. Proper driving requires education and practice just as any other skill. However, society has never required suitable education for those who drive. Most people view driving as a right rather than an earned privilege. This results in a societal attitude that "*everyone* knows how to drive." Such an attitude is often carried into the EMS profession even though the act of driving an ambulance entails greater responsibility and skills than those of the average driver. As a result, EMS agencies have not given as much attention to driving skills as they have to prehospital medical skills.

In many cases, ambulance driver education was better several years ago than it is today. At that time, most ambulance services were privately owned. The owner of the ambulance certainly did not want his shiny coach-type vehicle wrecked. Since few knew how to care for the patient anyway, the senior person drove. This policy allowed the new employee a chance to learn alongside someone who had most likely been around for a while. This policy also helped the new attendant to get over those "adrenalin rushes" that affect people lacking field experience. Today the roles are usually reversed. We are now better oriented to the medical attention required by the patient and able to render that care. With this advance, the new EMT will often be assigned to drive while the senior EMT continues to care for the patient being transported. Unfortunately, all too often there isn't adequate driver training available for the new driver.

Prehospital medical technology and continual training have moved emergency medicine to new heights since the early 1970s. This text is intended to bring the driving component of the EMT's job to a level similar to that medical education. To accomplish this, we must examine the overall aspects of driving. Just as basic CPR is a vital component of advanced life support, before a successful emergency run or a proper patient ride can be delivered, the EMT or EMT-Paramedic must have a thorough knowledge of the basics of driving, the dynamics that affect the vehicle's control and the laws governing ambulance operation. It is the intent of the authors to deal with all aspects of driving and not just those specific to ambulance operation. Certainly any vehicle operator will have acquired much of the material covered within the text. However, it is uncertain how much an individual driver obtains or retains since there is no standardized training available. For this reason, we felt compelled to include as much pertinent information as possible.

Unfortunately, there are those in EMS who seem to be in it for the excitement and power they perceive their position gives them. They might use the lights and siren, not out of the necessity to progressively move traffic from their path, but to bully their way through traffic, often intimidating others with a sudden blast of the siren at short distances. Such a person can be seen transporting the most stable of patients to the hospital with at least the emergency lights, if not the siren, activated. By offering an alternative method of driving, which allows for a faster and safer response to calls, we may be better able to rein in those who would abuse the privilege.

The text is intended for use by anyone in the prehospital emergency medical field, and while writing it, we tried hard to meet that end. We recognize and welcome the growing involvement of women in the ranks of EMTs and EMT-Paramedics and were very concerned they be included in this book. Unfortunately, it is difficult to write so extensively without occasionally using the male gender to refer to both men and women. While the variance "he/she" can be used, it does become cumbersome. We acknowledge this deficiency and apologize since we intend the text to be all-inclusive.

We also recognized that the laws governing the operation of emergency vehicles vary from state to state. The legal information offered within the text is intended to be used only as general guidelines. For this reason, we strongly advise all EMS personnel to become familiar with the specific laws governing emergency vehicle operation within their jurisdiction.

It is, then, the purpose of this text to give those charged with the responsibility of driving an ambulance a sense of the right and wrong way of doing the job, and to bring that level of the profession up to the same level as the current prehospital medical care standards. We do this by presenting methods that may make the task easier, safer, and more professional.

Dedication

Many of the recollections I have, even going back to my early childhood, are of riding beside my father as he drove the ambulance. It was his guiding influence that led me into emergency medicine. For that reason I dedicate this book to my father, Charles Childs.

Brad Childs

To Chief W. H. "Spike" Durfee, father of rural EMS Systems development and a trusted mentor.

Don Ptacnik

1 YOU AND YOUR VEHICLE

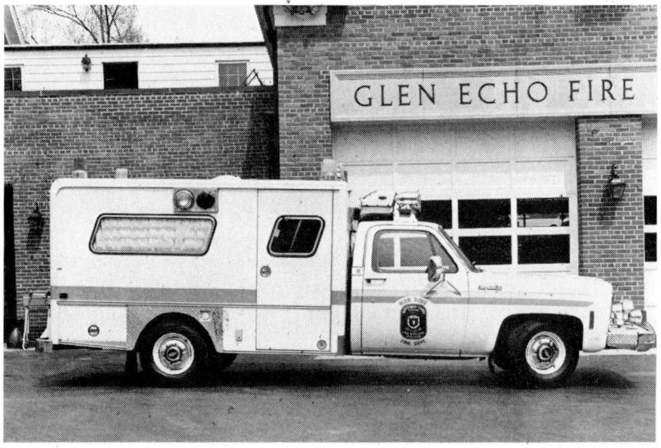

There is more to emergency driving than just climbing into a vehicle and driving away. In today's traffic, it is essential for the operator to be familiar with the vehicle to the point that he or she knows exactly how it will respond in a given situation and with a given driver action. To operate a vehicle with the utmost safety, one must become a part of the unit. The driver must be positioned securely where he can work all of the controls and see most efficiently. Many accidents are caused by an operator's unfamiliarity with the vehicle or because he can't exert proper control over it.

Emergency vehicles are routinely driven at variance to other traffic, a situation that requires confidence in the vehicle and dependence on its efficient operation. Lives depend on the ambulance arriving at the scene and then being able to get to the hospital safely.

Since accidents also happen because the vehicle malfunctions, or at the least functions inefficiently,the operator must also make sure that the equipment is mechanically sound. Most malfunctions can be avoided if the operator has a routine system of inspecting the vehicle and providing preventive maintenance.

Ambulances receive more abuse than most other vehicles. Consider how they must respond instantly, without time for a proper warm-up or even the chance for the engine oil to begin circulating and then the long periods of time the machine sits idling at the scene. The importance of a sound vehicle becomes clear. Reliability can only be accomplished by routine inspection and preventive maintenance.

Vehicle Inspection

Daily Inspection

The condition of a mechanical system such as an ambulance can change rapidly, and little problems can quickly become big ones. With the abuse an ambulance routinely receives, the chance of malfunction becomes greater. The only way the vehicle's ability to work properly can be guaranteed is for it to be inspected daily. While it is easy for an ambulance driver to assume the previous shift left a properly functioning vehicle, the responsibility for that vehicle's availability, operation, reliability, and safety lies with the present operator. The oncoming shift must complete a proper daily inspection.

Problems found while performing the daily inspection may require immediate attention and may force the vehicle to be taken off-line. Other problems may only require careful notation so they can be corrected in a timely manner.

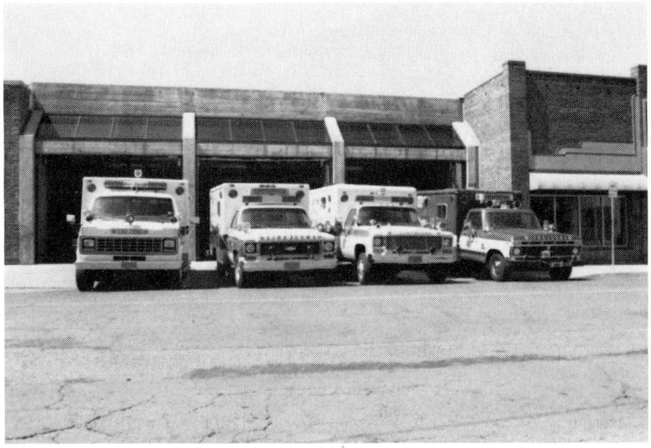

Fig. 1.1 Typical fleet of Vehicles at Station.

The daily vehicle inspection should be done as soon after the shift starts as practical, but during a time that is as free of interruption as possible.

Operators of large ambulance fleets may choose to stagger the times at which crew changes occur. This time difference combined with good dispatch techniques can allow for the completion of calls in progress and sufficient time for vehicle inspection without creating a backlog of calls.

The daily vehicle inspection has five components. The inspection begins with approaching the vehicle, followed by checking under the hood, entering the vehicle, and circling the vehicle. It ends with a drive. The inspection should progress in an orderly fashion with a check list available to assure that nothing is missed. (A typical daily vehicle inspection sheet can be found in the Appendix.)

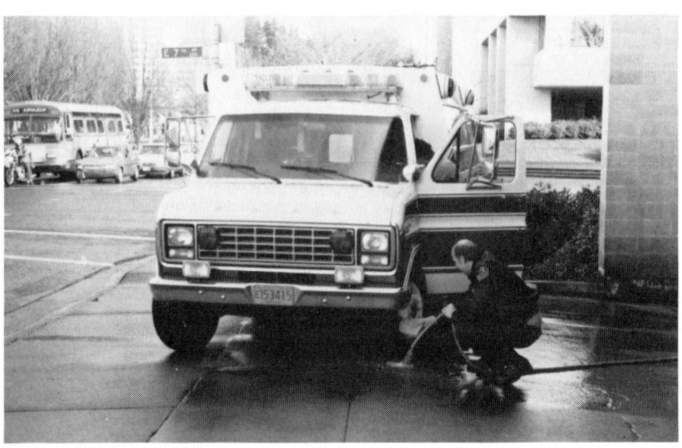

Fig. 1.2 To maintain a Public image as Professionals, a squad should have a clean unit.

Approaching the Vehicle

The inspection of the vehicle begins as you first walk up to it. How is it sitting? Is it level? If not, it may have a broken suspension component, or a flat tire. Are there any fluids under or around the vehicle? A puddle of fluid under it may be something minor such as the air conditioner defrosting. A puddle might also be leaking engine coolant, gasoline, or oil. Note if the ambulance is clean. It is important for the public's perception of you as a professional, as well as your service, to have a clean unit. Also look for any other obvious problems such as dents or loose body parts.

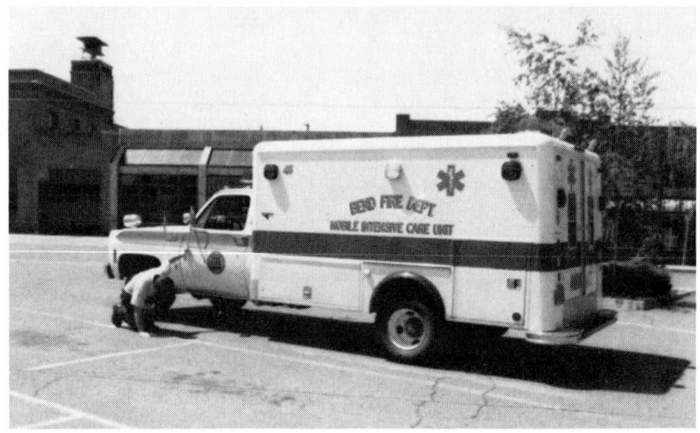

Fig. 1.3 Vehicle inspection starts with the approach. Is it level? are there any fluids under or around it?

Under the Hood

The best time to check under the hood is when the engine is cold. All fluids are in their reservoir, and the engine is cool enough to work around. If the engine has been running, allow at least 15 minutes after it has been shut off before starting the inspection to allow for the oil to drain back into the pan. While under the hood the following should be checked, working from one side of the engine compartment to the other:

Oil. The oil dipstick should be fully seated in its holder before it is withdrawn. Oil should appear between the full mark and the add mark. Since the oil pan carries a surplus, it is not necessary to keep the level right up to the full mark. Overfill may cause oil to be whipped into a froth by the crankshaft. This action causes air bubbles to get into the lubrication system reducing oil pressure and lubrication. Excess oil is usually thrown off by the engine.

Oil can give several different signs indicating a need for replacement. If the engine oil or transmission fluid has a gritty texture or a burned smell or appearance, it should be replaced. Old oil may begin to separate, another sign that replacement is needed.

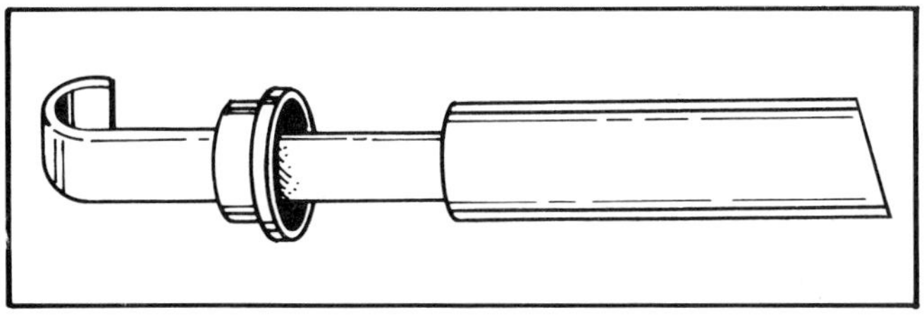

Fig. 1.4 Be careful when seating a dipstick in its tubing; often, the stick's guard or cap will hit the tubing exit preventing stick from fully seating. This will cause a low reading to be observed.

Power Steering Fluid. Power steering fluid is checked in the same manner as the engine oil. The power steering fluid reservoir is located at the front of the engine. Add clean power steering fluid until the dipstick registers on the full mark. If the dipstick does not register any fluid, the vehicle should be taken out of service until the reservoir can be refilled and the entire power steering system checked for leaks. Effect repairs as necessary before returning the vehicle to service.

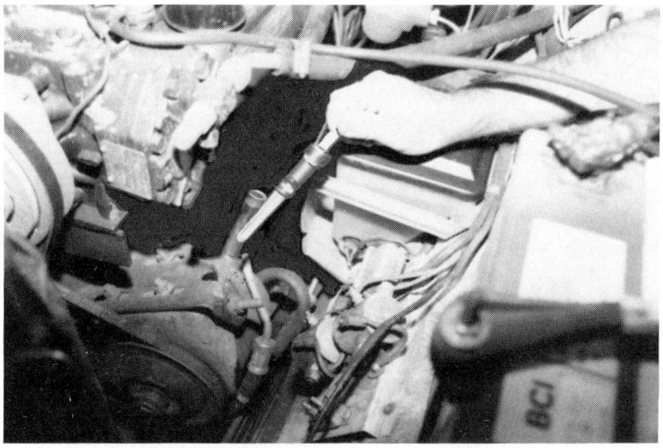

Fig. 1.5a Power Steering fluid level is checked at its reservoir in a manner similar to the oil.

Cooling System. The cooling system is under pressure when the engine is warm. Never remove the radiator cap when the system is warm because the potential for boiling coolant being sprayed about, causing burns, is very great. Most late-model vehicles have a separate reservoir that is translucent, allowing for a quick check of the fluid level without the need to remove the radiator cap. The fluid level should be between the two lines. Diluted antifreeze (see manufacturers recommendations) should be available to replenish the cooling system. A proper mix of water and antifreeze should be used year-round.

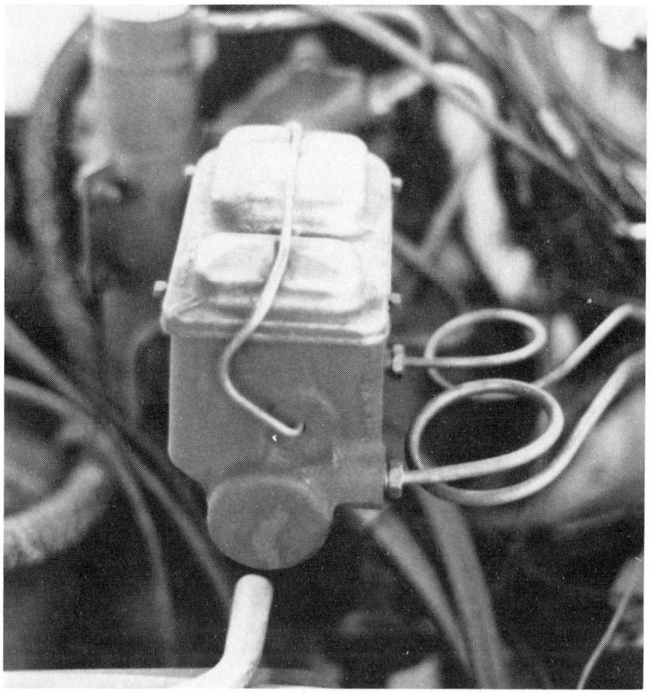

Fig. 1.5b Brake fluid level is checked in the reservoir, typically located on firewall.

Brake Fluid. Although brake fluid does not need to be checked every day, it should be checked quite regularly. The brake fluid level is checked at the reservoir located on the fire wall. Using a screw driver move the bale off the top of the reservoir lid. The fluid should be near the top of each compartment. Refill as needed with fresh brake fluid and carefully replace the lid and bale. Once the brake fluid has been replaced, an inspection drive of the vehicle is indicated with particular attention given to braking characteristics. If the reservoir is found to be completely dry, the brake lines should be bled by a competent mechanic after it is refilled.

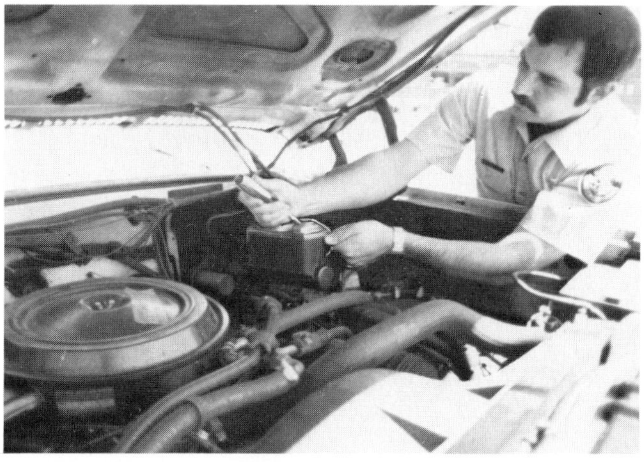

Fig. 1.5c Using a screwdriver, move the bale off of the top of the reservoir.

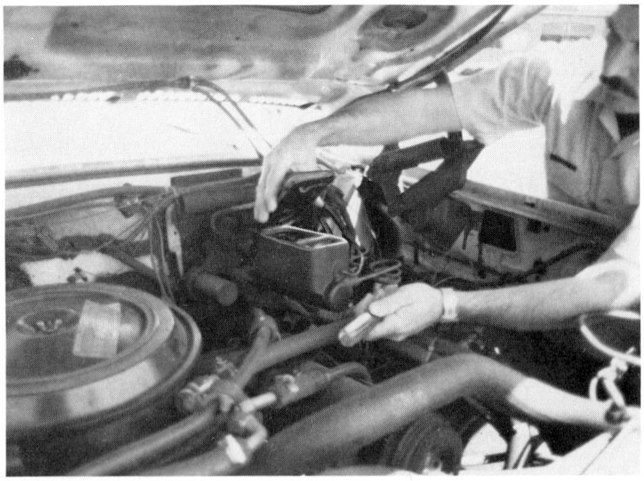

Fig. 1.5d Brake fluid should be near the top of each compartment.

Batteries and Battery Terminals. Check the battery terminals to make sure there is no acid build-up and that the terminals are tight. If acid is present it can be easily cleaned away with a solution of sodium bicarbonate and hot water. Avoid splashing the solution on your clothing. Eye protection is also recommended when working around batteries.

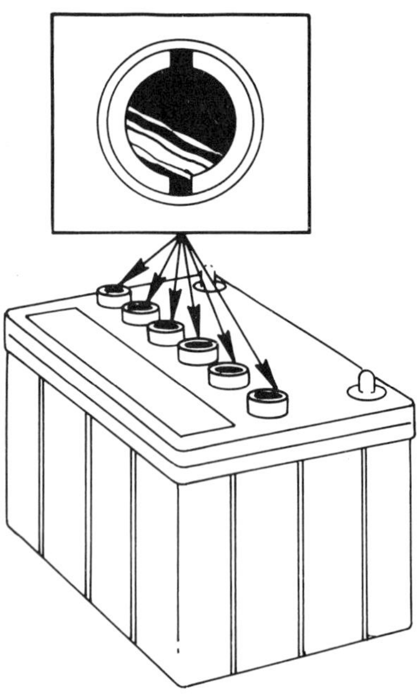

Fig. 1.6a Dilute battery acid should be at a level up to but not above inspection ring just inside the filler hole.

Fluid Level. Many of the batteries in use today require no check of their fluid and, in fact, the fluid is not accessible. If the battery has caps, remove them carefully without allowing the bottom of the cap to come in contact with the top of the battery or other contaminated areas. The cap should be turned upside down before it is set down . The battery fluid should be up to but not above the inspection ring just inside the filler hole. The battery fluid level is adequate as long as the vertical plates visible in each cell are completely covered. If the cell appears dry the battery should be taken out of service until the cell can be refilled and tested. When filling the battery cells, use only sterile water to avoid introducing harmful contaminates into the cell.

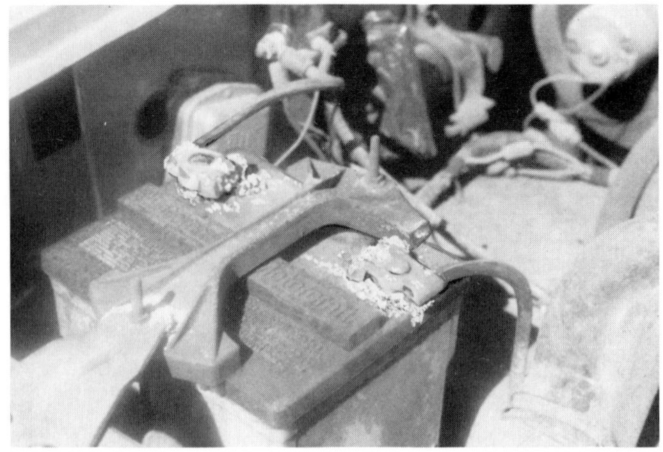

Fig. 1.6b Deposits built up around the top of battery, especially the terminals and securing bracket should be washed away.

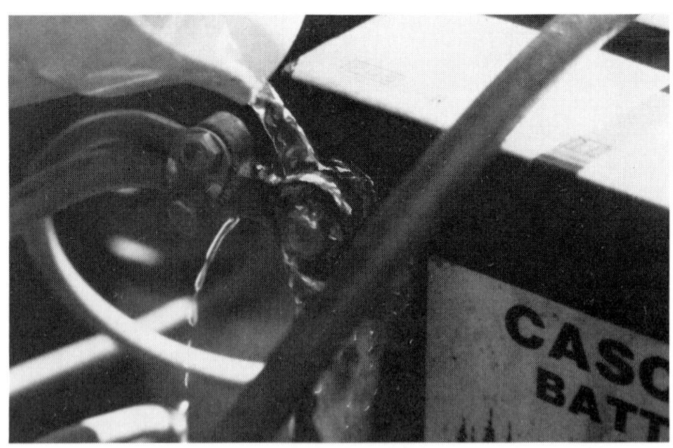

Fig. 1.6c Acid build-up on battery terminals can be easily cleaned away with a solution of sodium bicarbonate and hot water.

Specific Gravity Inspection. The battery's specific gravity should be checked once a week using a hydrometer. This is a simple-to-use instrument with a filler hose, glass cylinder, and suction bulb. The bulb is compressed prior to introducing the filler hose into each battery cell. The battery fluid is withdrawn into the hydrometer. The three floats within the glass cylinder should float, indicating adequate specific gravity of the electrolyte fluid. Failure of the floats to maintain their proper level indicates a weak cell. The battery should be replaced.

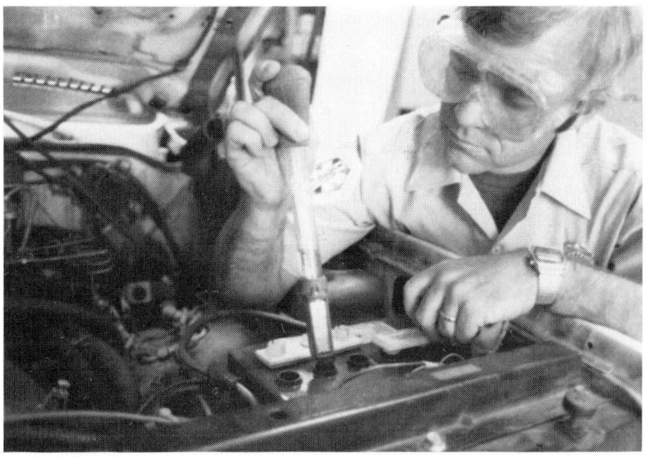

Fig. 1.7 Battery's specific gravity should be checked weekly using a hydrometer. Safety goggles should be worn to prevent acid splashing in the eyes. (Note battery cap turned upside down to avoid contaminating inside with debris from battery.)

As each cell is checked, carefully eject the battery fluid back into the cell prior to checking the next cell. Avoid splashing the fluid. Once the battery caps are replaced, flush any spilled fluid off the top of the battery and chassis using a soft stream of water.

Windshield Washer. The windshield washer fluid reservoir should be kept at a minimum of half full. When replacing windshield washer fluid, use a diluted solution specifically made for windshield washers rather than plain water. Such a solution helps keep the windshield clean longer and will not freeze in a cool environment. A container of diluted solution should be available for refilling the reservoir.

Engine Block. The engine itself should be relatively clean. This facilitates maintenance as well as making leaks easier to find. The engine also runs cooler when clean since it doesn't have an insulating layer of grease and dirt to hold the heat in.

Hoses. Radiator and heater hoses need to be inspected for pliability. Squeeze them firmly to make sure they have not become excessively brittle or soft or mushy feeling. While squeezing the hoses, note if something like a crust breaking can be felt on the inside of the hose. Such a finding may indicate that the cooling system needs flushing. Visually inspect for cracks or splits in hoses, especially near the hose clamps. If a hose is split, the vehicle should be taken out of service until the hose can be replaced. Look for any sign of leaks near each hose connection. Simple tightening with a screwdriver of the hose clamp may be all that is required to stop the leak. Occasionally, a hose may be trimmed back a few inches, and reconnected to control a leak from a spring-type hose clamp. Be sure you have an adequate amount of excess hose prior to cutting and refitting. The cooling system must be cold and the radiator pressure cap removed prior to this procedure. Some coolant will be lost and must be replaced after trimming cooling system hoses. It is important to remember that the engine will torque when running, requiring some play in any hose connected to the engine.

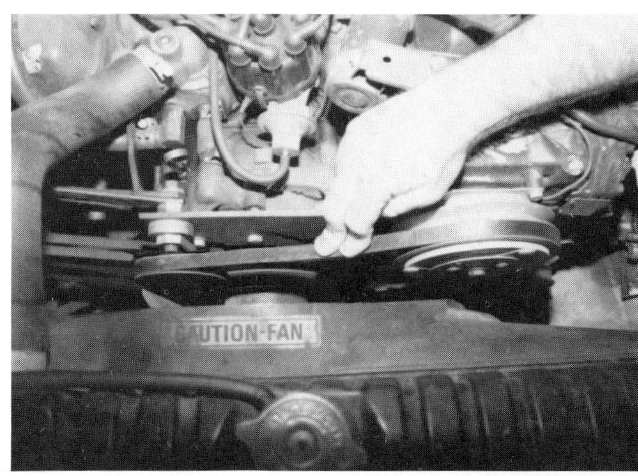

Fig. 1.8 Engine belts should be checked to ensure proper tension. You should be able to depress longer belts about ½ inch between pulleys and shorter belts a somewhat shorter distance.

Belts. The engine belts need to be checked to make sure they are tight. You should be able to depress the longer belts approximately one-half inch between two pulleys and the shorter belts a correspondingly shorter distance. It is important that the belts have some give since a tight belt will bind the bearings of the pulley shaft, cause drag on the engine, and cause rapid wear of the bearings and belts. Observe belts for cracks, splits, cuts, or a glazed appearance along with a lack of flexibility. Any of these findings indicates that the belt must be promptly replaced.

In-vehicle Inspection

It is always important to check for any obstacles that may present a problem when moving the ambulance prior to entering the vehicle. Even though you are only inspecting it at this time, the possibility exists that you may have to respond to a call or otherwise move the vehicle before the inspection is complete. Upon entering the vehicle, check to be sure it is clean and that all articles are stored properly and securely. Placing a patient's family in a vehicle that is dirty does little to instill their confidence in you or your service. Articles that are not stored properly become easily scattered while driving. Clutter contributes to an unprofessional appearance and unsafe working environment.

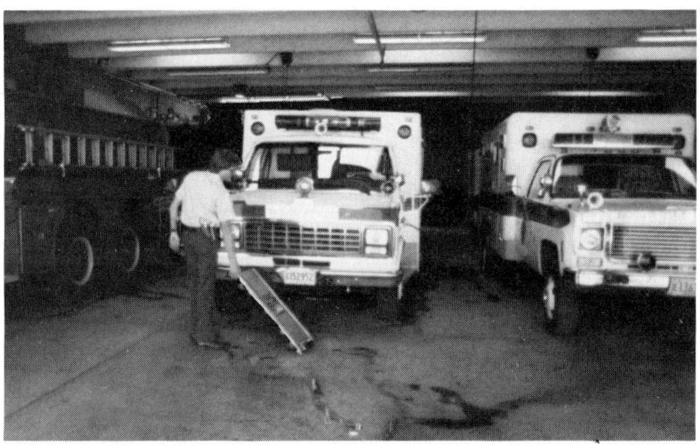

Fig. 1.9 Any obstacles around the vehicle should be removed prior to the in-vehicle inspection.

Once seated in the vehicle, the driver should insure that all accessories are properly adjusted:

Seat. The seat should be adjusted so the driver's legs have plenty of room but do not have to stretch to reach the pedals or foot activated switches such as the headlight dimmer switch. Once the seat is adjusted, attempt to move it back and forth. Insure the seat is locked in place.

Steering Wheel. If the vehicle has a tilt steering wheel, adjust it so that the driver's legs have a maximum amount of room and the wheel is comfortable to hold. Adjust the wheel so you don't have to look through it to see out the windshield. Also make sure all instruments can be seen adequately.

Headrest. Often overlooked, the headrests are adjustable in many vehicles. The headrest should be adjusted to a height at which it pads the middle of the back of the head. An improperly positioned headrest can contribute to whiplash-type cervical injuries should the vehicle be involved in a collision. A low headrest may stop the neck from moving backwards while the head is snapped back, hyperextending the cervical spine.

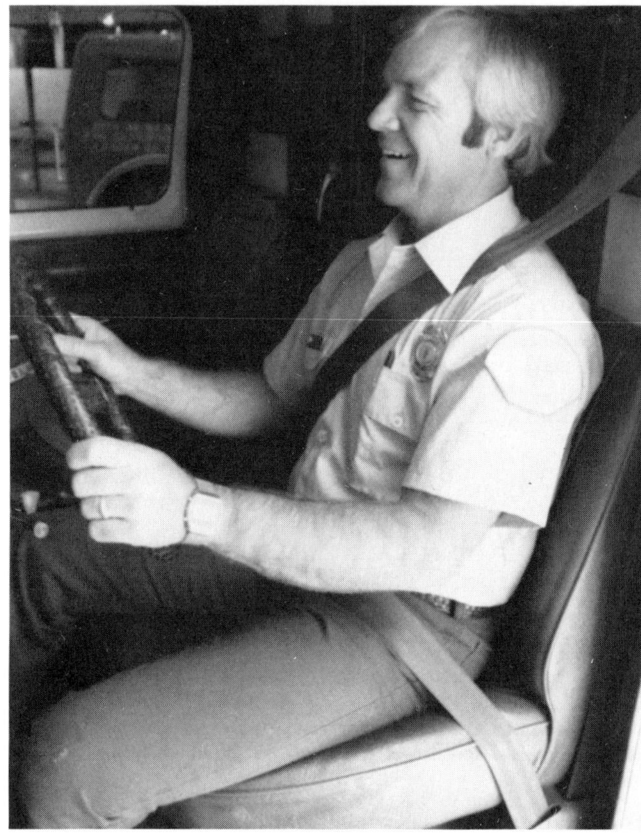

Fig. 1.10a Once seated, the driver should ensure that all accessories are easily reached and properly adjusted. (Note comfortable arm and leg position.)

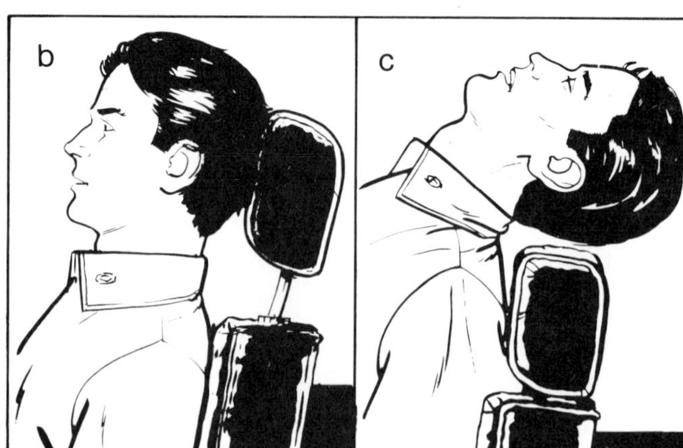

Fig. 1.10b The head rest should be adjusted to a height so it pads the middle of the back of the head.

Fig. 1.10c If the vehicle is involved in a collision, an improperly positioned headrest can contribute to whiplash-type cervical injuries.

Safety Belts. Two safety belts are usually available for use in today's vehicles. A seat belt and shoulder harness, often combined into one system, are available for both driver and passenger safety. The seat belt should be adjusted to fit snugly over the pelvis while the spine is well back against the seat. When the driver is seated in the same position with hands on the steering wheel, a properly adjusted shoulder harness should allow for one's fist to be placed between the belt and the chest.

Mirrors. Mirrors may be adjusted once the driver's seat and safety belts have been properly adjusted. Mirror adjustments should be made with the driver seated in a comfortable position with both the seat belt and shoulder harness fastened. With the vehicle parked on level ground, each side view mirror should be adjusted so the horizon appears in the middle of the mirror. The side of the vehicle should just be visible enough to provide a reference. This mirror position allows for maximum field of vision along each side of the vehicle and to the rear. The inside mirror is usually of no value to the ambulance operator other than to allow him to observe his partner in the patient compartment. At night the inside mirror may also reflect the patient compartment lights back into the driver's eyes, reducing some forward vision.

Systems Check

Once the driver accessories have been adjusted, start the engine and allow it to warm up for a couple of minutes. The equipment bay door or garage doors should be open to allow exhaust gases to escape. Recent reports have cited that dangerous carbon monoxide concentrations are commonly found in most ambulance garages, adjacent lounges, and offices. Begin a check of the various systems:

Gauges. Readings may vary from vehicle to vehicle. Learn what is normal for your vehicle. Any deviation from normal should be cause for concern since most engine problems can first be detected by a fluctuation in a gauge reading. The fluctuation may be either above or below the normal reading. If a reading appears to be other than normal, the vehicle should be taken out of service until the problem can be corrected. It is advisable to post the normal readings for each gauge of a particular vehicle as several different crews may operate any given vehicle.

Lights. Using your partner as a spotter, check all light systems on the vehicle. Check the front, each side, and the rear daily. Immediately replace any bulbs or repair any lights that are not working properly. Each light is important for safe and proper driving. Following is a list of all light systems:

Front:
- headlights (high and low beams)
- parking lights
- turn signals
- clearance lights
- hazard or four-way flashers
- emergency flashers
- emergency rotators
- spot lights

rear:
- tail lights
- brake lights
- turn signals
- back-up lights
- hazard or four-way flashers
- license plate light
- clearance lights
- emergency flashers
- emergency rotators
- loading lights

side:
- clearance lights
- scene lights
- side bar night light

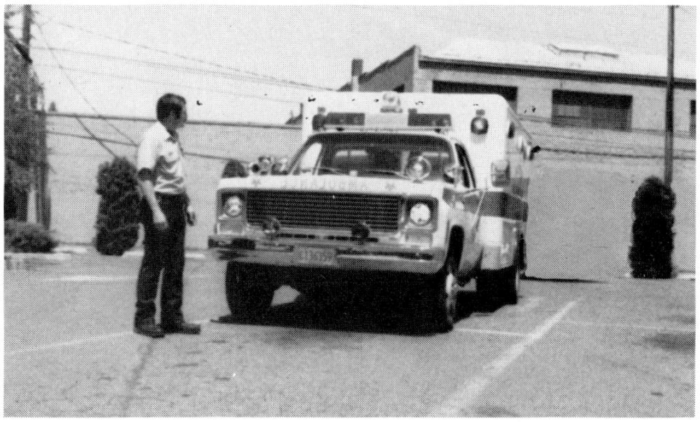

Fig. 1.11 Use your partner as a spotter for checking the light system to ensure proper functioning (especially for brake and back-up lights).

Brakes. Depress the brake pedal to see if it feels firm and does not travel too far. If the travel seems too far or the brake feels spongy, the vehicle should be taken out of service until the problem is corrected. Vehicles equipped with power brakes must have the engine running when the brakes are checked.

Parking Brake. Although often called an emergency brake, the parking brake should not be considered anything more than a brake to hold the vehicle while parked. Check the parking brake's holding power by first depressing the foot pedal until it feels solidly locked. While it is locked, place your left foot on the main brake, move the transmission gear selector to drive and slowly remove pressure from the main brake while pressing on the accelerator pedal with your right foot. The vehicle should be held in place with moderate pressure applied to the accelerator. Should the vehicle move forward, the parking brake should be adjusted.

Windshield. It is important for the windshield to be kept clean. A dirty windshield reduces visibility, especially at night or during adverse driving conditions. Check to see if a film has developed on the inside surface, and clean when necessary. Check for chips or cracks. Once a windshield is cracked, the crack will continue to grow until it involves the length or width of the entire surface, so it should be replaced in a timely fashion.

Windshield Washers. Activate the windshield washers to assure that the pumping mechanism is working properly and the jets are properly aimed. The windshield washer jets should spray fluid into the middle of each windshield wiper's path.

Windshield Wipers. While the cleaning solution from the washers is still on the windshield, activate the wipers to make sure they function properly. If any streaks of cleaning solution are left on the windshield after the wipers have passed a couple of times, the wiper blades should be replaced. Wiper blades should routinely be replaced each fall, since summer heat has a tendency to deteriorate the rubber edge. Faulty wipers are reason for taking the vehicle out of service until the problem can be corrected.

Radio. Perform a short check to make sure the radio is functioning properly. All frequencies should be checked daily. The vehicle should be taken out of service until radio problems can be corrected. An exception to this rule might be made if portable radios can be substituted. The portable must have adequate range to allow communications within your normal response area.

Heater and Air Conditioning. The heater and defroster should be checked daily for proper function of the fans. The air conditioners (driver's compartment and patient compartment) should be turned on once a week for a few minutes to keep the seals in the units from drying.

Horn. The horn should be checked for proper operation. Some horn buttons or rings found on steering wheels of ambulances have the option of activating either the horn or siren. If so equipped, each function should be briefly tested.

Fire Extinguishers. Ambulances are generally required to have two fire extinguishers on board. One is typically located in the driver's compartment. The extinguisher should be checked for its presence, charge and secure mounting.

Siren. Generally, it is not necessary to put a siren through a complete test of each mode. Electronic sirens can be tested by simply "bumping" the switch once. The Public Address mode may be checked by selecting the PA mode on the control head and clicking the PA microphone key. Wind-up or Class Q sirens need only to have the switch bumped and the siren brake rapidly applied. If the siren does not function properly, the vehicle should be taken out of service until the problem can be corrected.

Walk-around Inspection

Once the in-vehicle inspection is completed, it is time to take a walk around the vehicle to inspect the other components. As you move around the vehicle, look closer to make sure it is clean and waxed. Wax preserves the luster of the paint and protects body metal. Examine for any dings, scrapes, or dents. Examine the mirror brackets and the body seams for the appearance of rust or weakening of the metal. Check exterior compartments for rust or weak floor panels.

Doors. Doors get hung on, slammed, and objects caught in them fairly regularly. This abuse tends to knock the door out of alignment. As you walk around the vehicle look at the doors to see if there is equal spacing between the doors and jambs. Open each door and close it. Make sure each door closes easily, without excessive drag, and latches securely. Most loose door problems can easily be corrected using simple hand tools.

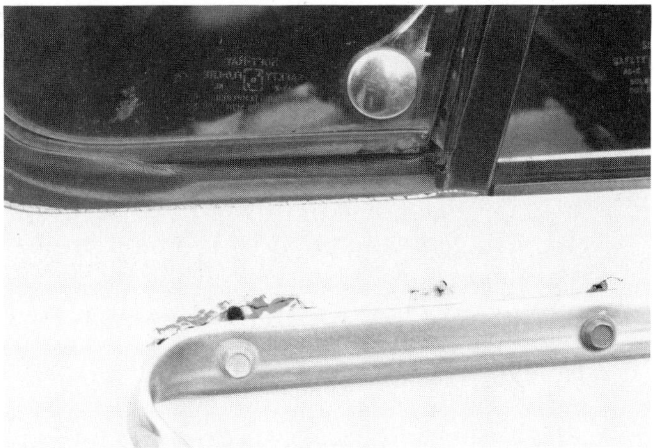

Fig. 1.12 Examine mirror brackets and body seams for evidence of rust or weakened body metal.

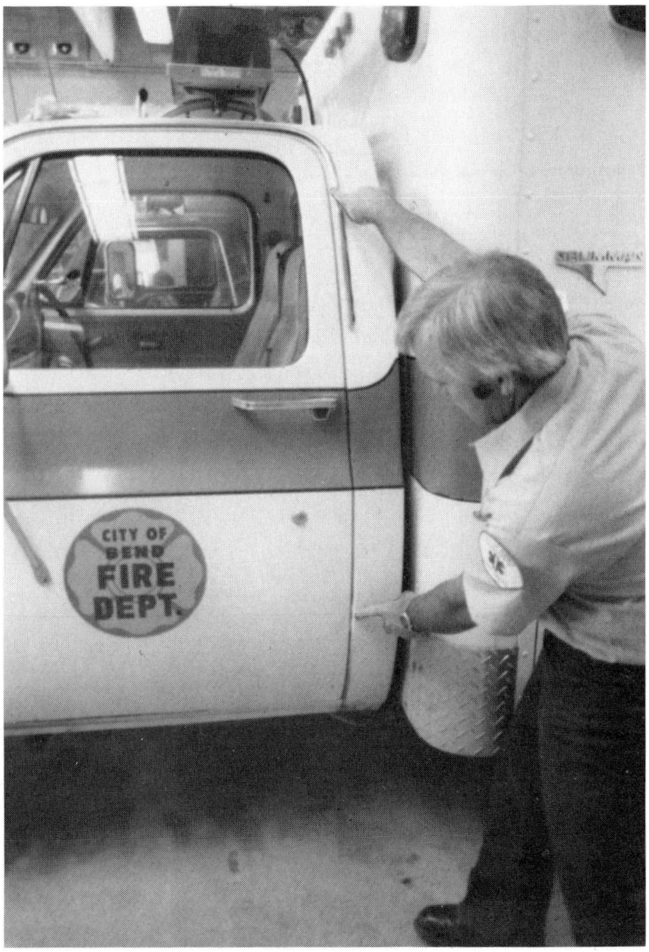

Fig. 1.13 Observe for equal spacing between doors and jambs.

Shock Absorbers. Shock absorbers perform a vital role in vehicle handling and control; they also influence tire wear and occupant comfort. Without adequate shock absorbers, a vehicle will bounce uncontrollably down the road. Visually inspect each shock absorber for any sign of fluid leaking from the cylinder. Should a leak be detected, the shock absorber should be replaced immediately. The method of bouncing each fender of a vehicle up and down to check shock absorber travel is not practical with today's heavy truck and van ambulances.

Front Alignment. The system that enables your vehicle to have proper steering and reduces uneven tire wear is the steering system. Because of the vibrations received from traveling down the road, wear on chassis parts, and our propensity for hitting bumps and curbs, the front-end alignment must be adjusted from time to time. The best way to detect alignment problems is by observing the front tires for uneven wear. Run the palm of your hand across the tread of the front tires. If you find the tread smooth in one direction but rough in the other, the front end is probably out of alignment. Performing this check frequently will catch misalignment soon enough to prevent significant tire damage. Visual tire wear (tire shows more wear on one side of the tread than the other) will show only after the wear has gone on for a considerable time. Unless severely out of alignment (heavy tread wear or drifting), wheel alignment is not critical on a short-term basis. The vehicle should be scheduled for maintenance soon after an alignment problem is discovered.

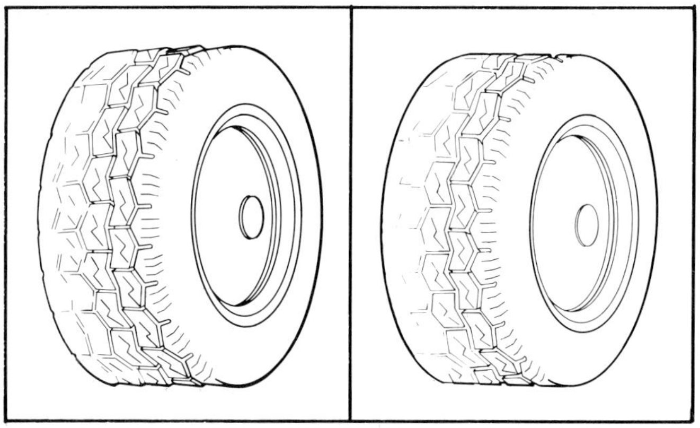

Fig. 1.14 The best way to detect alignment problems is by observing the front tire for uneven wear. Using the palm of your hand check smoothness of tread surface.

Tires. Once the front tires have been examined for uneven tread wear, examine for tread depth on all tires. The tire is constructed with wear bars that run across the tire tread, buried close to the base of the tread. It is time to replace the tire when the wear on the tire is to the point these wear bars have reached the surface, joining the tread pattern. Ambulance tires should be replaced well before this occurs.

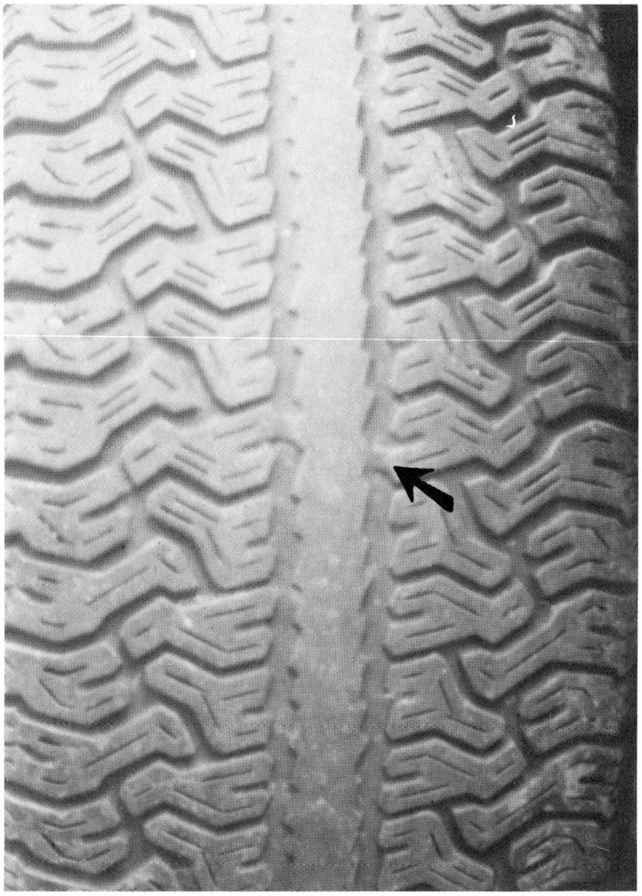

Fig. 1.15 Tires should be replaced before the tread becomes even with the wear bars that run between tread lines.

You should also feel around the tire for any irregularities or lumps on the tread or sidewall. Such a finding indicates a separation of the layers of the tire which will significantly weaken the tire. Layer separation is reason for immediately taking the vehicle out of service. The tire must be replaced.

Tire wear and ride comfort are determined largely by air pressure. Overinflated tires will produce a bumpy ride. Underinflated tires give a smooth ride but handling becomes more difficult and tire wear increases. Tire pressure should be checked while the tires are cold since heat from driving can raise the pressure as much as 5 pounds per square inch (psi). Tire pressure should be within the recommended limits posted on the sidewall of the tire. If the tire needs to be inflated in excess of this limit, the tire is too light for the weight of the vehicle. Generally, it is preferable to inflate the tire to a pressure closer to the stated maximum. Recommended tire pressures may vary significantly from front to back tires. If the vehicle is equipped with dual rear tires, it is important to check both the inside and outside tire pressure. Difficult handling characteristics may be encountered if pressure from one side of the vehicle to the other varies more than a couple of pounds per square inch. Specific tire pressure for each vehicle should be posted somewhere easily seen by the crew, such as on fenders above each wheelwell. Improper tire pressures can produce drastic wear. An overinflated tire run for an extended period of time will have marked wear along the center of the tread with minimal wear along the edges. In contrast, an underinflated tire will show cupping, or significant wear to the outer edge but minimal wear in the center.

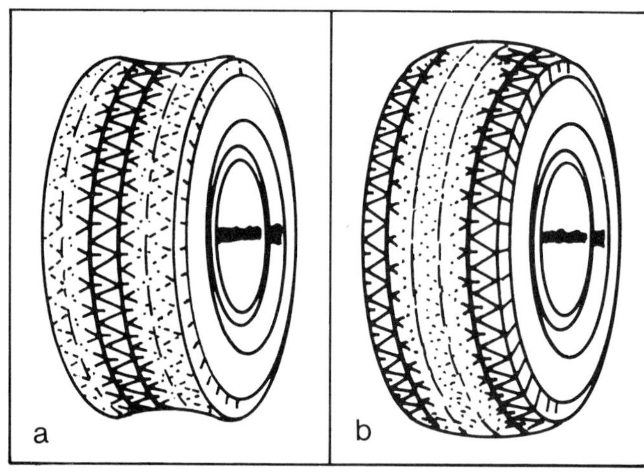

Fig. 1.16a Underinflated tires will show cupping or significant wear to outer edges with minimal wear in the center.

Fig. 1.16b Improper tire pressure can increase tread wear drastically. an overinflated tire will show marked wear along center of tread, less wear along edges.

Wheels. While examining the tires, also check the wheels. Tires are normally manufactured a little heavier in some areas than others, thus requiring weight to counteract the tire/wheel imbalance.

Should the wheel weights be lost, the vehicle will actually bounce down the road, creating handling problems and undue tire wear. Missing weights can be detected by a discoloration in the wheel where the weight used to be, or by a small line of residue outlining the weight's former position.

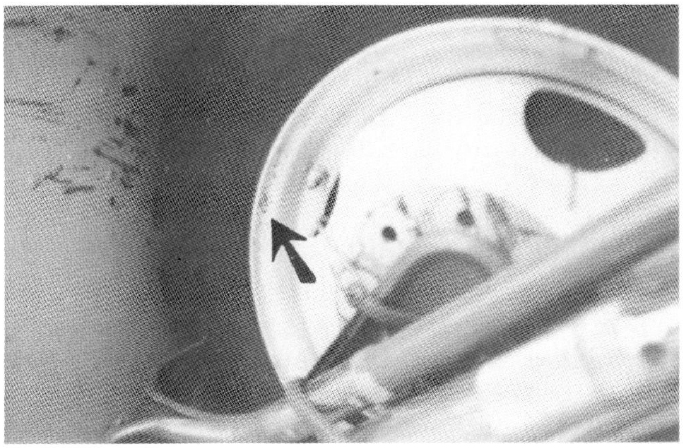

Fig. 1.17 Inspect wheels for evidence of missing wheel weights. (Dirty residue near valve stem indicates missing weight.)

Occasionally remove the hubcaps and check to make sure all lug nuts are tight. Lug nuts can loosen from road vibration, sometimes causing the wheel to leave the vehicle without warning. While the hubcaps are off, inspect the wheel itself to make sure no fatigue fractures have developed around the lug holes, rivets, or joints. Also inspect for dents or bends in the rim itself. Any irregularities noted with the wheel are cause to take the vehicle out of service until the wheel can be replaced.

Spare Tire. Since the spare tire occupies its own area, its condition is routinely overlooked and a frequent source of embarrassment for all vehicle operators. The spare tire should be routinely checked for proper inflation and adequate tread life. It is also a good idea to inspect the spare tire wheel rim for damage which can occur from miscellaneous items stored in the spare tire compartment. Also check for the presence of an appropriate jack, jack handle, and wheel lug wrench.

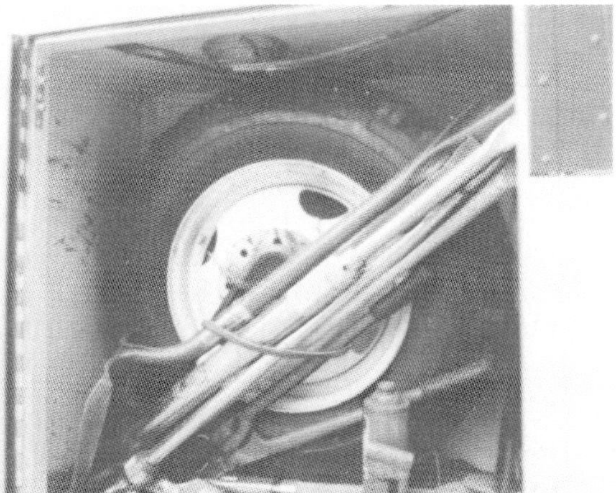

Fig. 1.18 Typical ambulance spare tire compartment

Dynamic Vehicle Inspection

Once all other inspections have been completed and any noted discrepancies corrected, the vehicle should be driven. Initially, the vehicle should be driven in an area relatively free from traffic and at slow speeds. By the end of the test drive, vehicle speeds should have been increased to the posted limits found on expressways or the open highway. This, of course, would be done on such a road as a freeway. The following components should be evaluated during the test drive.

Engine Performance. The engine should run smoothly and stay running. If the engine seems to run rough once it has warmed up, or if you can't keep it running, or if it dies on acceleration, the vehicle should be taken out of service. The engine will knock while accelerating under a load if improperly timed or if low-octane gasoline is used. The engine may also continue to run after the ignition is turned off. This knocking and any other unusual noises should be noted and checked out by a mechanic immediately. Squeals, especially on acceleration, often indicate a belt needs tightening or replacing. Hissing may mean engine coolant is leaking or that a vacuum leak may be present.

Brakes. Any pull or fade noted when the brakes are applied is extremely hazardous to safe vehicle operation. Two early signs of brake failure are spongy pedal action and excessive pedal free travel. Brakes should be tested in an area free of traffic and at speeds of 10 to 15 miles per hour. Release your grip of the steering wheel without removing your hands from the wheel and apply the brakes abruptly. If the brakes grab or pull to one side, or if they feel spongy or have excessive pedal travel, remove the vehicle from service.

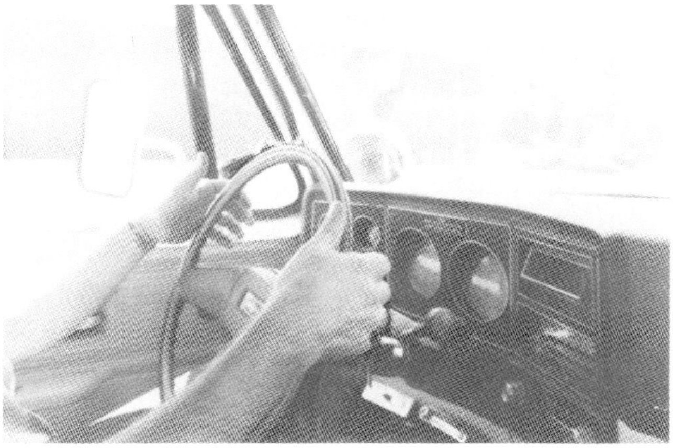

Fig. 1.19 Test brakes in an area free of traffic and at speeds of 10–15 mph.

Steering. In the same area where the brakes are checked, again release your grip on the wheel without taking your hands from it to see if the vehicle tracks straight. Most roads have a natural crown, and the vehicle will naturally drift down this crown to some degree. While driving, observe the vehicle for easy steering or a tendency to wander which requires constant correction. Check the steering wheel for excess play by turning it back and forth, and note the amount of input needed before the vehicle starts to turn. Steering wheel play should not exceed one-eighth of a turn. Listen for any noises during turning and feel for jerking in the wheel, either of which can indicate problems with the power steering. Any steering problem dictates that the vehicle should immediately be taken out of service until the problem can be corrected. Recheck the power steering fluid level and refill as necessary. If fluid must be added after the test drive, reinspect all power steering hydraulic lines for possible leaks.

Suspension. While driving, check the suspension system by feeling for unusual heavy leaning during cornering, floating sensations after negotiating high spots in the road, or some lack of steering response. Observe how the vehicle handles bumps. Does it continue to bounce up and down more than once after hitting a bump or dip in the road? Any of these findings indicates that the vehicle should receive service in the immediate future.

Tire Balance. Out-of-balance tires are usually not noticeable at slow speed; however, at speeds between 40-50 miles per hour, a definite shimmy can be felt. If a tire is out of balance, it should be corrected promptly.

Transmission. While driving, feel for how the transmission shifts. If it seems to slip while shifting gears or the engine RPMs seem to increase before shifting, an automatic transmission may need fluid or adjustment of the transmission itself. Another ominous sign is the transmission not staying in gear.

After the test drive is completed, the final check of the vehicle should be the level of the transmission fluid. Automatic transmission fluid levels should only be checked while the transmission is warm, with the engine running and the transmission gear selector in neutral (park in some models).

Exhaust System. The exhaust system should be checked for any leaks while the engine is idling. Most exhaust leaks can be easily heard by simply placing your head under the chassis and listening for pinging sounds or air leaks. On cold mornings, one may be able to see exhaust vapor leaks under the chassis. Should an exhaust leak be discovered, the vehicle should be taken out of service until repairs can be made.

Listen and Feel. Generally, any vibrations that become noticeable, or any rattles, should be noted and investigated.

Monthly Inspection

In addition to the daily inspection, the vehicle should undergo a finer inspection monthly. A detailed cleaning is also required once a month. The cleaning should consist of emptying each cabinet and cleaning and inspecting for torn wrappers on supplies, unsafe or damaged equipment, and expired or otherwise unsafe drugs. During the cleaning and inspection, look at each compartment in detail and note any problems with doors, shelves, or any other areas not inspected daily.

Patient compartment door seals should also be checked once a month. Using a hose with a nozzle, spray water around each door and attempt to spray water past the door seals. If a leak is observed, the seal should be replaced as it may allow exhaust fumes into the patient compartment.

Ambulance Modifications

Ambulances are modified to some extent from what the original truck or van chassis manufacturer produced. Some of these modifications deserve attention:

Dual Batteries. Most ambulances are equipped with two batteries. To make maximum use of each battery, they should be wired through a selector switch such as a Cole-Hersee switch. Such a switch allows use of either battery, both batteries together, or for both batteries to be turned off completely. Dual batteries are typically wired in one of two ways.

One type of dual battery system has the engine starter and basic chassis operating off one battery. The rest of the electrical systems, including the patient compartment and emergency lights, operate off the secondary battery. This arrangement keeps the battery for starting the vehicle isolated from any other system that might drain it. However, if the battery feeding the starter develops a bad cell or a loose connection, the vehicle cannot be started. This system may also utilize two alternators, one for each electrical system.

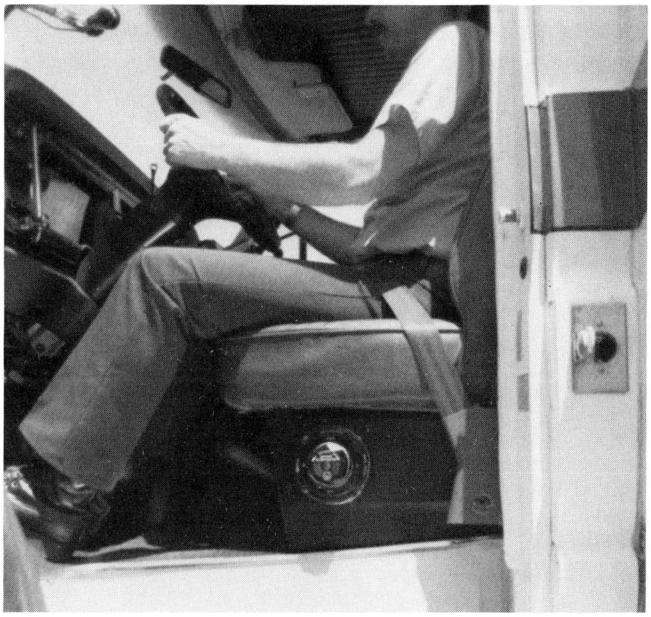

Fig. 1.20 For best results, batteries should be wired through a selector switch such as a Cole-Hersee switch.

The other method of wiring the batteries has the total electrical system wired to operate from either battery. With this type of system, the batteries are typically labeled 1 and 2. Battery 1 is then used on all days with odd calendar numbers, while Battery 2 is used on the even-numbered days. This practice keeps both batteries equally exercised. Under this arrangement, a totally charged battery is available in case the other fails. If the vehicle will not start, you may simply switch to the other battery. If neither battery will turn over the engine, switch the selector to the "Both" position. Immediately after starting, switch back to the normal battery, allowing it to recharge. If the vehicle is operated with the selector on "Both," the weak battery can, through the switch, drag down the strong battery.

Important: Never switch the batteries through the off position while the engine is running or while any electrical load is present. Such action can easily burn out the voltage regulator.

Gauges. By monitoring oil pressure, engine temperature, and the electrical system, a good driver can often see a problem developing and take appropriate steps to correct it before it leads to trouble. Unfortunately, many vehicles do not come with gauges but instead have lights that only serve to let the driver know once the trouble has developed. With the type of use ambulances receive, it is important for them to be equipped with gauges in order for the critical systems to be properly monitored.

Volt Meter. The electrical systems may be monitored by either the amount of amperes or the amount of volts being delivered to the battery. Monitoring the number of volts delivered to each battery is a more accurate system when dual volt meters are used.

Alternator. The electrical load of an ambulance is unusally large, far above that of the normal vehicle. For that reason, it is necessary to have an oversized alternator. Use of larger alternators or dual alternators necessitates more frequent tightening of their drive belts.

Tires. The tires that come with the stock chassis may not be large enough to carry the load once the weight of the cabinetry, equipment, personnel, and several patients' weight have been figured in. When purchasing a new ambulance, the person responsible for ambulance maintenance should double-check the tire specifications to make sure they are adequate.

Suspension. Just as the original equipment tires may be undersized, the stock suspension system may not be adequate for a fully loaded ambulance. When purchasing an ambulance, it is important to make sure that the suspension is adequate for the expected loaded weight. When driven in a straight line, such a suspension system will deliver a rougher ride than a stock system. An under-suspended vehicle can be dangerous to drive since control will be limited by improper handling characteristics.

Side View Mirrors. Because of the increased visibility required for safely driving an ambulance and because of chassis modifications, accessory mirrors are often mounted on the vehicle. When accessory mirrors are selected and mounted, care should be taken to place them so they do not create additional blind spots. It is not uncommon for a mirror to be placed so high it blocks the driver's view of traffic at side streets. For that reason, it is not uncommon for a driver to look into an improperly mounted side view mirror, mistake the traffic he sees in his mirror (the traffic *behind* the ambulance) as stopped, and then proceed into the path of the cross traffic not seen in the blind spot. Such mistakes can be reduced by utilizing square mirrors mounted below eye level.

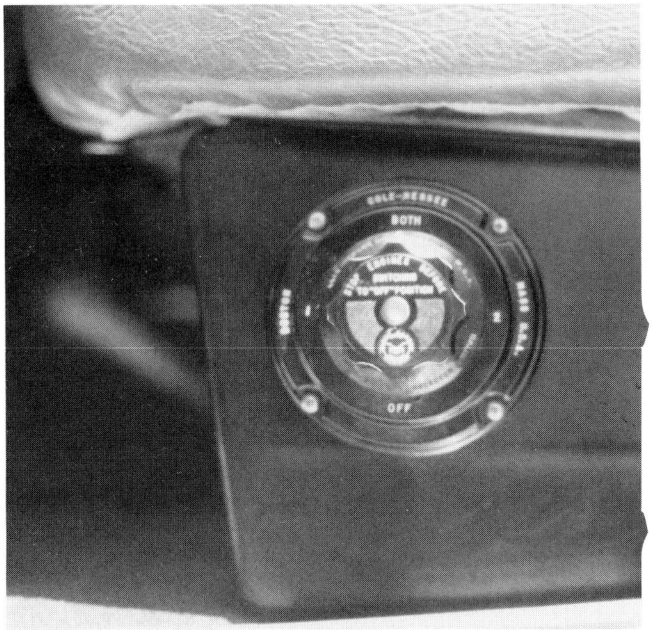

Fig. 1.21 Switch allows use of either battery, both together or batteries to be turned off altogether.

Convex Mirrors. Convex mirrors are quite popular as aids to better side vision. Although they are an excellent adjunct, they cannot replace standard flat mirrors since they distort the depth of field. For this reason, convex mirrors should be mounted in such a fashion as to not interfere with the standard side view mirrors. Avoid mounting stick-on convex mirrors to existing mirrors. A convex mirror, mounted separately with a

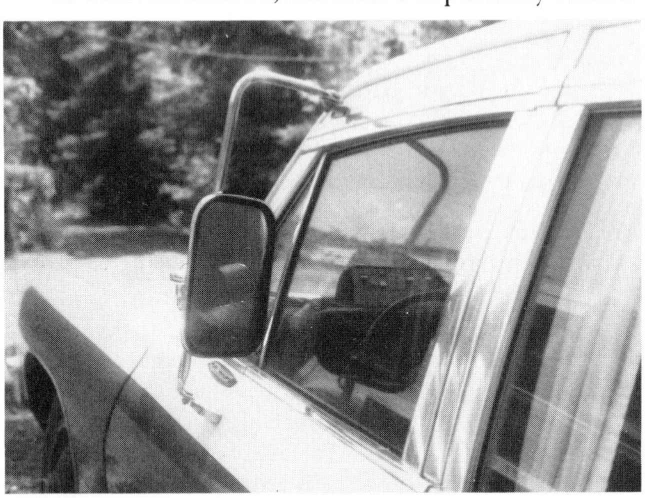

Fig. 1.22a When mounting optional mirrors, take care not to create blind spots.

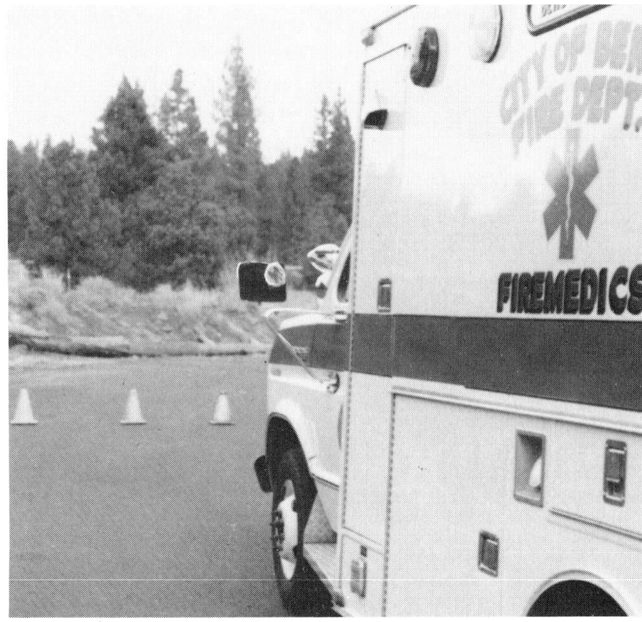

Fig. 1.22b Ideally, mirror should be mounted below eye level.

bracket attached to the framework of existing mirrors is preferred. Avoid raising the standard mirror as it will interfere with the driver's vision at cross streets.

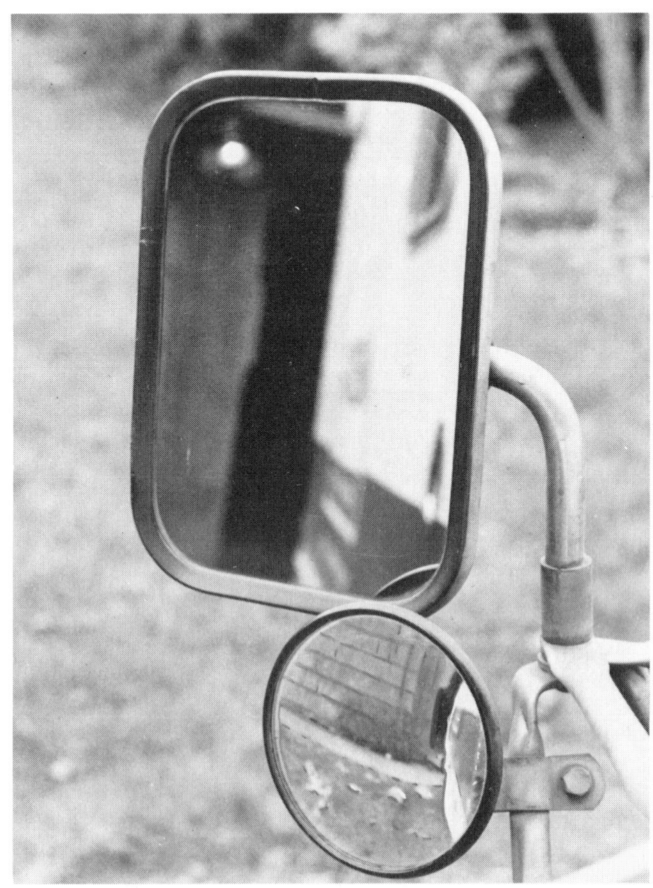

Fig. 1.23 A separate mirror is preferred to avoid limiting use to the standard mirror. (Photo courtesy of **jems.**)

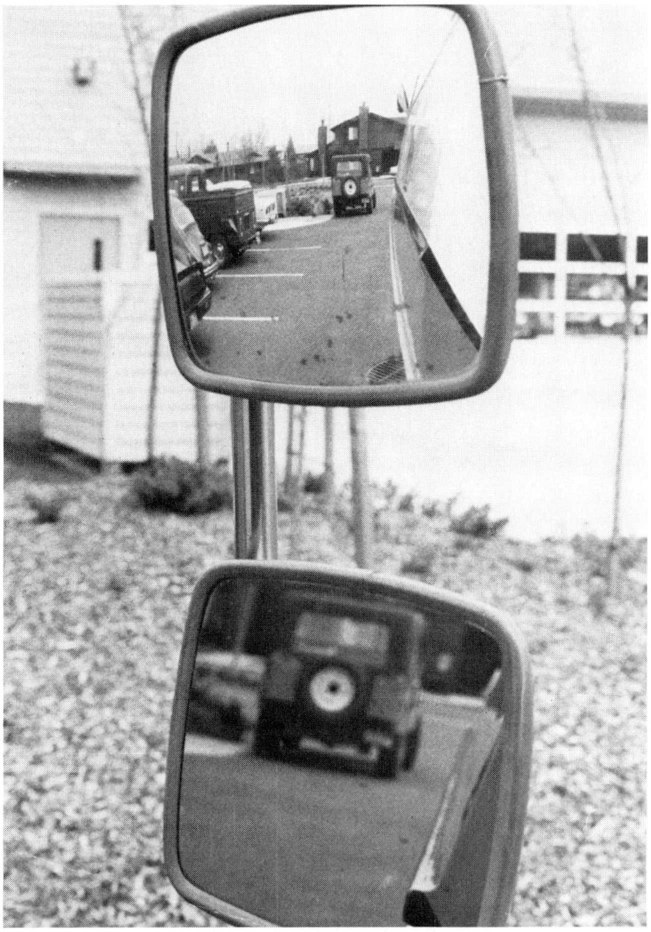

Fig. 1.24 Convex mirrors open up the field of vision but distort depth perception. (Photo courtesy of **jems.**)

In the Driver's Seat

Driver Positioning. The basic element of vehicle control is the stability of the driver behind the wheel. The driver must be positioned properly so he or she becomes a part of the vehicle being driven.

The driver should position himself to allow maximum freedom of movement. The thighs should be resting on the seat, the knees slightly flexed, the spine well back against the seat back. It is important to have plenty of leg room without having to actually stretch to reach the pedals. This leg room will allow for smooth, rapid transitions between foot pedals.

The arms, too, should be well out in front with the elbows slightly bent to give maximum freedom of movement. For optimum control, imagine the steering wheel as the face of a clock and place the hands at the 9 o'clock and 3 o'clock positions. This allows the hands to turn the wheel with ease and sets up an automatic counterforce between the two hands. This counterforce helps keep the wheel from being jerked too hard in a crisis situation, such as a skid. In some situations, you may have to turn the vehicle without having the time to change hand positions. With the hands in the 9 and 3 positions, the wheel can be turned a full 180‘ before the hands have to be repositioned.

The seat belt does more than just hold the driver in the seat in the event of a collision. It can also prevent that collision. In hard counter-steering situations, a lot of force is placed on the driver. The driver will find some of the effort that should be going into steering is actually being used just to hold himself behind the wheel. This effort can be reduced if the seat belts are properly used and adjusted.

Tension and fatigue also reduce a driver's ability to control his or her vehicle. Proper driver positioning can help reduce these conditions. With the driver properly seated and seat belts used to maintain that position, the driver will be more relaxed and better able to operate the vehicle.

Starting the Vehicle

Far from being just a matter of turning the key, starting the engine is a complex procedure requiring certain activities to be carried out.

Prior to Starting. Starting the vehicle actually begins with a careful check around it to insure all obstacles are removed or at least mentally noted. Make sure the transmission is in park or, in a manual transmission vehicle, that the shift lever is in neutral. Quickly check the electrical system to make sure all major systems such as the air conditioner and lights are off. (These will not be affected during actual cranking of the engine since the starter switch overrides them; however, if difficulty in starting is encountered, these accessories may help to drain the battery of its charge.) Depress the brake pedal a couple of times to make sure it functions properly and then keep it depressed while starting the vehicle.

Starting. The engine should normally be started quickly, before the seat belt is fastened or other functions take place. This allows an extra few seconds for the oil to begin to circulate before the vehicle is moved. The vehicle should be started according to the manufacturer's recommendations and the experience the driver has with the particular vehicle. Starting procedures will vary depending on whether the engine is cold or warm.

Cold Starting. When starting a cold engine, push the throttle to the floorboard once and release. Turn the key until the engine starts. Some engines may require the accelerator to be pumped two or three times while cranking the starter. Do not crank a starter for more than 20 seconds at one time.

Warm Starting. Push the accelerator halfway to the floor and hold. Turn the key until the engine starts and release the accelerator pedal.

Flooded Engine. Once in a while, the engine will become flooded with too much fuel, making it harder to start. In such a situation, push the throttle to the floorboard and hold it there until the engine starts.

Difficult Starting. Never crank an engine starter for over 20 seconds at one time. This will cause the starter to overheat. If the engine fails to start within 20 seconds, switch the ignition key off, while keeping the throttle to the floor. Allow the starter to cool for 10 to 15 seconds and try again. If the engine does not start after being cranked for 20 seconds, allow the starting motor to cool a full minute before again attempting to start the engine.

Once an engine has started, it should be allowed to run a minimum of 3 minutes before being shut off. This period of engine operation will allow the cylinders to be recoated with oil and the battery to regain some of the charge lost during the engine starting.

When shutting off the engine, let it idle momentarily and then turn the key off.

Avoid accelerating the engine and then turning the key off. Such a practice injects gasoline into the cylinders but does not allow for combustion. The gasoline then dissolves the oil coating protecting the cylinders. When the engine is next started, it will run momentarily without adequate cylinder lubrication.

Diesel Engines

Diesel engines have become quite popular with today's motorist because they are so economical to operate. Their use in ambulances has been somewhat limited until very recently. One major ambulance manufacturer expects diesel engines to be in nearly 40 percent of all the ambulances manufactured in the future. The main improvements in diesel vehicles which now make them more practical for ambulance applications include improved transmissions and better idling characteristics. Diesel fuel systems are more prone to freezing during the winter than gasoline systems, so clean fuel is a must. One word of caution: Be very vigilant of fuel level to insure that the vehicle does not run out of diesel. Once the fuel injectors are dry, they must be reprimed in order to start the engine—a very time-consuming process.

Starting Procedure. Diesel engines do not operate under the same principles as gasoline engines. Instead of a spark plug to ignite the fuel/air mixture, diesels rely on the heat generated by high compression for fuel ignition.

Many diesel engines only require turning the key to start. Other diesel-engine vehicles require the key to be turned to the "on" position and then a waiting period until a dash light goes out. The light indicates a "glow plug" heating either the intake air or combustion chamber. It is necessary to wait for the glow plug to come up to the proper temperature before the dash light will go out and the engine can be started.

Propane-fueled Engines

Propane-burning engines are being used in some parts of the country. Essentially, propane-fueled engines operate much the same as gasoline-powered ones since the only real major changes are the carburetion system and the mounting of a compressed liquid gas tank. Starting and operating procedures are the same as for gasoline-fueled engines. There have been some reports of propane freezing in the fuel lines when propane engines are operated under a heavy load on extremely hot or cold days. Such an occurrence would obviously not be desirable, especially if it happens to an ambulance.

Post Starting

The post starting procedures can be divided into primary and secondary procedures:

Primary. Once the engine is started, insure all passengers are seated and properly belted in. Check that the doors are closed and locked. The doors are an integral part of the body structure. Door locks are designed to hold the doors closed during a collision, thereby maintaining better body integrity. Make a quick check of the mirrors, steering wheel, and headrest to assure that nothing has been inadvertently moved.

Within the first minute of engine operation, the gauges should be checked to make sure all systems are functioning properly.

Secondary. Once you have completed the primary procedures, check the systems you will specifically need, such as lights, wipers, or heater. To drive, place one foot firmly on the brake, place the transmission gear selector in the appropriate gear, and release the parking brake before moving.

Station Doors

Before driving the ambulance out of the equipment bay or garage in which it is kept, always look up at the overhead doors to insure that there is adequate clearance for the vehicle to pass. It is not uncommon for radio antennas and emergency lights to be torn off the ambulance as it passes under a partially opened overhead door. It is also important to be aware of station doors equipped with automatic timers designed to close the door after the vehicle has left the station. Should the engine stall or you lose track of the time you have to clear the door, you may find yourself filling out additional paperwork and receiving a great deal of attention from your coworkers, the kind of attention none of us wants.

Preventive Maintenance

A vehicle is a tool and as such should be kept in proper repair. While accident statistics reflect relatively few accidents caused by mechanical malfunction, many experts believe mechanical malfunctions contribute to a far greater share of accidents than reported. Consider the driver who sideswipes another car. He is cited for failure to maintain control of his vehicle, but it is never officially recorded that contributing to the collision was a severely unaligned front suspension system which caused the vehicle to wander.

Mechanical inefficiency and breakdowns can be minimized with proper preventive maintenance. Every part of a machine is subject to wear and, if allowed to, will eventually fail. Wear can be reduced and the life of the part prolonged with proper servicing. The life expectancy of each component can be determined. With preventive maintenance, a schedule can be established for routine servicing and replacement of each component prior to the part reaching its life expectancy.

Preventive maintenance actually saves the ambulance service money. Fleet operators have found that it is more economical to pay for servicing than for repairs when a part fails unexpectedly. When parts are due for replacement, it is more economical to schedule that replacement and the associated maintenance time than to respond to a mechanical breakdown on the road. Properly performed preventive maintenance can lessen the EMS agency's liability due to the inability of an ambulance to respond to an aid call.

The ambulance is the basic tool of the trade. As such, preventive maintenance for the vehicle should be of primary concern for every ambulance operator. While the driver/EMT may not be directly responsible for the maintenance of the ambulance, he or she should be acquainted with the maintenance schedule and when the vehicle is next due for service.

Maintenance schedules are nothing more than minimum guidelines for predicting required service. The stress and wear each vehicle receives are governed by many elements. Vehicles in the same fleet may require differing preventive maintenance schedules depending on the type of driving to which each ambulance is regularly exposed. An ambulance driven in hilly or mountainous terrain receives more stress on the transmission than one driven on city streets. A vehicle used primarily in an urban area may require more frequent tune-ups as the vehicle spends much more time idling in heavy traffic than perhaps a vehicle used in a more rural setting. The life expectancy of engine oil cannot be adequately predicted when used under such extreme service conditions. Many communities have testing laboratories that can evaluate a sample of your engine oil to help determine at what interval the engine oil should be changed for each vehicle.

Mileage alone is a poor indicator of the actual wear on the engine since it spends much time idling at the scene. A variety of drivers will also affect the expected wear on the ambulance. Although preventive maintenance schedules should be developed specifically for each ambulance vehicle in service, a few generalizations can be stated.

If the engine oil is not tested at a laboratory occasionally, it is advised that the oil and oil filter should be changed at 2,000-mile intervals. The chassis should also be lubricated and the fluid level of the differential checked at the same time. Brakes should be inspected every 5,000-8,000 miles or any time a problem is suspected. While the wheels are off the vehicle for brake inspection, the wheel bearings can be inspected for pitting and then repacked. A good preventive maintenance program will reduce breakdowns and, with adequate service records, insure a higher vehicle resale value.

Minor Maintenance

While the ambulance crew is usually not responsible for major maintenance of the vehicle, each driver should be able to take care of minor maintenance problems. Minor maintenance performed by the crew will help reduce the burden on the maintenance department of the ambulance service or the costs associated with utilizing an outside service. It will also keep the unit in service. Minor maintenance easily performed by the crew could include:

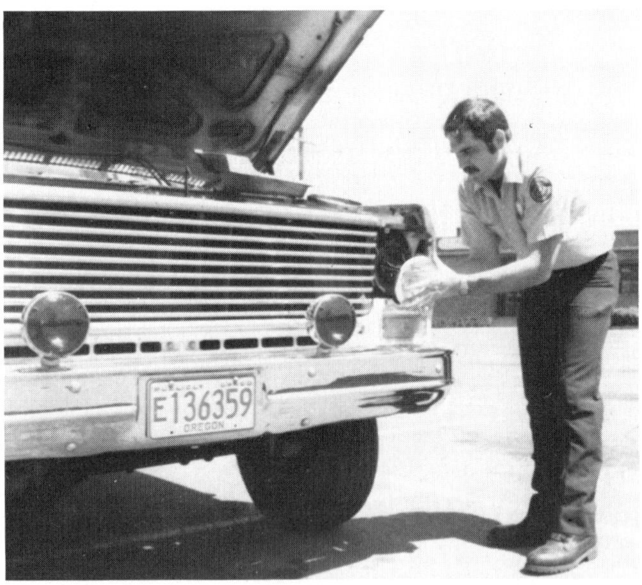

Fig. 1.25 Crew can perform minor maintenance to help reduce the burden on the maintenance department or reduce outside service costs.

Battery Cleaning. The batteries can build up a thick layer of acid around the connecting terminals. This buildup can easily be cleaned away by pouring a solution of sodium bicarbonate and hot water over the acid buildup. Once a month remove the cables from the battery and brush both the cable ends and the terminals until shiny metal is exposed. Remove the ground cable first and replace last to avoid arcing the battery. The battery selector switch should be in the off position when removing battery cables.

Belts. The belts (fan, power steering, etc.) have a way of working loose. Each can be easily tightened by the crew with a minimum of tools.

Fasteners. The vibration given the vehicle by the moving drive train parts and the road will eventually cause many of the fasteners that hold the cabinets together to loosen. The crew can periodically go through the vehicle with a couple of screwdrivers and check each screw.

Lights. Burned-out lights can usually be replaced by the crew.

Fluids. Almost all fluids that may need to be replenished in the vehicle can easily be cared for by the crew.

Maintenance personnel may identify other small tasks that can easily be accomplished by the crew.

Wear and Tear

Ambulances typically receive more abuse than the ordinary automobile. This abuse unfortunately causes mechanical inefficiency or part failure long before normal scheduled maintenance or replacement would be expected. Most abuse can be avoided. For instance, people leaving the vehicle give the door a flick, letting it slam shut on its own. Ambulance crews are notorious for this since they always seem to be in a hurry. This action can break hinges and, at a minimum, increase wear on the latching mechanism. The door may also be knocked out of alignment. It is best to close a door gently using the door handle as a pushing point until the door is latched.

Steering and suspension systems receive a tremendous amount of wear. Much of this wear comes while the vehicle is being stopped or traveling at very slow speeds. Avoid turning the wheels when the vehicle is stopped, as this creates undue strain on the suspension and steering components.

If you hear a squeal coming from the engine when turning hard at slow speeds, the power steering has been turned further than it can respond. The wheels do not turn any further once the squealing is heard. Back off some of the turn-

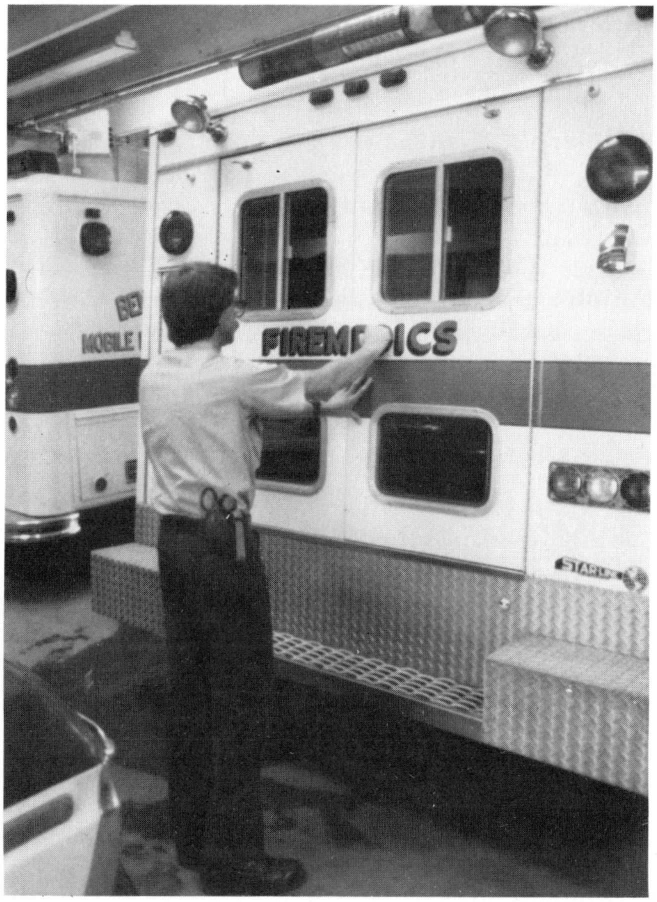

Fig. 1.26 It's best to gently close doors using door handle as a pushing point.

ing until the squeal ceases. If the steering wheel is not released at this point, undue strain will be placed on the system, reducing component life expectancy.

The suspension system also receives abuse when hitting bumps. Certainly you should avoid any bumps that you can. Some bumps, such as railroad tracks, cannot be avoided. Typically, when a driver sees tracks in his path, he will slow down by braking while crossing them. This motion puts a lot more weight over the front suspension as the vehicle pitches forward upon slowing. A better way to approach this situation is to brake before the tracks and then coast over them with the foot off the brake. This procedure allows the weight of the vehicle to be distributed more normally over all of the vehicle wheels when the suspension encounters the bumps.

Brake life seems to be a big concern in ambulance operation. Several agencies report only getting 10,000 miles from a set of brakes. The normal life expectancy of brakes is in excess of 20,000 miles. With proper maintenance and driving techniques, some agencies are able to get as much as 30,000 miles out of a set of brake shoes. Extending the life of brakes can amount to sizable savings. It does require the driver to exercise some restraint. Don't use the brake for simple slowing; backing off the accelerator will sufficiently slow the vehicle. This practice may be hard for many drivers to adjust to, as there seems to be a security in having a foot on the brake pedal. This practice also requires the driver to be more attentive to the traffic around him and to quickly anticipate changes in speed.

Left-foot braking also increases brake shoe wear. The left foot is usually found to be resting on the brake pedal, causing the brake pads to heat up and wear. This practice also keeps the rear brake lights illuminated even though the vehicle is not being slowed or stopped.

The park position of the transmission tends to be used to hold the vehicle when the parking brake should also be set. This practice can cause problems. When the transmission is placed in park, a small pawl (locking mechanism) in the transmission is moved against a mechanism to keep the system from functioning. This pawl can become bent, worn, or even fractured. Failure rates are increased when the pawl must hold the weight of the vehicle against gravity, e.g., parked on a hill. To avoid strain on this pawl, first engage the parking brake before placing the transmission in park.

There are many other ways to reduce wear on the engine. Starting the engine before fastening the seat belt gives the engine a few extra seconds to lubricate and warm. It is up to the crew to think before acting and try to reduce strain and component wear whenever possible.

Driver Health

When operating an ambulance, not only must we consider the condition of the vehicle but also the condition of the driver. The vehicle is only as safe as the person who is driving it. If the person is not able to see, exert physical control on the vehicle, or concentrate on the task at hand, the drive becomes unsafe. Certain physical criteria must be met for a driver to be qualified to drive an emergency vehicle.

General Health. The operator of an ambulance should not have an established history of any medical disorder that might impair his or her ability to safely operate a motor vehicle. Pre-existing health conditions such as high blood pressure, uncontrolled epilepsy, diabetes mellitus, and heart disease may prevent an otherwise fit driver from operating an emergency vehicle. The decision as to whether or not such a person will be allowed to operate an ambulance should be based on the recommendations of the ambulance company's physician and any restrictions stated by the ambulance company's insurance carrier.

The ambulance company should not allow a person to drive the ambulance if they have any psychiatric disorder or organic or functional disease likely to interfere with his or her ability to operate the ambulance in a safe manner.

Vision. Clearness of vision is called visual acuity. As a person gets older, acuity diminishes. This decrease in acuity may be so slow the person does not realize it is taking place. For this reason, it is important for the driver of an ambulance to undergo regular eye examinations. An ambulance driver should have an acuity in both eyes of not less than 20/30 with corrective lenses, or not less than 20/40 for one eye and 20/50 for the other.

Four percent of the drivers today are color-blind. Color-blindness may not keep a driver from performing competently; however, it should be known by a driver and his employer. A driver must be able to differentiate between red, amber, and green.

Hearing. The prospective ambulance driver must be able to perceive a whisper at not less than five feet. If an audiometric device is used, a loss greater than 25-30 decibels at 500 Hz, 1,000 Hz, and 2,000 Hz would disqualify a prospective emergency vehicle driver. The driver may be accepted if his or her hearing can be corrected to within these standards through the use of a hearing aid.

A driver must also be aware of his emotional state and drive accordingly. If fatigued or ill, he or she should be relieved of duty.

Anger and other emotions also affect driving performance. Anger can preoccupy a driver, distracting him from the task at hand. An angry driver may not perceive situations developing as quickly as he would normally. The angry driver also tends to easily lose patience and, therefore, take risks. An ambulance driver must be mature enough to effectively deal with his emotions or recognize that he cannot, thus removing himself from behind the wheel.

Driving History

How a driver will perform in an emergency situation can be determined, to a certain degree, by looking at his past driving record. A driver of an ambulance must possess a driver's license allowing him to drive an ambulance within that particular state. The driver should also have a clean driving record. A history of several driving citations indicates a possible attitude problem and a disregard for traffic regulations. This potential attitude problem can become a major concern when the person is responsible for maneuvering a vehicle through traffic safely while at variance to other traffic.

When a driver is being considered for use as a volunteer driver or employment as an ambulance operator, his or her driving record should be requested from the state motor vehicles division. The report should not reflect any major violations or reveal any citations or accidents not previously disclosed to the employer. Your ambulance company's insurance carrier may have specific guidelines that might automatically disqualify a driver found to have several violations. The carrier might also increase your insurance premiums if drivers possessing poor driving records are utilized as ambulance drivers. It is also a good idea to review each driver's motor vehicles department record every year or two to determine if citations have been issued which might influence insurance coverage or indicate a poor driving attitude. A poor driving record reduces the chances for a successful defense in court should there be involvement in a motor vehicle accident.

Driving Experience

Individual driving experience should also be researched prior to allowing someone to operate an ambulance. Has the applicant received special driving instruction? Does he or she have sufficient driving experience to comfortably operate a motor vehicle? Has the driver operated a vehicle similar to the ambulance type he or she is to operate? Not all drivers obtain a driver's license on their sixteenth birthday and then drive 10,000 miles per year in a variety of driving conditions.

Driving is a skill which should be highly developed by the ambulance operator. It is all too common for motor vehicle operators to become lax and less attentive after years of driving. All ambulance drivers should successfully complete a defensive driving course and receive driving technique refresher classes on a regular basis.

The professional ambulance operator must be competent and confident when driving the vehicle in any weather condition or traffic situation.

Ambulance Familiarity

In order to drive any vehicle well, the driver must be totally familiar with the characteristics of that particular vehicle. The driver must know stopping distances, turning radii, and the agility of the specific vehicle. He or she must also develop a feel for the space the vehicle occupies on the road. The driver must be aware of his proximity to other obstacles and his or her vehicle's relation to them. This familiarity can only come about with experience, both in the specific type of vehicle and in the vehicle in particular.

Vans, often used as a basic chassis for ambulances, provide a unique driving challenge to people not familiar with driving them. Because the driver sits almost over the front tires, instead of behind them as in other vehicles, one not familiar with driving a van will have a tendency to initiate turns too early. This proximity to the front wheels also makes it harder to judge how much shorter a radius the rear wheels will turn in a curve compared to the front wheels.

The short hood also proves difficult for drivers not familiar with vans. Without the hood out in front to sight down, drivers often find it more difficult to keep the vehicle centered in the traffic lane.

Persons new to driving a particular type of vehicle need practice. Some of this practice should come about off the road where they can learn the perception necessary to keep track of the vehicle's relationship to other objects. Other practice must come about on the road just to become familiar with the vehicle's individual driving characteristics. Drivers already familiar with a certain type of vehicle need only to gain experience on the open road. Specific idiosyncrasies of that particular vehicle may then be noted. Driver/vehicle familiarization must be accomplished before the driver takes the vehicle on an emergency call or tries to drive with patients on board.

2 LEGAL ASPECTS OF EMERGENCY DRIVING

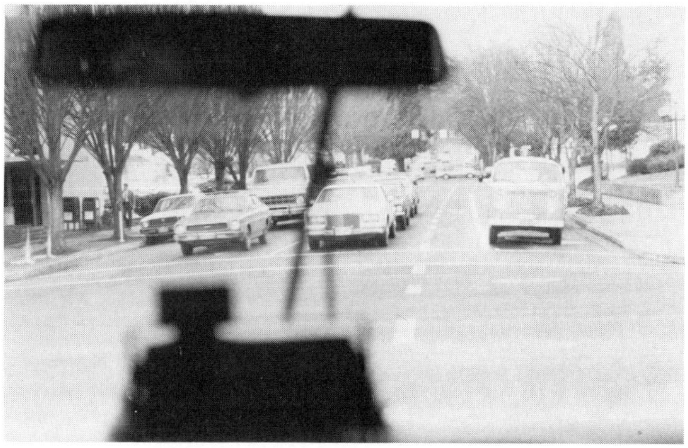

Any time you discuss the operations of an emergency vehicle, you must also address the laws that affect that vehicle's operations.

In this chapter, we will present an overview of the basics of law and some of the traffic law exemptions and obligations an ambulance may be privileged to exercise. We will also go into some depth on the moral and legal concerns of operating the ambulance in an emergency mode and at variance to other traffic. Additionally, we will give recommendations on how the EMT/driver and his employer can reduce the degree of liability exposure they each share.

What is Law?

Law consists of the written, enforceable principles and regulations established by a government, applicable to all people.

Law comes from many sources. "Common" law or "case" law is the sum total of court rulings on similar cases within each state and the United States. The law of negligence is an example of common law.

Statutory law is created by legislative (lawmaking) bodies. Congress, state legislatures, and some federal and state administrative agencies can create statutory law. City and county ordinances also fall into the category of statutory law. Whereas common law is less easy to define, statutory laws (e.g., motor vehicle laws) are usually crystal clear.

Regulations are laws enacted by an administrative agency such as the Department of Motor Vehicles or Bureau of Health to regulate a profession or trade. Ambulance operators and EMTs are certainly ruled by such agencies in each state. The administrative agency is enabled by legislation and will generally have three powers:

1. The legal authority to make regulations;
2. The authority to enforce the laws or "administrative rules" under its jurisdiction;
3. The legal authority to revoke or suspend certificates, licenses, or permits it had previously issued (hearings are required for this act).

Since a regulation's power is derived from an enabling statute, it cannot contradict any existing statute. Regulations have the full force of law and must be strictly followed.

The last source of law is from the U.S. Constitution. Constitutional law also has bearing on the operation of an ambulance in the way EMTs handle patients, their property, and their right to privacy.

Since the relationship between the different types of laws can be confusing, here are a few ways you can reduce the confusion and protect yourself and your patients.

- First, you or your employer should obtain copies of all statutes and regulations concerning ambulance operation and emergency medical care.
- Next, you must become familiar with the respective requirements of each of the laws.
- Finally, you must keep informed about new statutes or administrative rules affecting your industry.

There is one more source of "law" EMTs should be aware of and operate within. That source is your EMS agency's "policies and procedures" manual. Although you might view operation within the manual's parameters as strictly limited to maintaining your employment, that isn't entirely the case. In recent court decisions, violation of a company's written policies or operations manual has been considered as evidence of employee negligence.

Understandably then, to protect yourself from lawsuits as well as maintaining your employment, you must also be familiar with any of your agency's policies which affect the operation of the ambulance or patient care.

What is an "Emergency Vehicle"?

An "emergency vehicle" is generally defined as "a vehicle equipped as required by Statute and/or Administrative Rule which is used by a publicly maintained fire or police department or a vehicle of a federal agency which is designated as an emergency vehicle by that agency, or other publicly or privately owned vehicles designated by the Administrator or Commissioner of an appropriate State agency." The importance of this definition may not be evident upon first reading. Reread the definition. Are you sure that your ambulance is, in fact, a properly licensed emergency vehicle in your state? There are jurisdictions within the United States that have specifically left ambulances out of their definition of emergency vehicles. If this is the case in your state, the ambulance will fall into a special category when compared to fire suppression or law enforcement vehicles. An example: In one state, emergency vehicle speeds are not regulated as long as the driver does not endanger persons or property. The same state regulates that an ambulance (specifically not defined as an emergency vehicle), traveling in an emergency mode, will not exceed the designated speed limits by more than 10 mph and must not endanger persons or property. Why the difference? Historically, ambulance operators in that state were perceived as reckless drivers, often racing one another to the scene.

Public Perception

The example just given should seem senseless to today's EMS providers. Unfortunately, call jumping and concerns for a "razzle-dazzle" approach to the scene still exist. Each member of the public perceives EMS providers in a slightly different manner. It is your moral and legal responsibility to operate the ambulance in accordance with all state and local laws. It is also important to drive in a courteous, nonthreatening manner, whether traveling in an emergency mode or not. If EMTs abuse the rights given to them as operators of emergency vehicles, those rights will be withdrawn, either by legislation or public indifference to the presence of the ambulance. Once these privileges are lost, it will take many years to regain them, as is the case of the state limiting the speed at which an ambulance can exceed the designated limit.

Privileges Granted to Emergency Vehicle Drivers

Generally, when responding to an emergency the driver of an emergency vehicle will be exempt from many of the traffic laws controlling normal civilian vehicle operation. Even with an exemption, the operator of the E.V. can be found criminally or civilly liable if he is involved in an accident. Additionally, when the E.V. driver exercises an exemption to a traffic law, there is always an obligation or special requirement associated with the exemption.

Examples of Typical Exemptions

Drivers of authorized emergency vehicles may:

1. Proceed past a red traffic signal or stop sign, usually only after slowing as may be necessary for safe operation;
2. Park or stand in disregard of a statute, regulation, or ordinance prohibiting that parking or standing;
3. Exceed the designated speed limits so long as he does not endanger persons or property;
4. Disregard regulations governing direction of movement or turning in specific directions.

Some typical "obligations" required when the emergency vehicle is operated in an emergency mode and the driver exercises his exemptions (privileges) include:

1. The vehicle must be equipped with and have in use visual signaling equipment meeting the specific requirement of the appropriate statutes and administrative rules.
2. The vehicle must also be equipped with and have in use an audible exhaust whistle, siren, or bell. **(Important: Each state's laws must be checked as to whether or not the audible device *Must* be in use while traveling in an emergency mode.)**
3. The operator of the authorized emergency vehicle must have reasonable grounds to believe that delay of the E.V. will jeopardize human life or cause significant property loss.
4. The operator of the authorized emergency vehicle shall drive with due regard for the safety of all persons.
5. The exemptions shall not be a defense to the E.V. driver in an action brought forth for criminal negligence or reckless conduct.

In short, the privileges (exemptions) granted to the driver of an authorized emergency vehicle shall only apply when:

1. *A TRUE EMERGENCY EXISTS,* and
2. *THE DRIVER EXERCISES DUE REGARD FOR THE SAFETY OF OTHERS.*

True Emergency

A "true emergency" can be defined as "a situation in which there is a *high probability* of death or serious injury or significant property loss and that the actions of the E.V. operator may reduce the seriousness of the loss."

Obviously, information provided by and *solicited from* the dispatcher will help make the nature of the emergency more clear in the E.V. operator's mind. In many areas of the country, it is common for the EMS dispatcher to direct the ambulance operator as to whether he shall respond to a call in an emergency or nonemergency mode. Other agencies will have a policy of responding to all medical calls in an emergency mode. Such a policy may be inappropriate and may only be recognized as such after an accident which leads to lengthy litigation. Your emergency response to a nonemergency (remember the earlier definition) patient may be brought forth as evidence by the opposing counsel, placing you in much greater liability for an accident which occurred while you exercised your privileges as an emergency vehicle.

Due Regard

In a strict legal sense, the concept of due regard for the safety of others is somewhat more difficult to define than that of a true emergency. Simply stated, a determination as to whether or not someone exercised due regard would be to compare the actions of "a reasonably careful person, performing similar duties, under similar conditions, to the acts of the person in question."

Example: If an ambulance blazed through a red traffic light at 40 mph and was involved in an accident, the question would be brought forth as to whether the ambulance driver exercised due regard for others.

Here are some of the questions that would arise from this collision. "Was enough notice or warning of approach given to others before the collision was inevitable?" "Was warning given in accordance with the laws and were the appropriate devices used?"

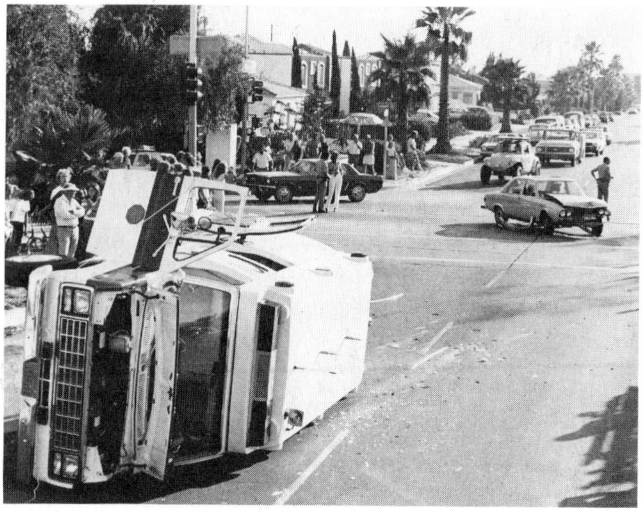

Fig. 2.1 When involved in an accident while traveling in emergency mode, the driver will be asked whether or not he exercised due regard. (Photo courtesy of **jems.**)

These questions will be asked when determining due regard. You can also safely assume that the question will come up as to whether or not a "true emergency" existed. Any unfavorable discoveries will hurt your case, whether it is in a civil or criminal trial, an in-house review board, or an investigation by your insurance carrier. Although law enforcement personnel are somewhat lax in citing ambulance operators for minor violations of the emergency privileges, should the ambulance be be involved in an accident, the police will not be in a position to extend a "professional courtesy" to you. Gross violations will certainly lead to criminal liability while less obvious errors will probably lead to civil litigation.

Negligence

Negligence can be recognized by most people, but few except attorneys can adequately give its definition. However, simply defining negligence as "carelessness" or "failing to do what is required" will suffice for this text. Charges of negligence can be easily imposed in a motor vehicle accident because each driver has a duty to other motorists and pedestrians within a radius in which they could be injured. If an injured party can demonstrate the existence of a law and its intent, that you violated the law, and that your violation caused him injury, you can easily be found guilty of negligence.

Example: While traveling in an emergency mode, an ambulance using its red lights but not its siren collided broadside with a car in a somewhat blind intersection. Although the traffic signal was red in the direction of the ambulance, its driver only slowed to 15 mph before proceeding through the light. The state traffic law requires all emergency vehicles to stop at controlled intersections before proceeding.

Can you determine if one or more laws were broken? Did the driver exercise due regard? Unfortunately, this type of scenario occurs daily in the United States. The laws are violated, and E.V. operators do not exercise due regard for others. This type of misconduct can certainly lead to a civil suit and perhaps even criminal charges.

Consider these additional potential problems. Your insurance company may not be required to honor their policy when the statutes are not obeyed and an accident results. A government-operated ambulance service may have governmental immunity if sued. You, as an employee, may have to face the entire liability issue as an individual.

Liability

Liability can be defined as the state of being obliged or bound by law to do something. One party which is automatically involved in a liability suit against an ambulance driver will be the EMT's employer. The reason the employer is found to be liable for the employee's act is threefold. First, the employer is in a position to control the employee. Second, the employee works to further the interests of the employer. Last, the risk of loss should fall upon the employer. Of course, for the employer to be liable, the negligent act must occur within the scope of the EMT's employment. Obviously, driving the ambulance during an emergency response falls within the scope of employment. What if the EMTs were out getting a hamburger without the consent or knowledge of the dispatcher and became involved in an accident?

Unlike employers, supervisors of EMS agencies are less likely to be named in a negligence action. Even secure with this knowledge, supervisors can further reduce their potential exposure by:

1. Providing employees with proper training (e.g., advanced driving techniques class);
2. Screening applicants prior to employment (e.g., review driving record and references);
3. Occasionally checking the performance of the employees in their charge to insure proficiency, etc. (e.g., review driving record to see that it has not adversely changed since employment);
4. Developing policies and procedures manuals to insure consistent driving patterns;
5. Encouraging self and others to keep abreast of all pertinent literature (e.g., read driving textbooks such as this).

Another example of liability which could lead to civil or criminal litigation would involve improperly maintained vehicles. Obviously, if the vehicle lost its brakes and crashed, causing injury to others, the potential for a suit would exist. If the plaintiff's attorney could demonstrate that the master cylinder had not been checked in six months and that the brakes had been ailing, you could easily see negligence. Here is another example of liability which you might not think of right away. The ambulance fails to start because it has been 50,000 miles since its last *documented* tune-up. The result is that another ambulance, eight miles away, must be dispatched to the call, which is only four blocks from the disabled ambulance's base station. The resulting delay in treatment *can* be used as cause in a negligence argument.

Another example which might lead to a negligence case is that of an emergency trip to the hospital with a heart patient. Perhaps the patient or his counsel could demonstrate that the actual light and siren ride caused added anxiety, increased cardiac load, and further damaged the patient's heart. The possibilities are endless.

Reducing Liability

Faced with endless conditions which could lead to a negligence suit or perhaps criminal liability, what are some of the steps you can take to reduce your liability exposure?

First and foremost, the ambulance should not be operated in an emergency mode unless:

1. **A TRUE EMERGENCY IS PERCEIVED,** and
2. **UNDER ANY AND ALL CIRCUMSTANCES, YOU EXERCISE DUE REGARD.**

Several other activities which can help to reduce liability include:

1. Consistent, relevant records regarding:
   a. Hiring practices which include exclusion of any applicant who does not have a good driving record. (Written and practical driving tests are also recommended prior to hiring EMT/ambulance drivers.)
   b. Training programs which can be documented for content, attendance, and acceptability.
   c. Maintenance records which demonstrate responsible/timely care of the ambulance. Daily inspection sheets are among the records to be retained.
2. Activities before an accident occurs:
   a. Developing a reporting/action system for unsafe conditions. If an ambulance keeps dripping oil on the floor and the second crew slips when they go to their vehicle, the oil can be cleaned up, the leak repaired, and an incident report can be filed. Evaluation of the incident report may indicate that the parking configurations should be altered to allow for a different path to each ambulance so such "slips" are avoided.
   b. Observing EMTs for compliance with company policy or commonly accepted principles. A New York Supreme Court ruled that an employee driving an ambulance at speeds in excess of the company policy was guilty of misconduct. How do you suppose such a finding would influence the driver/employer's percentages of liability if a suit evolved from an accident in which excess speed was a factor?
   c. Establishment of preventive maintenance programs are a must.
   d. Hiring good drivers and pulling bad drivers from behind the wheel can also lead to reducing the EMS agency's degree of liability should a tort action be instituted.
   e. Maintaining a thorough knowledge of the laws (exemptions and obligations) is crucial for every ambulance driver. (A current copy of the laws affecting ambulance operation may be requested from your State Department of Motor Vehicles.)
3. If an accident or loss occurs, it is important for the EMS agency to:
   a. Determine the cause of the accident.
   b. Once the cause is determined, institute preventive actions to reduce the possibility of a similar accident or loss. Such preventive actions will reduce your exposure to repeated loss and your degree of future liability.
   c. Should the accident prove to be an employee's mistake, corrective actions such as training are indicated. From each accident, all employees/drivers should learn ways to reduce the potential for a similar accident occurring in the future.

Keep in mind what the job of the EMT/ambulance driver entails.

The ambulance is to respond first to the request for aid without undue delay and, second, to transport the patient in a safe and timely manner. At all times, the ambulance must be driven with due regard for the safety of others. If it is driven in an emergency mode, a true emergency must be perceived because the EMT is capable of caring for all but a small percentage of patients without rapid transport. Most trips to the hospital are *NOT* true emergencies. Also remember that anything which causes delay or impairs safe operation of an ambulance can give rise to a potential lawsuit.

3 COMMUNICATIONS

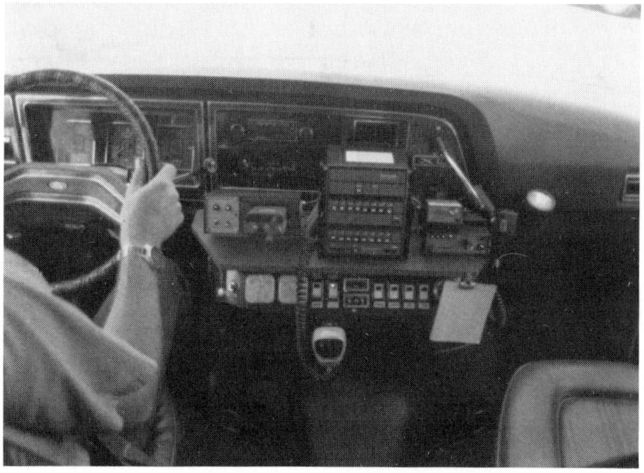

Emergency medicine has made tremendous strides since the early 1970s. One of the primary reasons for this surge has been the increased ability of the EMT to communicate with base station hospitals. It was radio communications which allowed a few brave programs in the forefront of prehospital care to take the principles Dr. Pantridge developed on defibrillation into the field. Radio communications enabled some specially trained ambulance personnel to provide advanced life support while being directed by a physician.

It was not so many years ago that ambulances had "RADIO DISPATCHED" boldly advertised across the sides of the vehicle. To actually write "RADIO DISPATCHED" on the side of the ambulance must have been some big deal. Indeed it was! With the inclusion of a radio in the ambulance, the crew could receive a call no matter where they were. The crew didn't have to wait to get back to the station to find out another call had been received. They could be notified directly by radio. When trouble with an address or a potentially violent situation arose, help was at their fingertips.

The use of radios has dramatically affected the way care is rendered in today's EMS system. With the use of the radio, the physician is almost at the side of the EMT or paramedic. It is this radio link with the physician which allows those same technicians to provide advanced life support, administer medications, and perform invasive procedures in the field.

It is unknown how many lives have been saved through the use of the radio. Radio communications allow the crew to be kept abreast of events developing at the scene even before they arrive. It is radio communication that allows the closest crew to be sent to the call whether they are near a phone or not.

Radio communications allow the first-on-the-scene fire crew to warn the ambulance technicians that the normal way into the scene is blocked by traffic. Communications allows the hospital to be informed of a patient and his condition long before he arrives, allowing the Emergency Department time to fully prepare for the patient's arrival. Communications plays a vital role in the work performed by EMTs and paramedics. It is also an important component of driving the ambulance.

Communication System

In an Emergency Medical Services system, the ambulance is but one cog in the overall machinery which comprises the system. For all of these EMS cogs to fit together and work smoothly, they must be in communication with each other. A network to provide this type of communication link may range from very simple to extremely complex. Certain elements must exist for the EMS system to work. Any EMS system should contain at least some of the following communication capabilities:

Access for the consumer into the EMS system;
Dispatch, for the proper crew and continual contact throughout the call;
Intercommunication between ambulance units;
Communications between ambulances and other agencies;
Hospital-to-hospital communications.

Equipment Basics

An EMS communications system requires a wide range of equipment. Ability to talk from the dispatch center to the ambulance will require at least two different transmitters and receivers, one in the ambulance and, of course, one at the base station in the dispatch center. The EMT over on the other side of an embankment will communicate with his partner with yet another type of transmitter/receiver (T/R). The hospital will have yet another type of communications unit. When the crew initially receives a call, they may be alerted through a small unit (pager) carried on the belt. It is important for the ambulance driver and other technicians to be familiar with the different communications delivery devices utilized within each EMS system.

Simplex. A simplex radio communication system requires nothing more than a base station T/R and a mobile T/R on the same frequency. Because a simplex system is the least complicated and relatively inexpensive, it is the most common type of system in EMS use today. Many ambulances have several frequency channels. One is utilized for base-to-ambulance communications, one for ambulance-to-hospital, and perhaps another for frequency extended use such as multicasualty situations. Such systems are still considered simplex if only one frequency can be broadcast on at a time and only one form of communication can be broadcast upon that frequency at a time while utilizing a single T/R. Typically, a fixed base station will be relatively high-powered and able to broadcast with between 80-150 watts of power. Mobile T/Rs have a broadcast power of 20-110 watts. This allows the mobile unit to transmit effectively over distances of 20 to 25 miles, depending upon the terrain and frequency.

Duplex. With the need to transmit electrocardiogram (ECG) by biomedical telemetry and at the same time be able to consult with a physician, many services have resorted to duplexing. Such a system utilizes two or more frequencies capable of simultaneously transmitting on both of them. One frequency is utilized for voice communication and another for patient telemetry.

Duplex systems are also frequently used in areas where a tremendous amount of voice traffic shares the same radio frequencies. In this application, all transmissions from the base station to the vehicle are made on one frequency while all transmissions to the base station are made on another frequency. This system requires that each ambulance have a transmitter separate from the receiver. It also means that ambulances cannot communicate between each other unless a third frequency is used for that purpose. The primary advantage to this type of system is that it does cut the amount of radio traffic on the main frequency in half. It also allows simultaneous transmitting and receiving, a great advantage for a busy dispatch center.

Multiplex. A multiplex system uses only one frequency but allows for at least two different types of communication at the same time over that frequency. To accomplish this, the multiplex system receives the information (e.g., voice and telemetry), encodes the information, and then transmits the coded message. When the message is received, it must go through a decoding process before it can be utilized. A functional multiplex system requires that the ambulance have an encoding device within the vehicle radio and that the hospital or other stations have a decoding device.

Private Line. A private-line feature enhances a radio system in a "radio-congested" area. With such a system, the radio receiver remains turned on but in a standby mode until it is triggered by a coded tone emitted by the transmitter. The advantage of a private-line feature is that the radio does not receive traffic that does not pertain to that unit or service unless specifically toned. Such a system typically has a dialer, or pushbutton keyboard, much like a telephone that is used to code the desired tones.

When private line is utilized in a motor vehicle, the microphone may have a special clip to hold the mike in a standby mode. When the mike is lifted from this clip, the radio opens the private

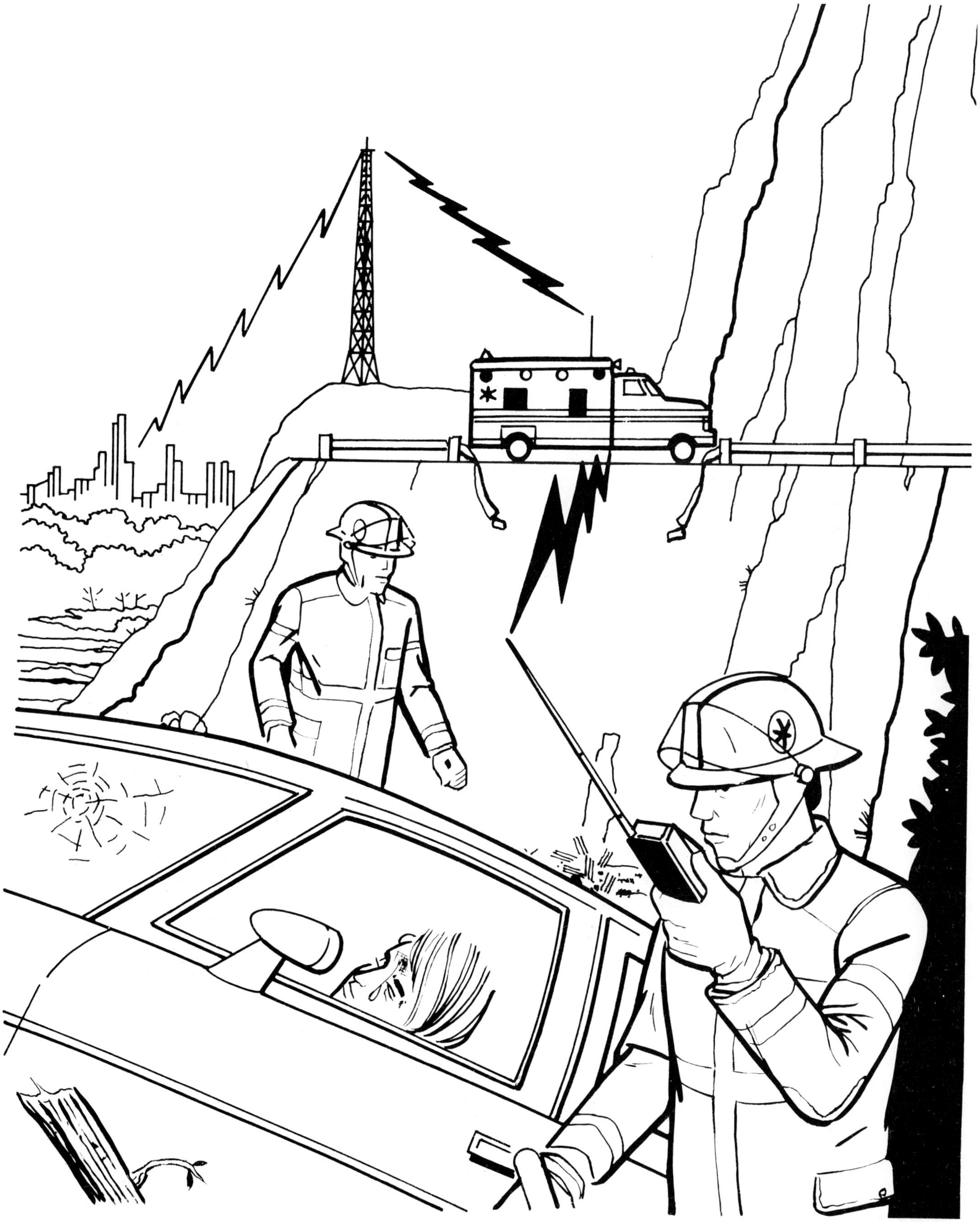

Fig. 3.1 In the emergency medical service, an ambulance is but one cog in the machinery comprising the system. All components must communicate with each other for the system to work smoothly.

line so all traffic can be heard. With the private-line feature, it is important that the operator listen for a moment after lifting the mike before transmitting tone to assure no one else is utilizing the frequency.

More sophisticated private-line systems will automatically emit a predesignated tone each time the mike is keyed. With such a system it is imperative that the operator depress the mike for at least one second before talking to allow this automatic encoding to be completed.

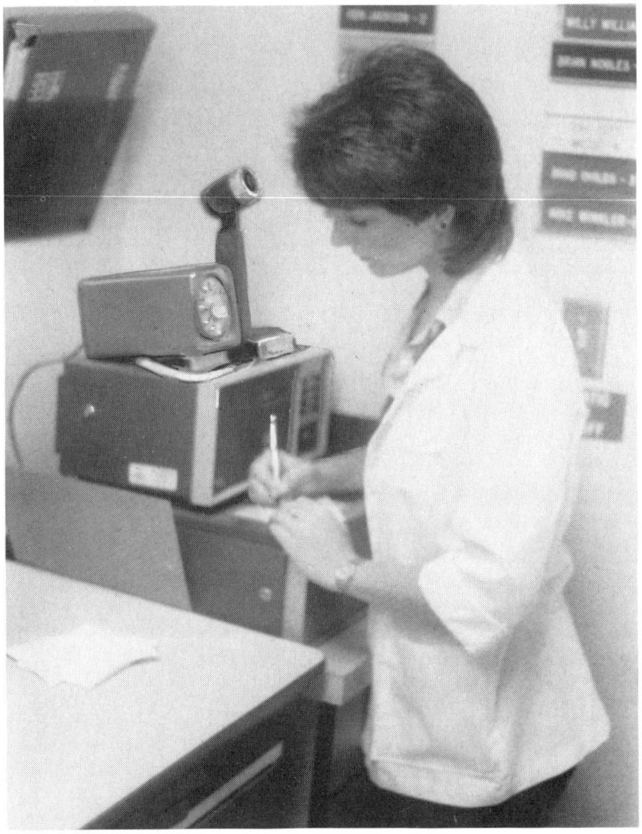

Fig. 3.2a Most hospitals today have communications with ambulances regardless of location.

Repeaters. Mobile radios used in the vehicle are not as powerful as the base station radio. The vehicle limits the size, weight, and power source of mobile radios. In areas where the ambulance radio must broadcast long distances, or where the terrain is rough, the ambulance radio may not be able to communicate with the desired station. In many such areas, this problem is corrected by the use of repeaters. Repeaters are radio stations, usually set high on a mountain or building, that pick up a signal and rebroadcast it. Mobile repeaters can also be placed in the vehicle. In-vehicle repeaters allow an EMT or paramedic with a hand-held radio to broadcast to the vehicle repeater where it is picked up and rebroadcast to either another base repeater or to a base station. Repeater systems are duplex, requiring two frequencies, one to receive and another for transmission.

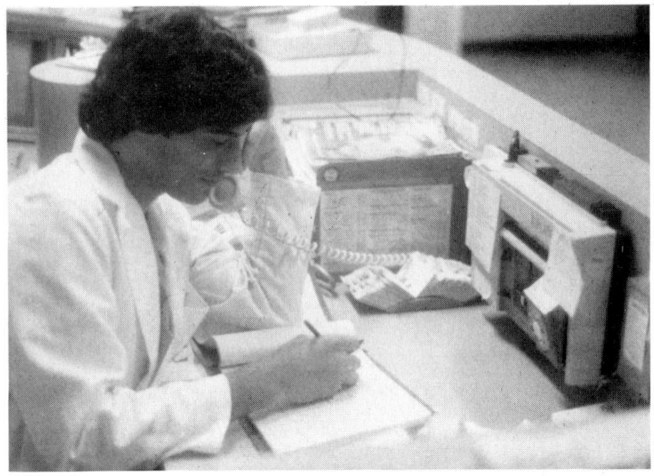

Fig. 3.2b Communications occur through a remote center linked to a base station several miles away.

Remote. Today, most hospitals have radio communications with the ambulances in the field. Often this is accomplished through the use of a remote center that is linked to a base station several miles away. For example, a hospital has a remote T/R that can communicate with the same power as the dispatch base station. This is because the remote T/R is connected to a base radio through telephone lines. The base radio may be at the ambulance operator's base station, or perhaps in another part of the hospital.

Portable Radios. With all of the equipment used today, it is impossible to initially take all of the patient-care equipment that might be needed from the ambulance to the patient's side. Therefore, only a basic amount of equipment is normally taken to the patient when the EMTs first arrive at the scene. This procedure can be a little more complicated when the patient is down over an embankment or up several flights of stairs. Enter the hand-held radio. With the portable radio in hand, one technician can go to the patient with the basic equipment, and then call back to the other crew member for any additional equipment that might be needed. The hand-held radio consists of a small unit. The typical portable radio usually has around five watts of power and can only use one frequency at a time.

Some portable radios are duplex or multiplex system-oriented and can transmit telemetry and voice between the scene and the hospital.

Pagers. Pagers are one-way radio devices that are worn on the clothing of the user. They generally receive a radio transmission that sets off a tone alert within the unit. Many pagers allow for one-way voice communication from the dispatcher. Pager use has significantly changed emergency response times. Volunteers can be contacted by the dispatch center at all times without having to worry what will happen if a call is received while they are away from a phone or stationary radio receiver. Many agencies have found that pagers are a reliable, relatively inexpensive way to contact crew members, whether on or off duty.

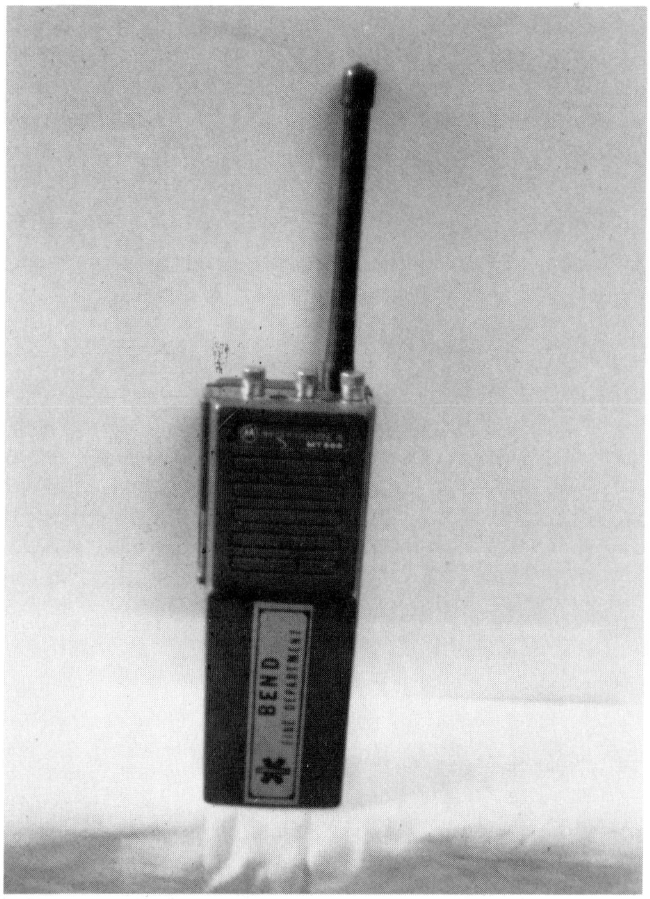

Fig. 3.3a Typical portable unit rated at about five watts of power output transmitted on one frequency.

Public Address (PA). A component of the EMT's communications system that is often overlooked is the PA system contained within the vehicle's siren unit. The PA setting of the siren can amplify and broadcast the mobile radio communication received in the ambulance so it can be heard while the EMT is away from the vehicle. The PA system also allows the crew to communicate with people at the scene, perhaps asking a crowd to move back or hailing other rescue personnel from some distance away. The PA can be used while en route to the scene to explain to a confused motorist exactly what you would like him to do. The PA system should not be abused. Do not yell at people or use this system excessively.

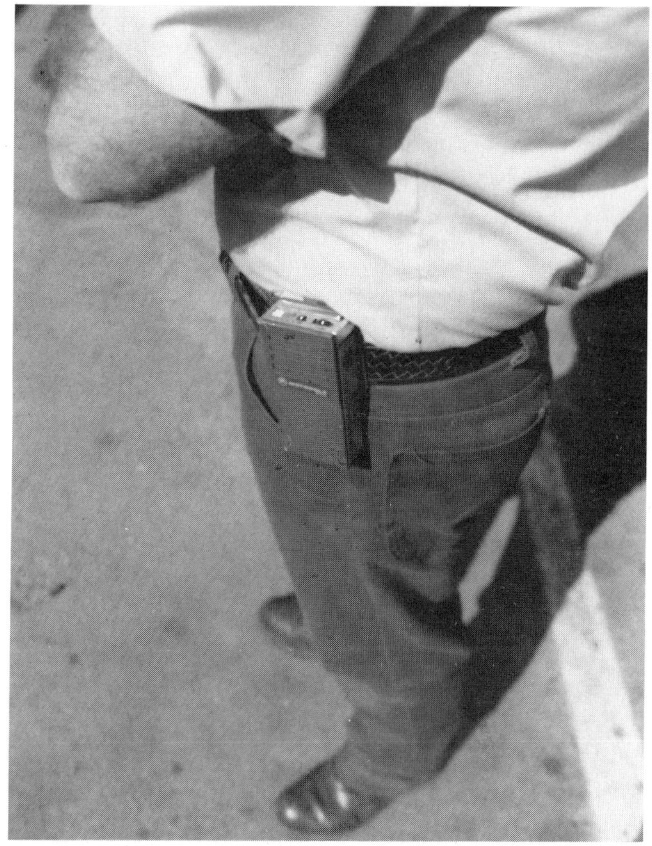

Fig. 3.3b Typical tone paging receiver.

Equipment Location

When fully equipped with siren, mobile radio repeater heads, portable radios, and other equipment carried in the driver compartment, the decision on where to locate all this equipment can become difficult. The typical place picked for mounting is the dashboard. This, however, is often the worst place to mount it. Equipment placed on the dash can increase the chance of accidents. It doesn't take much on the dash to create a blind spot for the driver. Visibility is engineered into the vehicle by the manufacturer. All too often, it is stolen from the driver by those deciding on where to place siren and radio equipment. Federal law requires dashboards to be padded to protect the vehicle occupants in a collision. This padding cannot do any good when it is covered with metal or hard plastic structures with sharp corners. Obviously, radio equipment and siren controls mounted on the dashboard can be injurious to your health.

The engine cowling on Type II (van) and Type III (van cab) ambulances acts as a good alternative to dash mounting. Here the equipment is readily accessible to all technicians, yet still out of the way. Some concerns have been expressed by maintenance personnel over such positioning. Placement of equipment on the cowling makes it more difficult to reach the engine, entailing the need to disconnect several wires before the cowling can be removed. Some of this difficulty can be overcome by placing plug connectors on the wires that come out of the unit (siren and radio) heads. Equipment can then be disconnected rapidly without fear of fraying or fracturing the wires. The equipment can also be located out of the way of the windshield by building a bracket to suspend the radio equipment from the dash. The bracket should suspend it below the dash level, low enough that it won't be struck by occupants in the event of a collision.

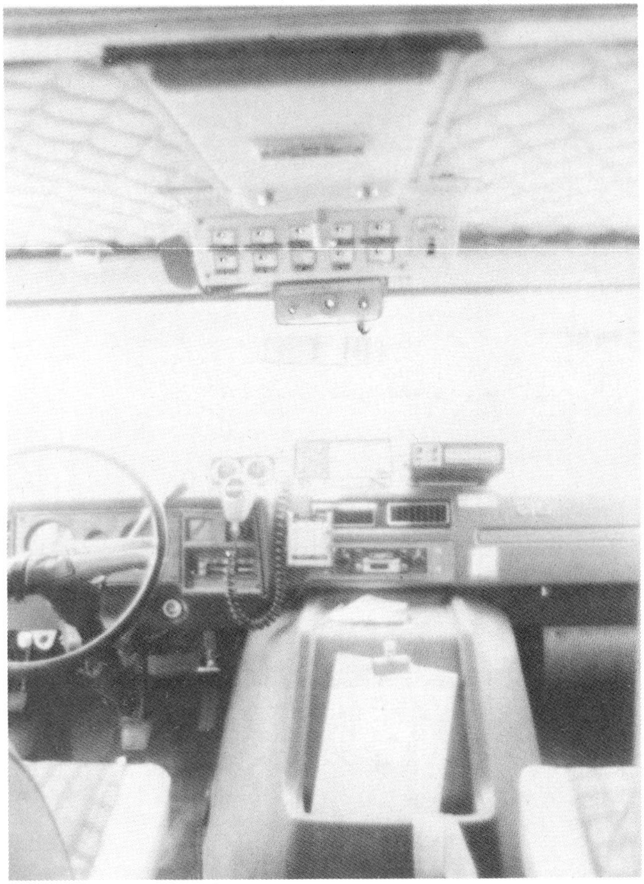

Fig. 3.4a The dashboard—a typical mounting site for radio equipment but it can create blindspots and a potential collision hazard.

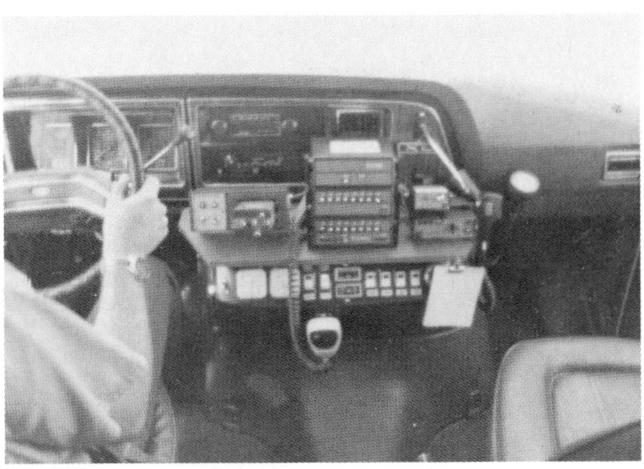

Fig. 3.4b The engine Cowling of type II or III vehicles is a good, safe radio mounting alternative.

Communications On the Radio

For many people, talking on the radio can be difficult. The idea of having to do so may frighten operators because they are unsure of how to conduct themselves. To others, talking on the radio is no problem; it's just like talking on the telephone. Such diverse attitudes point out the lack of understanding of the function, purpose, and limitations of the radio.

On the phone there is generally an unlimited time to convey a message. If the party on the other end wants a clarification or to interject a thought, he has only to do so. He can interrupt the conversation. With a radio, the same luxuries do not exist. The frequency is shared with others. Once the mike is keyed, we exclude others from communicating. Imagine then the frustration of a dispatcher who must convey vital information to one ambulance crew but cannot because another crew is occupying the frequency giving a wordy or unnecessary message.

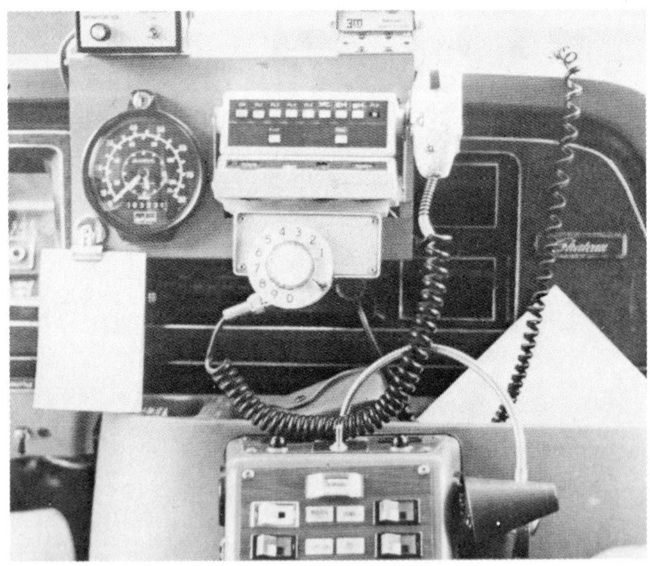

Fig. 3.5 Suspend radio equipment on a bracket mounted to the dash to keep it out of the way of the windshield.

Talking on the radio need not be difficult. It does require a certain amount of deliberation. The following guidelines should be followed when broadcasting information over the air.

Plan all Communication in Advance. Before keying the mike, take a moment to collect your thoughts on what needs to be said. A brief, concise message is always best. Where applicable, use standard formats (e.g., standard "10-code") for delivery. Everyone concerned will know what is being said and the message will be delivered in as brief a time as possible. Use proper terminology. Select those words that can be best understood. "Affirmative" comes across the radio much clearer than the word "yes." The word "yes" tends to get lost during radio transmission. By planning our message in advance, we can eliminate time-consuming fillers such as "Uh, . . ." or "Well, . . ."

"Advise" is a preferred word for radio use over "find out," "how do I," and "do you want." "Obtain" is used instead of "get" and "desire" is used instead of "want." "Traffic" is a radio message, while "copy" indicates that the speaker has understood a given message.

Listen to the Frequency for a Moment Prior to Transmitting. This assures that the frequency is clear for traffic. If others are talking, wait for them to sign off before using the frequency.

Depress the Mike Key for One-half Second Prior to Speaking. It is not uncommon for someone to key the microphone and immediately start talking. As a result of this hasty action, the beginning word or syllables of the transmission get cut off. To avoid such a situation, the operator has only to wait a moment before talking. Private-line systems require a full second pause for self-encoding.

Keep your Mouth Close to the Mike. By keeping the microphone two to three inches from the mouth, the operator has a much better chance of being understood. As the microphone is moved away from the mouth, some voice modulation becomes lost. Background noise may also drown out voice communications if the microphone is not held closely to the mouth.

Enunciate Clearly. Each word must be spoken clearly and without emotion to be easily understood. Don't clip words. Say each word in full instead of cutting off the last letters as in "goin'" instead of "going." Lazy speech patterns must be corrected. Don't talk with food in your mouth.

Repeat all Directions. It is very easy to confuse words spoken over the radio. Seven may sound like eleven. Two similar street names may also become confused. To help avoid confusion, all directions should be repeated by those receiving them. All physician orders should also be repeated to insure accuracy. In some states, this is required by law.

Clear the Frequency. Others may be waiting to use the air. When you finish your transmission sequence, you can help them access the air more quickly by giving a standard sign-off at the end of your last transmission.

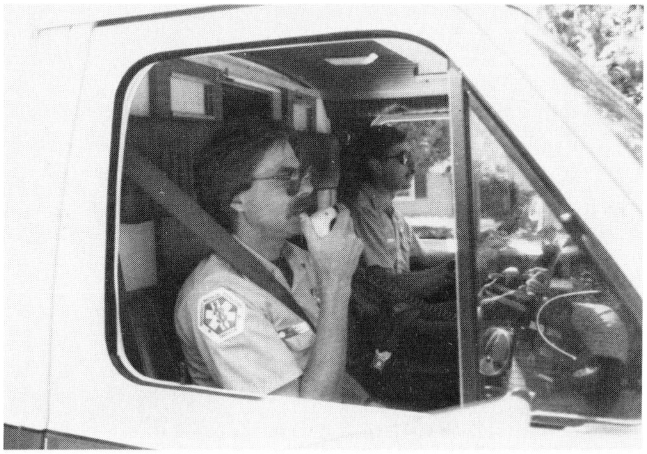

Fig. 3.6a Driver's priority is to drive safely; the other crew member makes radio transmissions whenever possible.

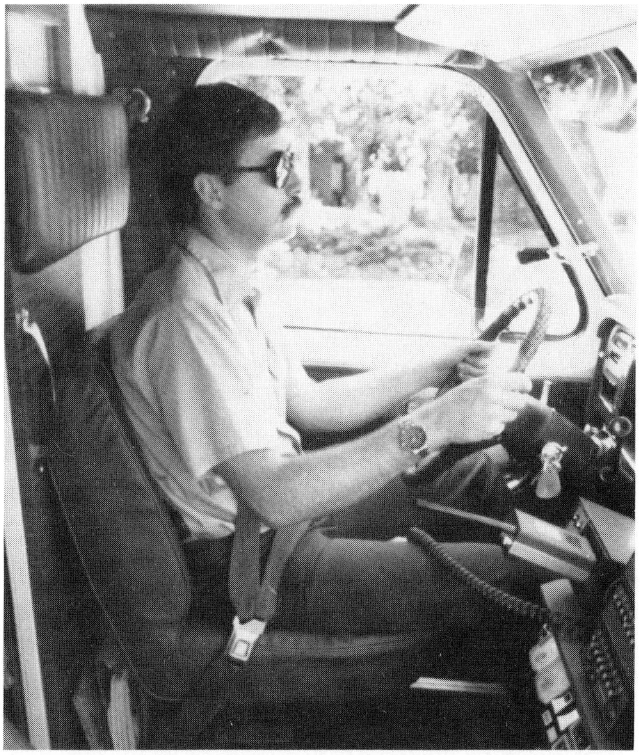

Fig. 3.6b When driver has to use radio, he should consider dropping microphone in his lap between transmissions to keep it within easy reach and avoid distractions.

The driver of the ambulance must exercise caution when using the radio. His priority is to drive safely. Whenever possible, the driver should allow the other crew members to make radio broadcasts. This, of course, cannot always be done as the crew may be very involved in patient care. Brief radio transmissions will reduce the time a driver is distracted from his or her primary mission, safe vehicle operation. Rather than returning the mike to its clip each time, the driver might consider carefully placing the microphone in his lap between transmissions. This practice keeps the microphone within easy reach and reduces driver distraction. It also avoids the problem of having to wrestle the mike from a tight or sticky clip.

Routine Reports. Most ambulance radio communications can be categorized as routine. Types of communications used on nearly every call include: Dispatch, en route reports, arrival at the scene, patient status reports, and the like. Because these communications are given frequently and in each case contain similar information, concise message formats can be developed. Through the use of the same format, the EMT will be less likely to overlook pertinent data or deliver extraneous information over the radio. Below is an example of radio traffic between a dispatch center and an ambulance ready for service but away from the station.

Dispatch: "Unit three four, Dispatch, ready to copy, code three."
Ambulance: "Unit three four, ready to copy, First and Oak."
Dispatch: "Unit three four, respond, two, nine, seven, three Maple, possible heart."
Crew: "Copy two, nine, seven, three Maple. Responding code three."

The dispatcher may also assign a "case" or "run" number at this time.

Following this call along further, we hear how the crew and dispatcher may communicate other routine messages.

Dispatch: "Unit three four, dispatch."
Crew: "Seventh and Oak."
Dispatch: "Be advised engine five is responding with you from their station."
Crew: "Three four, copy."

Crew: "Dispatch, unit three four."
Dispatch: "Dispatch."
Crew: "This address has a previous history of violence. Advise PD."
Dispatch: "Copy. Will advise PD."
Crew: "Twenty-first and Oak."

Crew: "Three four on scene."
Dispatch: "Copy three four."
Crew: "Three four changing to hospital frequency."
Dispatch: "Copy three four" and then gives the radio station call sign.

By analyzing these broadcasts or radio "traffic," we can see the format this agency has developed to give maximum information within a minimum of air time.

Every time a radio conversation is initiated, the designation of the unit being called is given first, followed by the designation of the calling unit. This serves to immediately alert the party for which the broadcast is intended and at the same time let others on the same frequency know that they are not needed.

Note that the dispatch gives the ambulance crew a moment to grab a notepad and pen to take down the dispatch information. This courtesy takes a few moments longer but saves the crew from having to ask the dispatcher to repeat the information.

Unit three four is in the field when called by the dispatcher. When they answer the call, unit three four gives its location at the end of the broadcast sequence as a "sign off." This allows the dispatcher to visualize the crew's location in relationship to the scene. The dispatcher can also estimate the probable route of travel and approximate time of response. While this practice is looked upon by some crews as meddling, it does serve several important purposes. It is the dispatcher's job to coordinate the response. This can be done much quicker and with less radio traffic if he receives a continual update as to the crew's location. With this information, the dispatcher can assure that the closest unit is responding. The dispatcher can also determine if the response time will be so long as to require a first-response unit, such as an engine company. He can also advise other agencies of the ambulance's approximate arrival time and probable route of travel. In the unfortunate event of an ambulance accident, it may be the ambulance not calling out at the scene that will tip the dispatcher off to the trouble. He can then isolate the ambulance location to a point between the scene and its last reported location.

All numbers are given in a singular form. That is to say, the address is given as two nine seven three instead of twenty-nine seventy-three.

Many numbers sound similar when delivered over the radio. In the case above, if the crew mistook seven for eleven, the ambulance would certainly miss the scene. Always pronounce the number "0" as zero.

All important aspects of directions should be repeated. In this case, the address is repeated by the crew to further assure that the message was received properly. Advisory messages do not usually need to be repeated. Advisory messages given in the above call include that it is a possible heart, that engine five is responding, and that the scene has had a history of violence. In the latter case, it is only necessary for the dispatcher to acknowledge the need for the police. If known, the dispatcher might also advise unit three four of the Police Department's estimated time of arrival (ETA).

Information such as engine five responding with your unit should also be routine. This informs the crew that they will have help at the scene. It will also tell the ambulance crew where that help is probably responding from. The ambulance crew can then determine the probable route to be traveled by engine five. With this information, the crew can be alert for other emergency vehicle traffic, especially where their routes of travel will probably merge.

When called by another party such as a supervisor or other agency, the ambulance crew should initially respond with its present location.

Supervisor: "Supervisor four, unit three four."
Crew: "Unit three four, Broadway and Jefferson."

When radio traffic is initiated by a mobile unit, the unit should give its location as a sign-off upon completion of the message.

Patient Information. The same principle of routine format and brief transmission should also be followed when radioing patient information to the medical control hospital. The information should include the patient's:

1. Age and sex.*
2. Chief complaint.
3. History of present illness or injury.
4. Level of consciousness and general condition.
5. Pertinent physical findings.
6. Vital signs.
7. Treatment in progress.
8. ETA at the care facility.

*Most EMS systems discourage divulging the patient's name over the air.

It is easy to see how much information can be delivered in a clear, concise manner, if preplanning of messages and standard radio formats are utilized.

Radio Codes. Using radio codes along with established formats for routine transmissions can pack an amazing amount of information into very short periods of time. In areas where radio traffic is relatively heavy or where more than one ambulance is on the same frequency, such codes get the information to everyone in a smooth manner and reduce the amount of time another crew may need to wait to use the radio. Radio codes can be awkward for those who don't use them regularly. Infrequent radio operators may find that the use of codes can actually consume more time than if words were spoken. The infrequent code user must mentally sort through the list of codes to select the appropriate code. Infrequent use may lead to the wrong one being used. Therefore, it is up to the individual agency to determine whether or not they will use codes. An example of a typical "10-code" can be found in the appendix.

There are certain patient conditions that are best transmitted through the use of a code. While some of these patient conditions may not be encountered frequently, there are only a few so code memorization should not be difficult. Special circumstances generally include patient-compromising situations that you don't want people at the scene to understand. Special codes can be used to communicate information on patients suspected of drinking, having a mental disorder, or being under the influence of drugs. Other patient conditions that you might want to disguise include attempted suicides and perhaps patient death. These special codes should be posted by the radio in an Emergency Department for ready reference.

An agency might also want to consider a code designating "public in the area." Such a code can be used on an occasion when requested information can't be easily given over the radio because someone close by doesn't have a need to know.

Phonetic Alphabet. The phonetic alphabet should be used to spell out street names or other pertinent information that cannot be easily understood when given over the radio. A standardized phonetic alphabet should be adopted by each EMS agency. It should be the same for all parties utilizing any one radio frequency. Proper use of the phonetic alphabet dictates that only the phonetic word is used. Example: X, Y, Z is X-ray,

Young, Zebra. Do not say X as in X-ray, Y as in Young, etc. A standard phonetic alphabet can be found in the appendix of this text.

Special Circumstances. Routine reports are relatively easy to give. They are delivered as common events occur and fall easily into a format that becomes a "system." Special circumstances are the situations that develop outside the routine. The first order of business is to determine whether the circumstance is worth reporting. An abandoned auto off the side of the road, not obstructing traffic, is not relevant to ambulance operation or immediate public safety. Rarely would such a case require comment over the radio. On the other hand, a police officer might notify his dispatcher as part of his duty. If the vehicle were stranded and the driver seemed unable to fix it, the ambulance crew might notify the PD so assistance can be obtained by the motorist.

Federal Communications Commission (FCC) rules dictate that radio stations licensed to ambulance operators or rescue squads only be used for the transmission of messages pertaining to the safety of life or property. It is advisable to consider whether your message is urgent or if you can wait until you reach a telephone before delivering a message. Good public relations can still be maintained by the crew when offering aid to the public by utilizing telephone lines instead of the ambulance radio.

The radio might be used to notify the police about an inoperative traffic light, the Water Department about a broken water main, or the Highway Department about a broken section of guard rail, as each could adversely affect public safety.

Once it has been decided that a particular situation dictates radio transmission, the radio operator must plan what he is going to say. It is in this area that some people seem to have difficulty. They pick up the radio on impulse and begin talking. As a result of impulse, the message is usually not given with an economy of words and the broadcast is loaded with fillers such as "Uh, . . ." The radio operator should always try to think about what he or she is going to say *before* starting a message.

Dispatch Information. The dispatcher is the coordinator of all of the calls his agency is handling. It is the dispatcher's job to receive the call, obtain the pertinent information, determine which crew is best able to handle the call, and dispatch that crew. The dispatcher also alerts any additional assistance that might be needed such as law enforcement, fire suppression, water, or heavy rescue. He also helps the crew get to their destination. This task can become very difficult and stressful for the dispatcher. The key to good dispatching is to get good information in the beginning.

Obtaining information from a caller is more than just taking down the information they give over the phone. If left to their own, many callers are unable to give adequate information. They ramble on about how bad the patient appears and keep asking the dispatcher to hurry, frequently without giving the location at which the help is needed. To overcome this problem, the dispatcher can get quick, pertinent information by taking control of the conversation and then leading the caller through a list of predetermined questions. Important information to obtain includes:

Address. Where is the patient? It is important to establish where the patient is since many callers give their own address. If the location is a rural setting or on the open highway, any landmarks, the nearest intersection, or milepost markers should be requested.

Phone Number. Frequently, the address that is given is wrong. The numbers are transposed, or perhaps the address has recently been changed. When the crew is having a difficult time finding the location, a call-back number can save the day. This number can also be helpful in determining in which area of town a call originated. If two cities are close together and have streets with the same name, it may be the phone prefix that first alerts the dispatcher as to which city is involved.

Name of Caller. Should the dispatcher need to call back to gain more information, it is advisable to have at least the name of one person who is familiar with the situation.

Apparent Medical Problem. Information gained from a few quick questions can help the dispatcher determine the urgency of the call and help prepare the ambulance crew for what lies ahead of them at the scene. Medically trained dispatchers can also advise bystanders of basic first-aid techniques to be applied prior to help arriving. In many cases, such information has proven to be lifesaving.

Type of Accident. It will be of great value to know what type of accident (auto, aircraft, industrial) and the number of patients injured in order to dispatch the appropriate resources. A submerged car may require the resources of several agencies including police, fire, heavy rescue, harbor patrol, and emergency medical services. Known hazards such as chemical spills, fire, or downed electrical wires can also influence the resources required and the direction from which units approach the scene.

A vital member of the EMS team, a good dispatcher can truly save lives and help the ambulance crews operate more safely and efficiently.

Professionalism

Just as driving and other components of the provision of EMS require professionalism, so does radio use. The radio is not a toy. It is not to be used to joke over and make cute remarks on. It is another important tool of the EMT and paramedic. Today, many people have monitors to listen to police, fire, and ambulance calls. For these people, it is their only contact with you. Your radio conduct is a reflection on the EMS profession. Be courteous and professional when you use this great tool.

4 ATTITUDES AND HABITS

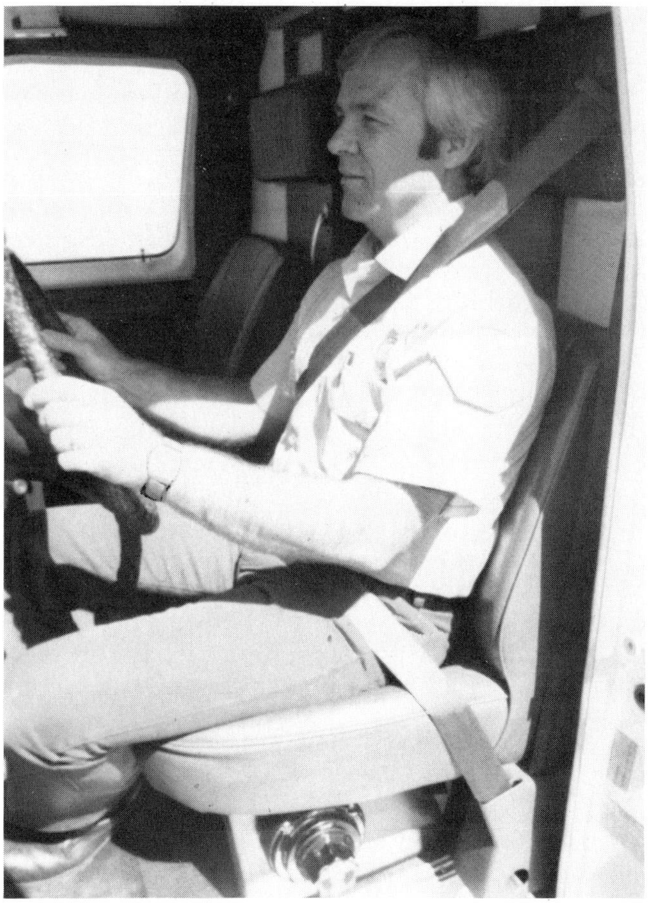

Lives depend upon how EMTs and paramedics handle the situations they encounter. Patient care and transportation is not for amateurs or thrill-seekers; rather, it's a responsibility for professionals. Being a professional does not mean that every EMT must earn his or her living from the provision of prehospital care. Paid or volunteer, every EMT must demonstrate the characteristics of a public health care professional.

As an EMS professional, the EMT must strive to perform all aspects of the job to the best of his or her ability and to improve upon that ability at every opportunity. Professionalism isn't a cloak to be worn while treating the patient and then cast aside while driving the ambulance. Nor is it to be worn like a uniform, only while on duty. A professional attitude must be a constant companion of any person providing health care to the public.

Driving has become commonplace in today's society. It is looked upon more as a right than as a privilege. Driving has become a habit many people take for granted. Because of this, many ambulance operators look at the task of driving the ambulance as incidental to the job of the EMT or EMT-Paramedic. EMTs may not look at their driving ability in the same light as they do their medical ability. Safe and efficient driving is a basic and crucial component of the provision of prehospital medical care.

The person who operates an emergency vehicle cannot take his or her driving ability for granted. A true professional will constantly build upon his or her driving skills.

Driver Attitudes

Modern traffic situations dictate that an ambulance driver must possess both driving skill and a proper attitude in order to drive safely and professionally. Of the two, attitude is by far the most important component. Records show that some drivers of exceptional skill are repeatedly involved in accidents. Other drivers, although less adept, have good safety records, a result of a proper attitude when driving. Attitude problems often show up when training operators to drive ambulances. Frequently, operators with years of driving experience do not learn the skills of emergency and patient driving as rapidly as others with lesser driving experience who are aware of their lack of experience.

Ability, combined with training, helps to develop skills. Driving skills, combined with a good attitude, make for good driving performance. Thus, attitude is the basic element that influences all other aspects of driving.

Professionalism in Driving

A professional attitude is one of maturity, responsibility, and courtesy. The professional driver feels no need to prove anything about his driving ability. He is confident and his actions can attest to that fact. The professional driver can demonstrate his or her ability by exercising caution and courtesy. Fancy driving, or utilizing the emergency equipment as an excuse to intimidate and bully others on the road, can be deadly child's play. While many drivers abuse their vehicles, a professional driver cares for his vehicle, because it is a tool of the EMS trade.

A professional attitude towards driving is exhibited by the following characteristics. The professional emergency vehicle operator:

1. Recognizes the ambulance as an important tool of his trade and, like all tools, cares for and properly utilizes the vehicle as a tool.

2. Respects and obeys all laws and traffic ordinances whether he agrees with them or not.

3. Recognizes that no one is perfect and, in doing so, anticipates and accepts that other drivers on the road will make mistakes.

4. Is always courteous, looking for where he can be of service to others.

5. Slows to allow other drivers to enter from side streets and signals his intentions to turn well in advance.

6. Utilizes his privilege of emergency status with discretion and does not intimidate others.

7. Recognizes adverse road and weather conditions and makes necessary adjustments in driving to insure continued safe vehicle operation.

Public Relations

You, the ambulance driver, are your agency's best, or worst, public relations agent. The crew is seen by the greatest numbers of the public while driving. Few people have the opportunity to observe the ambulance crew in quarters. Comparatively few people will observe the EMT at work at the scene. However, almost everyone will observe an ambulance crew as they are out driving. The crew may be seen responding to an emergency call or simply driving around a neighborhood familiarizing themselves with the coverage area. The ambulance operator's actions during these times will greatly affect how the public views them. If they are observed acting in a professional manner, the public will look upon them as professionals. This respect will, in turn, make the EMT's job in the field much easier.

Unfortunately, the EMT or paramedic does not have the same luxury as physicians and nurses do to develop a rapport with his patients. Instead, rapport must come from first impressions. How the patient first perceives you, the EMT, directly affects how much confidence they will place in your ability to help them.

Place yourself in the position of the patient. How would you feel if the only experience you could recall was the time you were forced off the road by a speeding ambulance? You were frightened or intimidated because the ambulance operator came up behind you and would not give you the chance to make a decision on how to get out of the ambulance's way. Instead, the driver kept blasting the siren at you. Now consider how the patient will view you if he or she recalls the ambulance driver who slowed to let him or her into traffic when he or she was trying to get out of a parking space. Such impressions will affect the attitudes with which the patient and society view you. It is much easier to get budgets passed and gain the respect of the community if you drive sensibly, exercising respect, caution, and courtesy to others.

Response Times

The EMT's attitude towards response times deserves comment. EMS really is a profession of minutes and not seconds; you must take the time to do the job properly. When the EMT becomes excessively rushed, a chain reaction is likely to occur which will continue to keep the EMT moving too quickly. Once preoccupied with response time, the EMT driver tends to become excitable. The EMT or paramedic will often run to the ambulance when the call is received. Walking briskly to the vehicle is adequate.

Once excited, the driver tends to drive the ambulance faster than he should, not recognizing that his excitement is influencing vehicle speed. At this point, it becomes difficult to reduce speed for more than a brief period, even when the problem is recognized.

The professional aspect of such a rushed response is suspect. The artificial building of speed and the pressures that go along with it rob the driver of the ability to properly analyze traffic situations. Later, this same rushed attitude may jeopardize patient care. The EMT may try to make the signs and symptoms exhibited by the patient fit into a preconceived diagnosis instead of allowing the diagnosis to be a result of the signs and symptoms. Taking such an approach, the EMT then becomes impatient and perplexed when the information does not fit together.

It is much better to have the attitude of deliberation and to think things through.

Attitude Pitfalls

Few people choose to have poor driving attitudes, but many do. Maintaining a proper attitude is difficult but recognizing some of the pitfalls that contribute to a poor driving attitude can help drivers correct any shortcomings. Conscious and continuous analysis of our own driving can help us to identify driving attitude pitfalls. Driving attitudes are not something we are born with, they are learned; and therefore can be improved upon.

Overconfidence. Drivers easily get into the habit of taking too much for granted. Equipment failure or an inappropriate response by another driver can lead to a collision. While driving an emergency response, the overconfident driver falsely relies on his emergency lights and siren to provide an invisible force field, making the ambulance impervious to other vehicles.

Faith in Experience. Many drivers believe that years of driving experience will see them through every situation. Most motorists consider themselves to be good drivers and will attribute their ability to experience. Experience alone is not enough. It must be supplemented by comprehensive, continuing education and constant self-analysis. Experience has a way of developing poor habits as well as good ones.

False Ideas. Many people have false ideas about what it takes to drive a vehicle. At the top of the list of false ideas are adequate stopping distances. Most people grossly underestimate the distance it takes to stop a vehicle. False ideas are also developed when intoxicated or fatigued.

Impatience. Probably the one pitfall that contributes more to a poor driving attitude than any other is impatience. People often suppress good judgment and take unnecessary risks just to save a few seconds. Such people become intolerant of others who are not as bold as themselves or who might not take a chance. The impatient "Go For It!" attitude has gotten everyone in trouble at one time or another.

Exhibitionist. Most people want to be noticed and tend to find a way to gain that attention. When attention-getting involves the use of a motor vehicle, the driver is really exhibiting immaturity. Subtle forms of exhibitionism, such as using speed to make passengers feel uncomfortable, may be hard to detect.

Tension

While some drivers can drive all day without much fatigue, others become exhausted after driving even a short distance. The difference can be tension. A driver who can relax while driving will be able to drive longer and remain more alert than one who is tense. When a person's muscles are tight, fatigue sets in quickly and the driver becomes less attentive. Most drivers experience tension at one time or another. For some, inclement weather causes tension. As the road becomes slippery, the driver may feel out of control and then become tense. Fog often causes a driver to become tense. With visibility reduced, the driver finds himself getting closer and closer to the windshield in an attempt to increase vision. Some drivers experience tension any time they drive.

Tension is detrimental to driver awareness. As tension sets in, the driver's visual habits can become impaired, causing the driver to begin to stare. The stare results in tunnel vision and a shorter depth of vision. The driver only perceives problems seen up close once they have reached a crisis stage. At this point, the driver must maneuver violently to avoid a mishap. What form of violent maneuver is most common? Hitting the brakes. When the driver does hit the brakes, his taut muscles cause him to exert excess pressure on the brake pedal, which will often result in a skid.

Tension also affects steering. Both hands on the wheel in a death grip and the muscles in our arms taut, we throw the wheel more rapidly, quickly and often further than necessary. This in turn creates a need for counter-steering, and we soon find ourselves out of control.

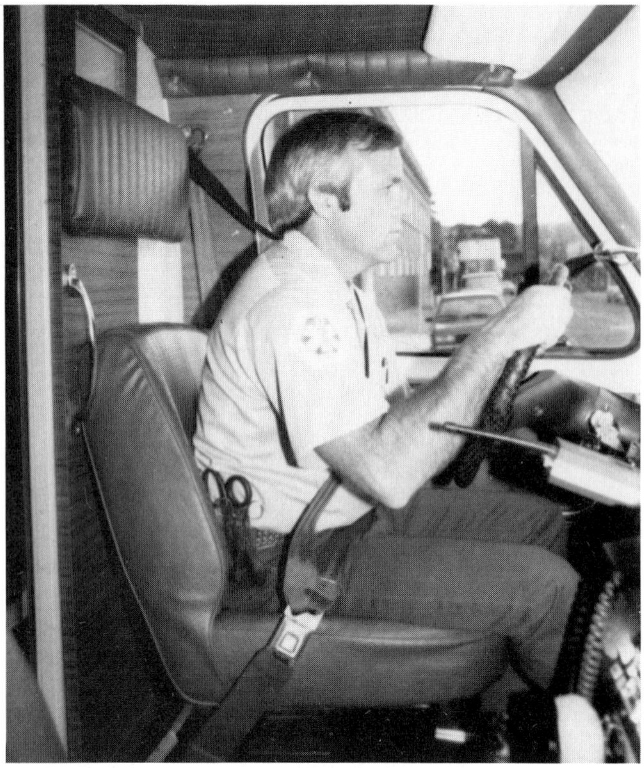

Fig. 4.1a When the muscles are tight, fatigue quickly sets in and a driver becomes less attentive.

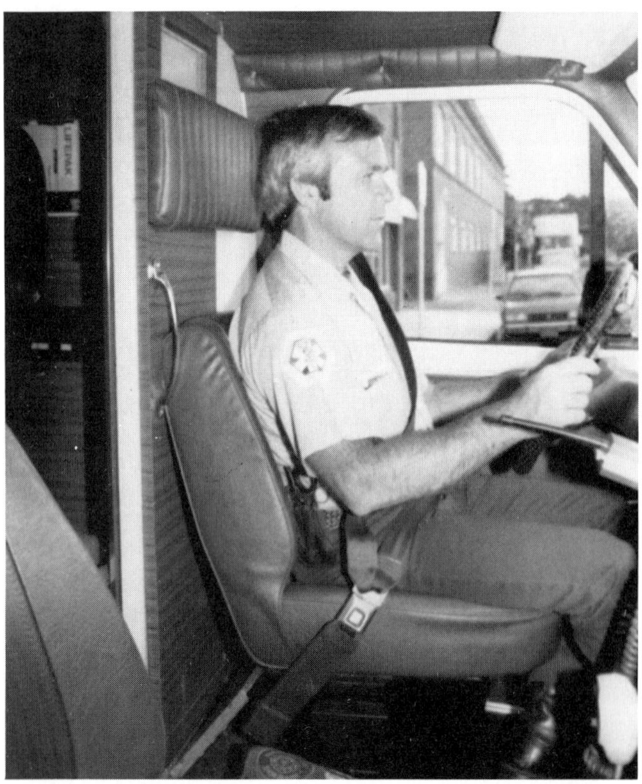

Fig. 4.1b Relaxed driver with proper posture will be able to drive longer and stay alert.

Tension can be reduced or avoided altogether. Listed below are some good driving habits which will reduce driver tension.

Posture. Sit with your spine firmly against the seat back, legs comfortably extended. A driver sitting in a slouched posture will find it more difficult to maintain control of the vehicle or to remain relaxed for long periods of time. Tension may also be exhibited by an exaggerated body posture. A tense driver often has a tendency to lean forward into the windshield and his driving. Tension may also cause the driver to grip the wheel more firmly. He might then notice that his hands become tired or cramped.

Confidence. The driver must have confidence in his vehicle and in his abilities. Confidence will help you to see problem situations early on and to handle the vehicle appropriately.

Restraint. A driver cannot remain relaxed if he is constantly having to brace himself against centrifugal force while in a curve. A seat belt does more than protect the occupants in a collision; it can actually prevent a collision by helping keep the driver securely behind the wheel. A properly adjusted seat belt eliminates the need for excess exertion in maintaining a comfortably seated position.

Recognition of Limits. Traffic, road, weather, and personal conditions limit the speed at which we drive. When driving faster than these limits safely allow, we become tense.

Factors Contributing to Tension. While most drivers can usually stay fairly relaxed, there are conditions that can lead to tension. It is important for the driver to be familiar with these factors. When encountering any of these conditions, the driver must consciously monitor his tension level to assure that he or she remains relaxed. Factors that contribute to tension can be divided into two categories: Driving Conditions and Mental Conditions.

Corrective Measures. When tension develops, it is up to the driver to recognize its signs and immediately take measures to relax. A few of the ways a driver can reduce tension follow.

Sit Back. The first step in reducing tension is to regain a proper posture. Sit with the spine against the seat back.

Breathe Deeply. A deep breath goes far in reducing tension. Breathe in deeply and exhale slowly. Several deep breaths may be needed.

Driving Conditions That Can Create Tension	Mental Conditions That Can Create Tension
Inclement weather	Anger
Slippery roads	Frustration
Darkness	Anxiety
Unfamiliar area	Excitement
Traffic congestion	Illness
Emergency driving	Fatigue
	Impatience
	Lack of confidence

Relax Your Muscles. As you exhale your deep breaths, consciously allow your shoulder, arm, and hand muscles to relax. This activity may require the assistance of several deep breaths to become effective. Imagine the tension being dispersed out of the ends of your fingers.

Aim High. Once you recognize any of the signs of tension, it is important for you to correct any vision or perception problems, such as staring. Aim high to see what is developing further down the road. Once you have broken the stare, your other good vision habits should return to normal.

Visual Habits

The prime determining factor of safe and effective vehicle operation is visual perception. With proper visual habits and good perception, the driver can anticipate a potential crisis and therefore have plenty of time to take appropriate action.

Seeing Habits. Probably the biggest cause of tension and lack of confidence is lack of proper seeing habits. Without proper seeing habits, the driver may miss events happening around him and so becomes nervous and tense. Have you ever been startled by a car passing you because you were not aware of its presence behind you? Proper visual habits are not gained through driving experience alone. Instead, they must be developed much the same as any other skill. A driver with poor seeing habits can go for a considerable length of time without having an accident and with only an occasional near miss. Sooner or later, these drivers will be involved in an accident. Unfortunately, many excuses are ready-made for such situations. Bad luck, a wrong move by the other driver, or maybe a distraction to the driver are common excuses. Traffic accident investigators know that rarely is one driver solely to blame for multiple vehicle accidents. Almost always, the other driver could have avoided the accident if he or she had only exercised proper visual habits.

Distractions

Few drivers dedicate full time to concentrating on the task of driving. Have you ever driven down the road and suddenly realized you do not recall traveling the last several blocks? Suddenly you become concerned whether the traffic light through which you just passed was green or red. We all become distracted at one time or another. With proper concentration, a driver will seldom make visual errors, or when they do they will snap out of them quickly. When strongly developed, proper visual habits will continue, even when distractions are present. Driver distractions are caused by many things, but they can usually be placed into one of the following categories.

Route Problems. So intent are we on looking for a street sign or address, we fail to concentrate on what is happening around us. The simple task of looking for or trying to get into a parking space can also cause distractions. Construction projects on a familiar road can really cause distraction.

Inattention. It is easy to become lost in personal thought. The weekend we are looking forward to or a loved one's illness can lead to driver distraction. Daydreaming is a serious driving distraction. If the mind is otherwise occupied, we may not see the whole picture. We may become so concerned over one hazard we fail to notice another, a common occurrence encountered when assessing a multiple system trauma patient. We see the fractured femur and overlook the fractured ankle. What about the driver who swerves to avoid someone pulling out in front of them only to run head-on into an oncoming car?

Scenery. Certainly, all of us read billboards and window shop as we drive. An obvious distraction. Many of us take a drive in the country to observe the beauty of the scenery. Other things can be classified as scenery or visual distractions as well. The motor vehicle accident to which you have responded is a distraction to other drivers. Often craning their necks to see what is going on, they suddenly pile into another car or perhaps even the rescue personnel.

In-vehicle Distractions. We have probably all ridden with a driver who talks a lot while driving. Frequently, this driver cannot talk without looking at the person he is addressing or without using his hands to talk. Have you ever watched a driver with a bee in his car? That bee gets a lot of attention as it goes flying about the car. All of these situations are distracting. So may be the simple task of reading the gauges or answering the radio. Distraction can be reduced if the driver has an awareness of where the equipment is and when and how to use it.

Unfamiliar Driving Tasks. Driving faster than normal becomes an unfamiliar driving task as we fight to keep our vision up with the vehicle's progress. Inclement weather can also be an unfamiliar driving problem. As we struggle to see further down the road, we get tunnel vision and give less attention to what is actually going on around us. Driving in a new neighborhood can be an unfamiliar task. If you are used to having the traffic lights suspended over the street, you may have problems adjusting to signals posted on a pole on the corner.

Proper Habits

Proper visual habits can be developed by increasing visual perception. Perceptual training requires more of the driver than just seeing objects. The driver must also be able to accurately and promptly recognize the meaning or implication of an object. For example, a slowing yellow bus is more than just a slowing vehicle. Its color and markings may indicate that it is a school bus. Is the school bus slowing because of traffic congestion? Is it slowing to pick up or let off children? Is there a chance that a small child may dart out into your oncoming path? All of these questions arise in the mind of a driver with good visual perception.

With increased perception, the driver can relax and drive with confidence. Several principles are involved in the process of seeing and perception:

1. Perception of traffic conditions is a process involving our senses and our mind. Once we sense something (most frequently through vision), our brain must then interpret the information.

2. Perception must be a selective process since we cannot perceive all that is observed; for this reason we best perceive information that is meaningful.

3. Perception is aided by concentration since the brain can only analyze information to which it gives attention. Should we be looking for one particular piece of information, we are not likely to see much else due to overconcentration.

4. Efficient and accurate motor skills are enhanced when the driver is more perceptive.

Development of proper visual skills takes time and practice. Proficiency does not come about just because a person wants to have good perception.

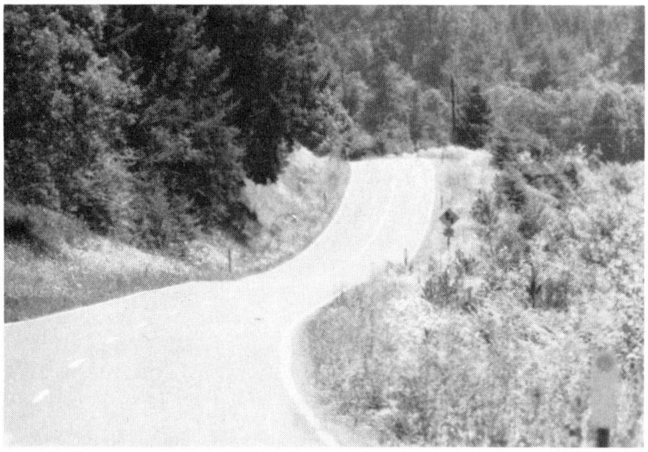

Fig. 4.2a You can often get an idea about the amount of curve ahead by watching the reflector posts along the roadside.

The Smith System®

The Smith System was developed to help drivers properly use their eyes while driving. Utilization of the five components taught by the Smith System Driver Improvement Institute will help insure that you are aware of all that is going on around you.

Aim High in Steering.® It is important to look far down the road in order to see what is ahead and have plenty of time to prepare for it. If a traffic light is ahead, the driver may want to adjust his

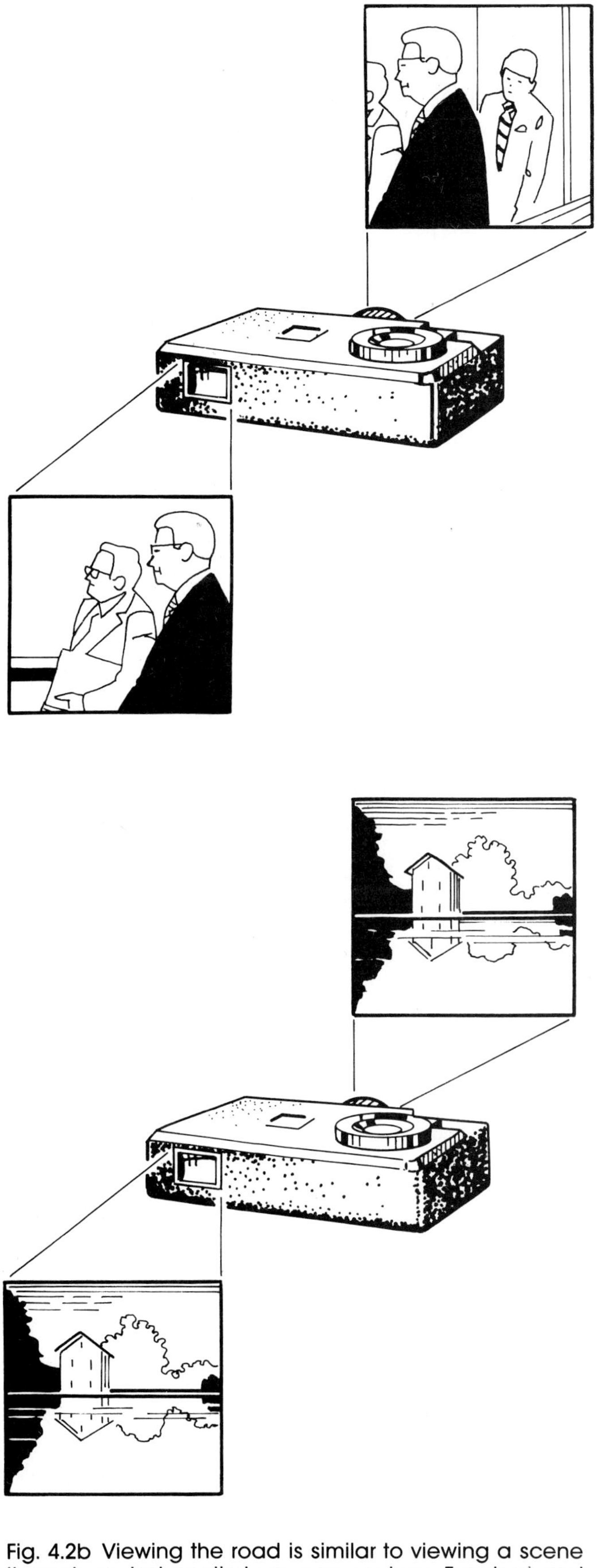

Fig. 4.2b Viewing the road is similar to viewing a scene through an Instamatic-type camera lens. For short and long distance photos, what the view finder "sees" and what's actually in the photo differ greatly.

speed or prepare to stop. If children are playing in a yard, the driver must prepare for the possibility of one of them running into the street.

There is more to aiming high than early awareness of what's happening. Driving a car can be compared to aiming an Instamatic camera. An Instamatic camera lens is separate from the viewfinder, similar to the driver sitting to the left of the center of the vehicle. When the camera is focused on a subject at a short distance, what is seen in the viewfinder and what the lens will actually take a picture of are dramatically different. When the camera is aimed at a subject in the distance, the photograph will more closely represent what was seen in the viewfinder. The same principle can be applied to driving. When we only look ahead a short distance, it becomes more difficult to aim the car properly because we get a distorted view of our vehicle's position on the road.

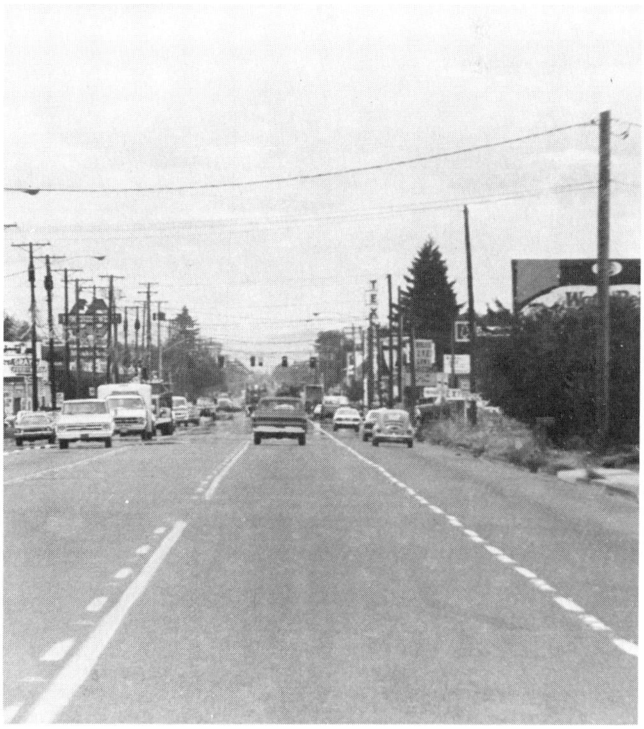

Fig. 4.3 Aim high while driving—it's important to look far down the road to see if potential problems lay ahead.

This principle can best be illustrated when driving down an expressway. With a retaining wall to the left and a tractor-trailer in the right lane, many drivers become uncomfortable. The task of driving suddenly becomes very difficult. The driver finds himself monitoring the truck and the wall, constantly adjusting his position between them. However, by aiming high, the wall and truck will be placed in proper perspective—they will no longer seem so near or perilous.

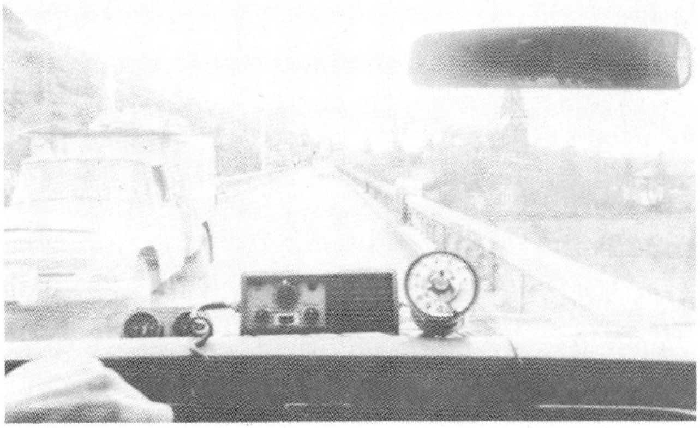

Fig. 4.4 In circumstances such as those shown here, many drivers become uncomfortable. Aiming high will put the wall and truck in proper perspective, making them seem less perilous.

The same principle can be applied in corners. Many drivers have to constantly correct their course in a turn. This occurs when the driver is only looking a short distance ahead and thus sees the curve in small segments. He then drives toward each segment, attempting to straighten out between each one. By aiming high, the driver will see the corner as a whole and drive accordingly.

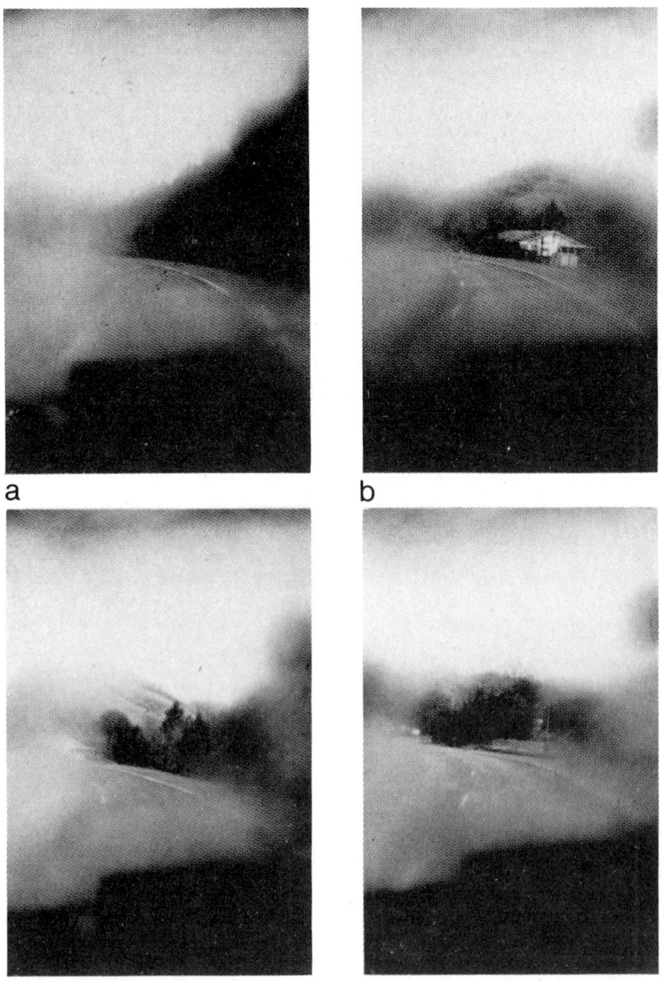

a b c d

Fig. 4.5a-d Aim high while driving on curves—looking ahead only short distances causes you to see the curve in small segments—this is inefficient as is seen in this sequence of photos.

Get the Big Picture® The car ahead is only a tiny part of what we need to see to drive safely. Unfortunately, many drivers tend to stare at the rear of the car in front or only a short distance ahead on the road. The safe driver needs to use his total vision to be aware of his surroundings. Using your total vision means you must also use your peripheral vision. It is peripheral vision that gives us information on objects moving into our focal vision. Through peripheral vision we also perceive such sensations as speed, both ours and that of the other vehicles on the road.

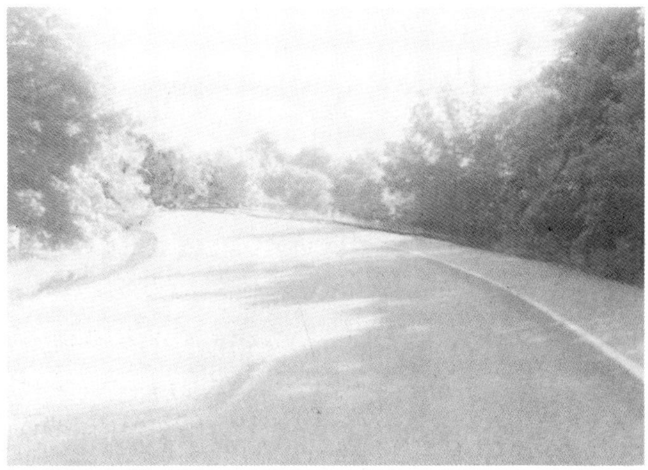

Fig. 4.6 Aiming high enables you to see the curve as a whole.

Proper use of our peripheral vision dictates that we can't focus on any one thing, especially something that doesn't deserve our attention. The more we focus our vision, the less our peripheral vision works and we develop tunnel vision (peripheral vision range of less than 140°). Staring at the vehicle in front of us causes a significant loss of peripheral vision.

Keep Your Eyes Moving® Our peripheral vision (normal is 180° in range) only introduces subjects to our minds. In order to better perceive information, we also need to keep our eyes moving so everything comes into contact with our very narrow focal vision (normally, only 3° in range). We need to check our mirrors, gauges, and the traffic around us to perceive properly. By keeping our eyes moving, we avoid the habit of staring. Consequently, we keep our peripheral vision functioning. It can be said that a driver who loses his

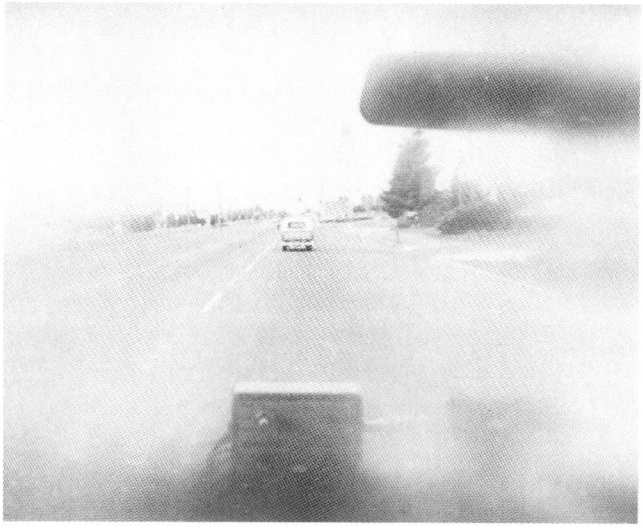

Fig. 4.7 Get the big picture—don't focus on any one object. starting at the vehicle ahead causes significant loss of peripheral vision.

attention for more than two seconds is staring. A staring pattern will continue until a strong influence breaks it. The vehicle in front of us often becomes very handy at capturing our focal vision, thus reducing our overall vision.

Leave Yourself an Out.® The perceptual driver will insure that there is enough room between his vehicle and all other traffic around so that he can avoid anything that may occur. He will maintain an empty space around his vehicle, following the car in front at a safe distance and allowing plenty of room between him and other situations taking place. Monitoring the rear view mirror, the perceptual driver will insure that there is enough room between himself and the vehicle behind. If there is not an adequate space present, speed is adjusted up or down to secure enough space. If the gap cannot be enlarged, he then makes room for the other driver to pass.

Also very important is an escape route, somewhere to go when things go wrong. An example of providing yourself with an escape route would be how you position your vehicle in traffic as you pass through intersections. You should try to have yourself positioned so that there are no vehicles to your immediate side, right or left. Should another driver start to cross in front of your vehicle, you may be able to avoid a collision by changing lanes or moving to the shoulder as the crisis develops.

The professional driver should always strive to keep as many options open as possible for his vehicle. Rarely while moving should a good driver be caught with traffic close in front, behind, or alongside. When a critical situation

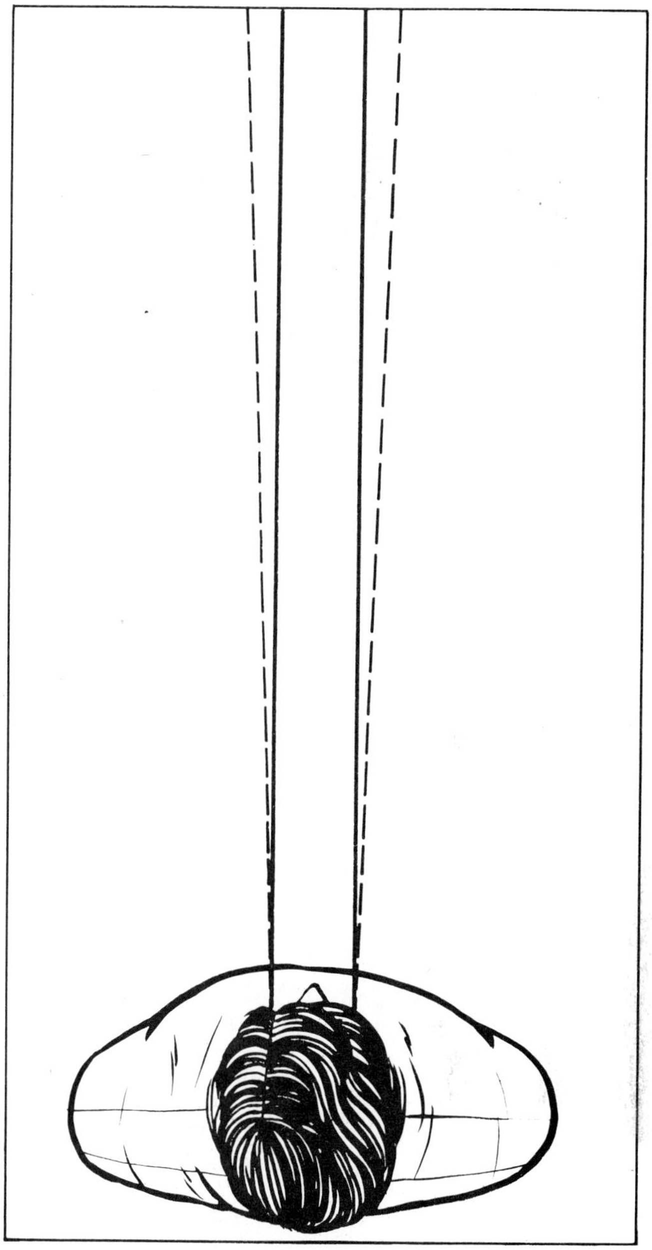

Fig. 4.8 Focal vision only allows your seeing at an angle of 3 degrees from straight ahead. to better perceive information, you must keep your eyes moving.

arises, the driver who provides himself with an escape route can usually avoid or reduce the severity of a collision.

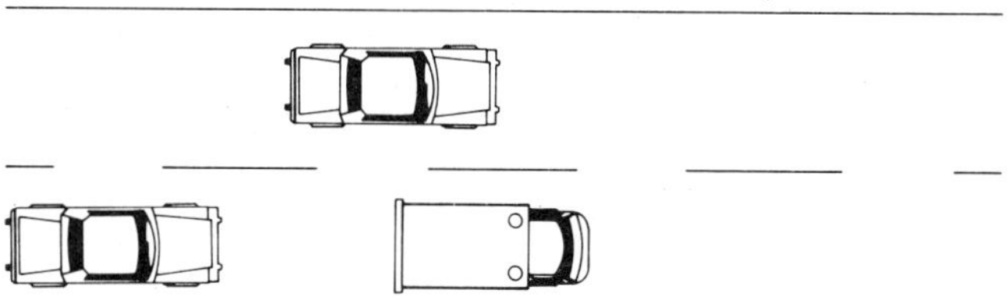

Fig. 4.9 Driving with a car on one side limits a driver's options to make evasive maneuvers.

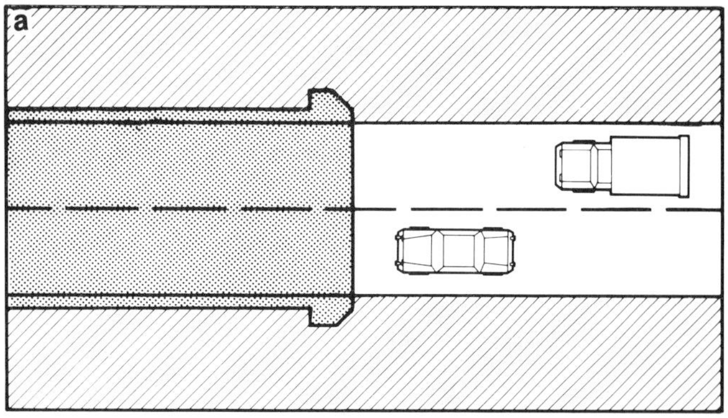

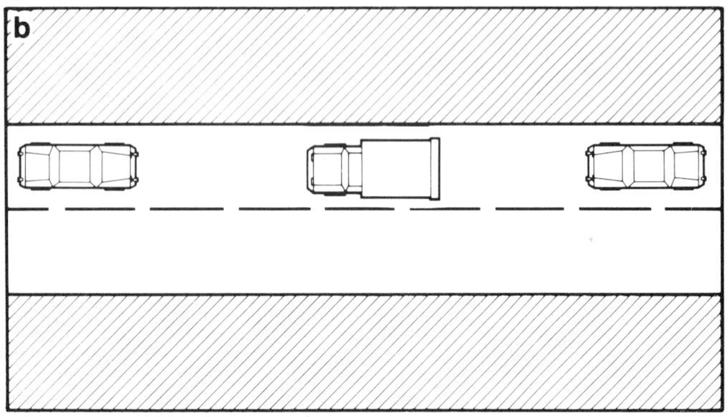

Fig. 4.10a Bridge abutments or guard rails limit escape route options.

Fig. 4.10b Always drive with a cushion of space between your vehicle and others to provide an "out" if needed.

The escape route needs to be maintained while stopped too. Many accidents occur when an inattentive driver drives into the rear of a car stopped at a stoplight. Frequently, a chain reaction occurs and the stopped vehicle is then pushed into another stopped vehicle.

Another example of insufficient forward escape route might be the instance of being stopped in a line of traffic and then receiving an emergency call. If you pulled so far forward that you cannot turn out of the traffic lane, you are essentially trapped. A good rule of thumb to help you determine how far away to stop from the vehicle in front of you is to be able to always see the rear tires of the car in front. This minimal space will normally allow you to drive forward, turning out of your traffic lane without any reversing. This same space may allow you to drive completely out of a pending rear-end collision, once you recognized the squeal of tires from the car behind. Be sure to check your mirrors and look for oncoming traffic before you try to outrun this type of collision.

Make Sure They See You.®Each driver on the road shares in the responsibility of making it safe. Everyone is at a disadvantage if he does not know another driver's intentions. It is every driver's responsibility to make sure all actions can be interpreted easily, and that they can be seen by everyone. The driver needs to signal his intentions clearly when slowing or turning and to position the vehicle so that it can telegraph his intentions. It is also very important not to drive in someone else's blind spot. Unfortunately, not every driver has good perceptual habits. When your vehicle moves into another's blind spot and stays there, the other driver may not even be aware of your vehicle's presence. Should the other driver decide to change lanes or turn, you may find yourself involved in an avoidable collision.

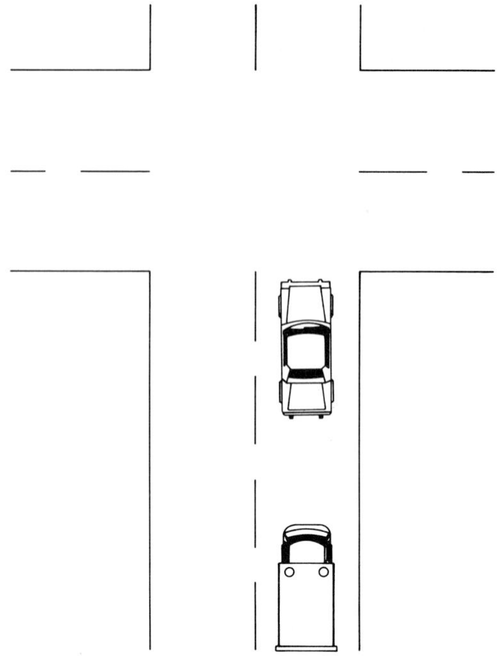

Fig. 4.11 Make sure a way out is always available even when stopped in traffic in case of another call or the car ahead stalling.

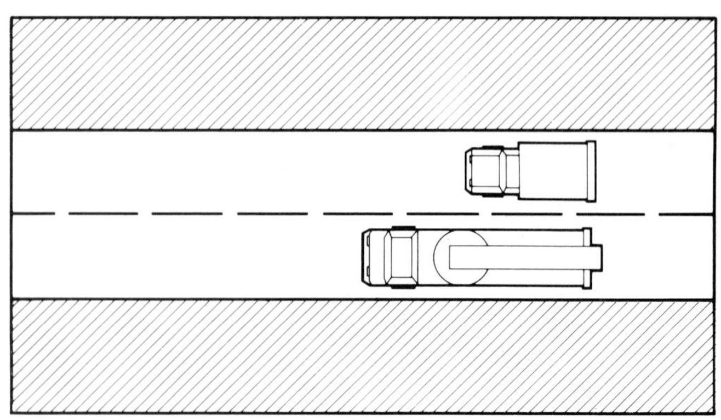

Fig. 4.12 Make sure other drivers see you—don't drive in some other vehicle's blind spot.

Typical blind spots include the right rear side of most passenger cars, the rear of trucks and tractor-trailer combinations, and the low sides of most high-cab vehicles. In order to be seen by drivers of trucks or vehicles with impaired rear vision, position your vehicle in the traffic lane so the other driver can see you in his left side view mirror. This positioning may require that you increase your following distance significantly. Good sense tells us that if you can't see the driver in front of you in his mirror, he can't see you.*

Seeing As a Defense

Along with developing proper visual habits, a driver must also have the ability to make proper decisons. With proper decision-making ability, a good defensive driver can interpret what is happening around him and make proper allowances to avoid collisions. Developing a defensive driving attitude and proper decision-making abilities requires a five-step process. The acronym SIPDE can be used to help you remember the process.

Search. The first step is to search. As you aim high, keeping your eyes moving, getting the big picture, one of the things you will be looking for is a potentially hazardous situation. Proper search can help you to determine what situations might develop before they actually do. Such things to look for could include children playing near the street, a car approaching an intersection, or a vehicle moving up alongside yours.

Identify. Identification refers to the process of identifying potential hazards. A car at a stop sign may or may not be a hazard depending on whether or not it pulls out in front of you. You must at least identify this car as a potential hazard so you can be prepared.

Predict. This step requires you to predict whether the identified hazard is real or potential and the "criticality" of the hazard. What are the chances of the hazard producing a conflict? It is important that the prediction step takes place before the situation reaches the point where the conflict is unavoidable.

Decide. Once a hazard is identified and its effect predicted, you must decide on what action, if any, must be taken to avoid the conflict.

*The five keys of the Smith System are copyrighted by the Smith System Driver Improvement Institute.

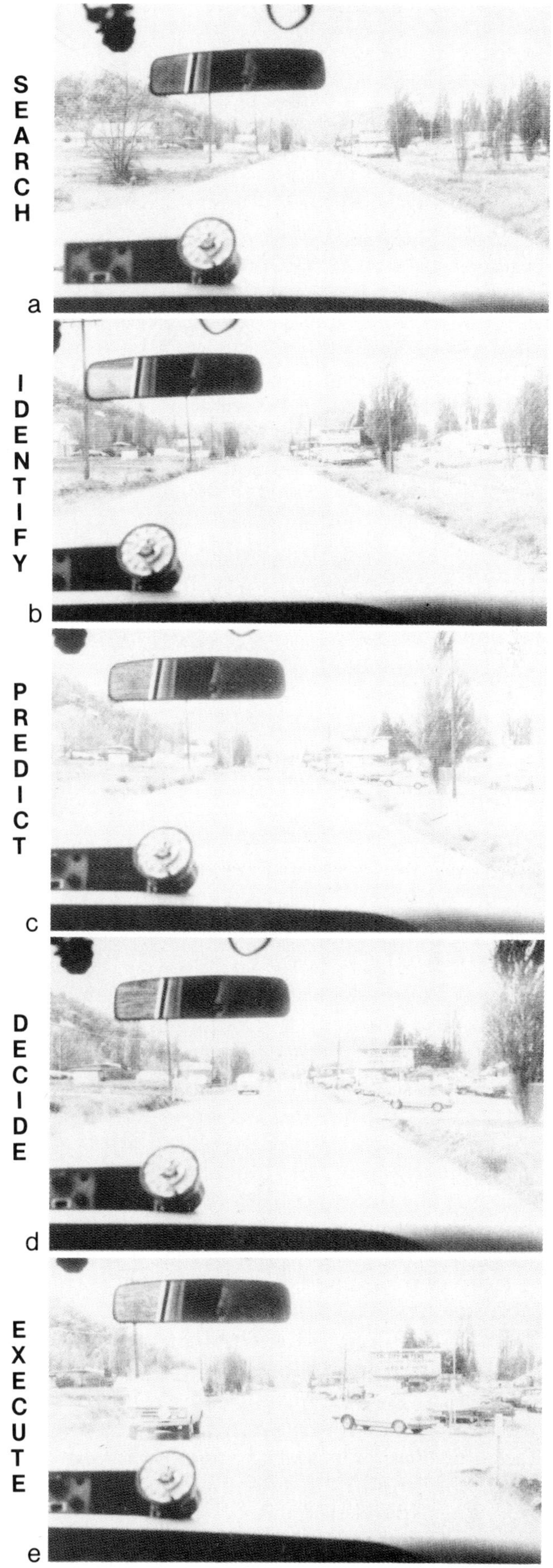

Fig. 4.13a-e Search for potentially hazardous situations.

Execute. Once the hazard has been found, identified, and an action decided upon, you must execute the needed action.

The "SIPDE" system must be executed rapidly with each situation that is encountered. The search must be constant to seek out potential conflict. While it is possible for the other driver to be at fault in a collision, it doesn't help you to be dead right!

The public views the driver of an ambulance as a professional. He is expected to be able to avoid conflict and to make allowances for others and do so courteously. This can only be done if the ambulance operator employs good visual habits and drives in a defensive manner. Knowing these perceptual systems and being able to incorporate them in everyday driving are two different things. It is not easy to develop some of these procedures, even when they are known. To help develop the proper perceptual habits, a system called commentary driving can be used. Commentary driving is described in Chapter 13, "Exercises You Can Do."

Following Distances

As mentioned earlier in order to drive safely, a driver must leave an adequate distance between his vehicle and that of the vehicle in front of him. This distance will allow the driver to avoid a collision if the vehicle in front suddenly stops. Clearly, from the number of accidents that occur each year, people misjudge this distance regularly. As speeds vary, so will the distance that has to be maintained.

What is an Adequate Following Distance? The distance is the sum of two elements: Reaction Time and Stopping Time.

Reaction Time. From the time a situation arises to the time the driver identifies the hazard, predicts its influence on himself, decides on an action, and begins executing that action is the period considered *Reaction Time*. For the alert driver, reaction time is about three-quarters of a second. It may increase if the driver is fatigued or inattentive. Reaction time also translates into distance traveled. At 60 miles per hour, a vehicle will travel 66 feet in three-quarters of a second.

Stopping Time. Once the brakes are applied, the vehicle will require time and distance to stop. The energy needed to slow a vehicle is significant and increases tremendously as speeds increase. There is no average braking distance for all vehicles. The distance will vary according to several factors, including the weight of the vehicle (or mass) and the speed of the vehicle (velocity). As the velocity of the vehicle increases, it requires more energy to stop. In fact it takes as much energy to quickly slow a vehicle from 90 mph to 70 mph as it does to slow it from 70 mph to 0 mph. When reaction time and stopping distance are combined, a heavy two-axle truck traveling 60 mph will take approximately 436 feet to stop.

It is clear that a truck cannot allow 436 feet between himself and the next vehicle. At that distance, the space would quickly fill up with other vehicles. How does a driver figure how long it will take to stop at a given speed and therefore what following distance he should use? It is only necessary to allow enough room to stop within the same distance as the car in front, minus their reaction time. The general rule used for this calculation is the miles per hour of the vehicle times two. At 55 miles per hour, a driver should allow 110 feet between himself and the vehicle in front. On the road, this distance can be determined one of two ways.

Car Length Estimate. This method is probably used most frequently if a driver actually considers following distance in feet. The driver should allow one car length for every ten miles per hour he is driving. A full-sized car is approximately 20 feet long. A driver would need to allow 80 feet between himself and another vehicle while traveling at 40 miles per hour. Few drivers can really picture the space required for four vehicles just like theirs between them and the vehicle in front. For this reason, the car length estimate system is cumbersome and less desirable than the three-second rule.

Three-second Rule (Ambulance). A less cumbersome system for determining safe following distance is the three-second rule. Most defensive driving courses teach the two-second rule for determining following distance for passenger cars. Due to the size and weight of today's ambulances, additional stopping time and distance is required.

Application of the two- or three-second rule is simple. Using this rule, the driver allows the rear bumper of the vehicle in front to pass a stationary object and then counts off three seconds (one thousand one, one thousand two, one thousand three). If the front of his vehicle passes the object before three seconds are up, he is driving too closely. Any stationary object can be used for such a yardstick; reflector posts, a discarded beverage can, anything easily seen can be used. The distance between vehicles will automatically increase as the speed of the vehicles increases.

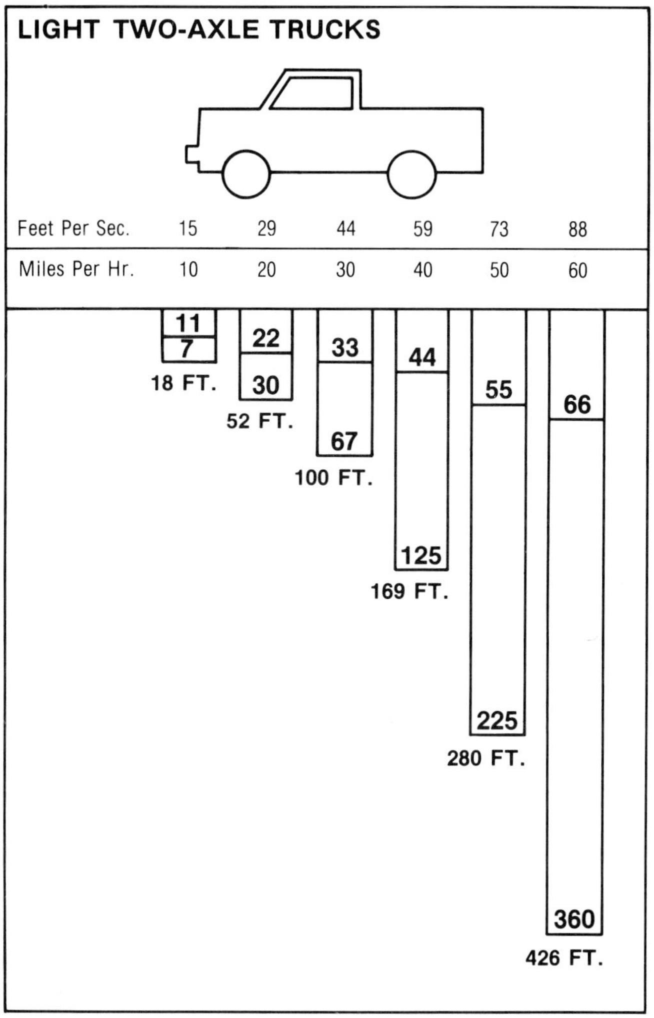

Fig. 4.14 Stopping distances at various speeds

Other factors can influence safe following distance. If the vehicle in front of you is smaller than the one you are driving, the distance should be increased. This is because a smaller vehicle can stop quicker and in less distance than a larger vehicle. If the road is slippery, or you are tired or ill, or if the load you are carrying is great, follow-

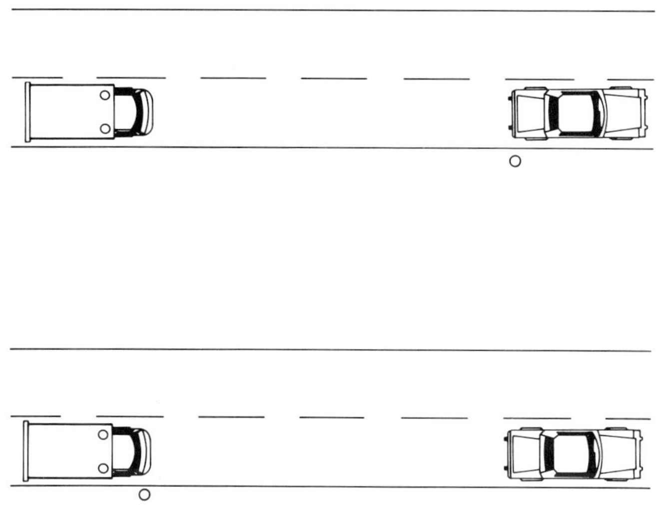

Fig. 4.15 Use the three-second rule to see that you're not following too closely—if front of your vehicle passes a marker object before three seconds elapse, you're following too closely.

ing distances must be increased to be safe. When any of these situations are encountered, the following distance should be increased perhaps to 3-1/2 or 4 seconds. If the vehicle in front of you is a sports car, 4-1/2 seconds may be required to insure a safe margin of distance.

The most important components of driving that you can improve upon are your attitudes and driving habits. With a proper attitude and good driving habits, you will truly be considered a driving professional. Without these assets, you will be handicapped and less likely to operate your vehicle in a safe and efficient manner.

5 FUNDAMENTALS OF DRIVING

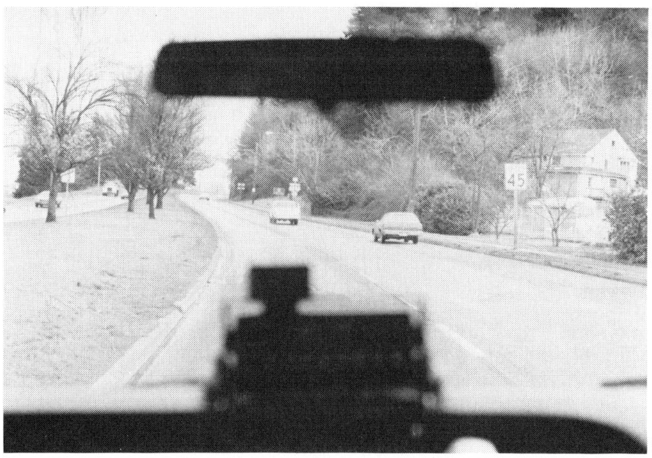

As with any profession, the basics are always important. In prehospital medicine, it is important to be able to do basic skills such as CPR well before moving into advanced skills such as endotracheal intubation, IV therapy, or drug administration. This simple philosophy applies to driving. In order to drive an emergency vehicle safely and efficiently on an emergency response, it is important to first understand and perform the basics well. Unfortunately, this proficiency does not come about just from having driven for five or six years. Even after having driven for 15 or 20 years, most people on the road today are not good drivers. A good driver must understand basic functions such as passing, backing, parking, and the various types of traffic that he will encounter. If a driver cannot perform these skills well when driving under normal circumstances, he will become dangerous when the pressure of emergency driving is encountered. In this chapter, we will examine some of the fundamentals of driving.

Passing

Watching others drive can become an interesting and educational pastime. The art of passing is one of the most interesting to observe. Have you ever noticed the impatient driver on a crowded highway on a holiday weekend? He finds it necessary to pass every vehicle on the road. He hurries to get around each vehicle, accelerating around them and then braking hard to get back into traffic before he gets hit by the oncoming traffic. When oncoming traffic clears, once again he is hanging out in the oncoming lane, passing the next car or even the next several. If he is approaching a blind corner, no problem is recognized by this driver. He only has to accelerate faster and hit the brakes harder to get back into line. What makes this common enterprise so interesting? It is that when and if this motorist finally arrives at his destination, he does so only a few minutes ahead of those who choose to stay in the flow of traffic. The risks this driver has taken—and subjected others to—do not seem worth the gain.

From time to time, passing is necessary. There are many reasons why vehicles are driven at different speeds. They may be transporting an unstable load. They may not have sufficient power to maintain speed on a long hill, or the driver may lack confidence in his or her ability to drive safely at a greater speed. When slower motorists are encountered on the open road, passing is an option to be considered.

Passing Considerations. A driver executing a pass has several factors he must consider before attempting to pass another vehicle. The overall distance involved, visibility, road conditions, vehicle characteristics and traffic must all be considered.

Passing Distance. When passing, surface distances are consumed at a tremendous rate. The vehicle is vulnerable to collision any time it is in the left lane. In a case where both vehicles are traveling at about the same speed, a passenger car will require approximately ten seconds to complete a pass at 55 miles per hour (mph). During that 10 seconds, the car will have traveled roughly one-sixth of a mile. A large vehicle such as an ambulance will require an even greater distance since the ambulance will not accelerate as rapidly as most passenger cars.

A driver executing a pass must also consider the distance of the vehicle coming toward him. Traveling at 55 mph, the oncoming vehicle will also travel roughly one-sixth of a mile. When the progress of both vehicles is combined, a safe distance of a minimum of one-third of a mile will be required at 55 mph.

Visibility. Many conditions can hamper a driver's visibility. If he is unable to see sufficiently down the road to assure himself a clear path, he cannot pass safely. Conditions that can limit visibility include:

Weather. Fog or heavy rain can reduce visibility to just a few feet.

Curves. A curve in the road ahead often hides oncoming traffic or perhaps a stalled vehicle.

Hills. The hill acts the same as the curve, blocking from view the vehicle that may be approaching from the other side of the crest.

Sunken Grade. It is not uncommon for a country road to dip, often several feet, before returning to its original grade. It can be difficult for a driver to see dips in the road ahead as it may appear to be straight and level. When the dip can be seen, it may be difficult to determine how deep it is and whether a threat may be hiding in it. The safe driver must become adept at spotting such grade changes and must avoid passing when they are present.

Sunken grades can be detected by observing the road edges. When viewed from a distance, the road edges will not form a smooth line if sunken grades are present. Instead, the edge will appear jagged. You may be able to see a large jag in the line if the sunken portion of the road extends for some distance.

Road Information. The road can tell a good driver a lot about whether or not he can pass. It is up to the driver to recognize and interpret this information.

Signs. A No Passing sign certainly should tell the driver that he shouldn't pass. Road signs such as Railroad Crossing, Congestion Ahead, Reduce Speed Ahead, and others should also be interpreted as saying "unsafe to pass."

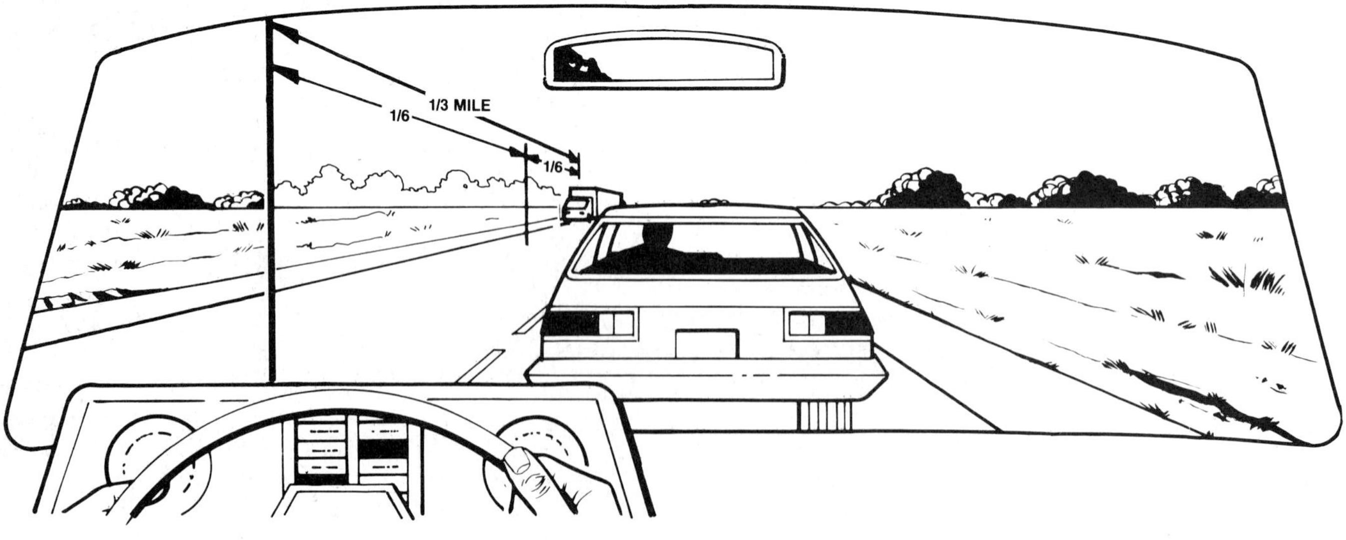

Fig. 5.1 Vehicles travel at least one sixth of a mile in the 10 seconds it takes to pass at 55 mph.

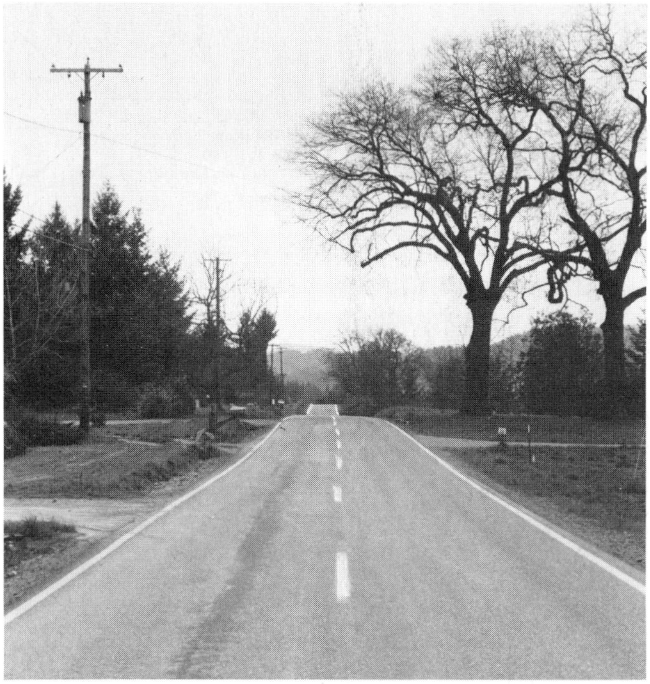

Fig. 5.2 Dips in the road are hard to detect and can even hide a truck. You can detect them by watching the road edges.

Road Marking. Double solid center lines indicate a no passing zone. A solid line appearing with a broken line on one side indicates passing from the side with the broken line is allowed. Of course, you can only pass when it is safe to do so.

Road Configuration. Besides hills, curves, and dips, a driver should be on the lookout for other road formations that might make passing hazardous. Narrow bridges, construction, and areas where the shoulder is narrow are unsafe passing zones. Such areas will reduce any possible escape route a vehicle might need.Passing while approaching an intersection should also be avoided. Even when traffic is observed, it is often difficult to determine the action of the cross traffic. It is not uncommon for a motorist to make a right-hand turn onto another street with that driver only checking traffic that is approaching from his left. This motorist turns right only to be looking head on into the eyes of another driver passing other oncoming traffic.

Occasionally, you may observe road markings or signs which forbid passing for no apparent reason. Normally, there is a good reason: A hidden side street, school zone, damaged road surface, or poor road design may have led traffic safety engineers to designate the area unsafe for passing.

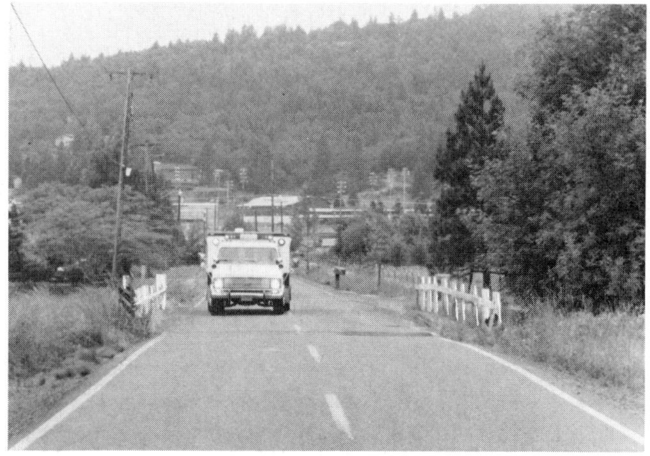

Fig. 5.3 Narrow bridges, construction and areas where the shoulder narrows are unsafe passing zones.

Vehicle Characteristics. Each vehicle performs somewhat differently from the next. For this reason, it is important for the driver to know his vehicle and how it will respond to any given input.

Ambulance drivers routinely drive several different vehicles for the same EMS agency. Therefore, it is important for the driver to familiarize himself with the assigned vehicle at the beginning of each shift. Characteristics that can affect safe passing include the vehicle's:

Ability to Accelerate. A driver is much more likely to consider passing when the vehicle he is driving can accelerate rapidly. Conversely, if the vehicle is very slow to accelerate, the driver should rarely consider passing as an option.

Steering Ability. How well the front wheels track affects the vehicle's steering. If the front end is out of alignment, the vehicle may have a tendency to wander, making it risky to pull alongside another vehicle.

Braking Ability. Brakes are important for passing. An unforeseen situation may force the passing driver to abort a pass or even to speed up to more rapidly complete the pass. In such situations, the driver may have to apply the brakes to quickly slow the vehicle. A vehicle with poor braking ability should not be passing other vehicles.

It is important for the driver to be familiar with all of these characteristics. If the vehicle's characteristics encountered are not those normally found, the vehicle should be taken out of service.

Traffic Situations. It has been said that it is usually pointless to attempt to pass traffic when it is congested. The result is rarely worth the effort. Additionally, it is generally illegal for a vehicle to pass another which is proceeding at the legal speed limit. If the passing vehicle must increase its speed above the legal limit to accomplish a safe pass, the passing vehicle is considered to be speeding.

Attempting to pass stopped traffic should be considered hazardous. You should only pass stopped traffic when the reason for their stopping has been determined and you can proceed safely. The traffic may be stopped because the lead vehicle is attempting to make a left turn. Passing in this situation is surely inviting a collision. The traffic may also be stopped to allow a pedestrian or perhaps an emergency vehicle to cross its path. Even if the traffic has stopped for your emergency response, passing a string of stopped vehicles can be hazardous. The traffic may bunch up and close off any escape route you might need if oncoming traffic is suddenly detected.

Another hazardous situation may arise when a driver attempts to pass on a vehicle's right side as it attempts to turn left. This practice places the passing vehicle in the turning vehicle's blind spot. Should the left-turning vehicle driver decide to proceed ahead or suddenly turn right, a collision is likely. Oncoming traffic may turn left across your path, unable to see you as you are shadowed by the vehicle in front of you. Passing on the right-hand side is illegal in some states.

The Act of Passing

Essentially there are two methods for initiating a pass. In one method, acceleration is done while turning from the normal traffic lane and continues while passing the lead vehicle. This method of passing requires a little more time than the second method since the passing vehicle must do all of its accelerating while in the passing lane.

The second method initially requires some additional distance between the lead vehicle and the one doing the passing. When the passing driver intends to pass, he begins accelerating while still in the right lane of traffic, anticipating the clearing of his intended path. As he approaches the vehicle in front and the path clears,

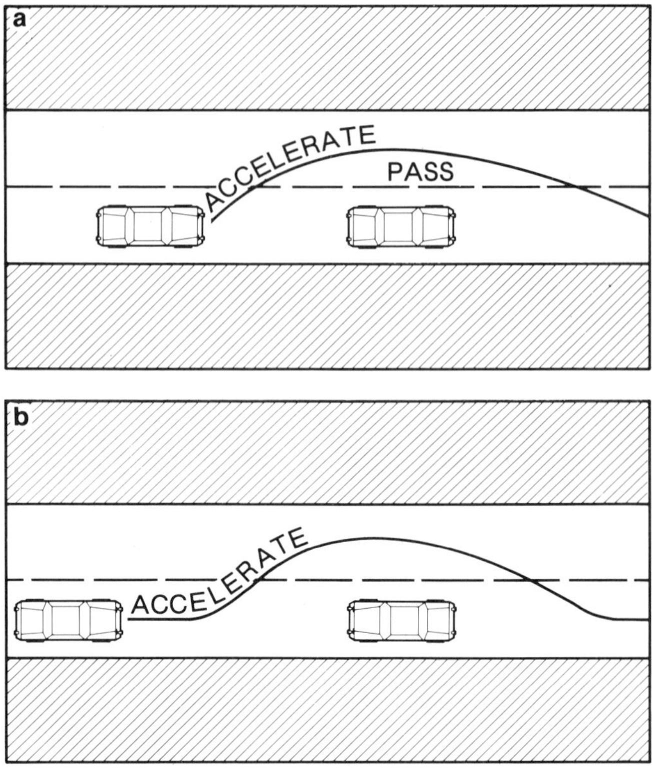

Fig. 5.4a One method of passing involves accelerating while turning from the normal traffic line and continuing while passing the lead vehicle.

Fig. 5.4b Another method of passing requires more distance between the lead vehicle and the passing one. The passing driver begins accelerating while still in the right lane, anticipating the clearing of his intended path.

he pulls out and around the other vehicle. This method utilizes a minimum of time and distance in the oncoming lane since passing speed is already attained. The speed of acceleration used before pulling into the oncoming lane must be carefully judged since a problem can develop if the driver in front slows or brakes.

Should a motorist decide to abort his passing attempt, he may not have sufficient distance to stop without running into the rear of the lead vehicle. This method, when applied safely, is a quick and effective means of passing.

Occasionally, it may be difficult to see around the lead vehicle because of its size. Under such circumstances, the driver intending to pass should pull as close to the center line as is safe to enable him to see around the oversized vehicle. This positioning may also alert the driver in front as to the intentions of the passing driver. Once alerted to the following driver's intentions, the lead driver might then pull over to make the pass easier.

Once the driver has made the decision to pass, he should not hesitate to execute the pass.

Any time spent hesitating allows for traffic conditions to change, often to a point at which the pass becomes unsafe. If any conditions indicate that the pass may not be completed safely, the driver should abort his passing attempt.

Several procedures should take place before the pass is initiated. First, check your left side view mirror to insure no one is approaching from behind or is in the act of passing your vehicle. Second, look over your left shoulder to insure no one is in your blind spot. Third, signal your intention to move into the next lane. This will alert the driver in front and any to the rear of you of your intent to pass. Finally, if all conditions still indicate safety in passing, initiate your turn into the next lane.

Once your pass has been completed, again signal your intent to change lanes. As soon as the overtaken vehicle can be seen in your rear view mirror or you have passed the first vehicle by about one full car length, promptly return to the normal lane of traffic. The return to the normal traffic lane should be executed in a smooth manner. Any jerky or rapid lane changes will be uncomfortable for your passengers.

Aborting a Pass. Occasionally, you will be faced with a rapid change in road or traffic conditions that will force you to abort your passing attempt. Since most vehicles can brake more efficiently than they can accelerate, it is usually better to brake and return to the original following position when aborting a pass. This rule holds true unless the passing vehicle is fully abreast of the lead vehicle. If accelerating rapidly while abreast, the driver may elect to complete the pass. Keep a close eye on the other driver as he may either brake or accelerate in order to "help" you get back in line safely.

Being Passed. There is an art to being passed which incorporates good judgment and courtesy. Do not become judgmental or upset with passing drivers, even if you are traveling at the designated speed limit. Such emotions can lead to increases in your tension level and adversely affect your driving performance.

Be aware of all traffic around you. Should you observe the following driver signaling that he is going to pass and you feel the conditions are unsafe, warn him. A simple arm signal, arm down, may be enough to warn the following driver of a dangerous situation.

Should the driver behind you attempt an unsafe pass, it is your obligation to help all vehicles avoid a collision. In such an event, you should pull as far to the right as possible to allow the passing driver additional driving room. You should maintain a constant speed until the passing driver decides on acceleration or braking to get him through the event. Once the passing driver's actions are observed, do the opposite. Example: He speeds up, you slow down; thus allowing him to return to the normal traffic lane more rapidly.

One common pitfall that is frequently observed during a passing situation is that the vehicle being passed speeds up. This acceleration may not be a conscious act of the driver being passed but rather a result of his poor seeing habits. Should the lead driver be staring, his peripheral vision will be greatly reduced. As a passing vehicle pulls alongside, his mind will try to equalize the motion in the peripheral vision. His subconscious mind will tell him to accelerate. A good driver will keep his eyes moving and not fall victim to this dangerous subconscious act.

Passing is a dangerous maneuver if not performed properly. It is important for the driver to evaluate all of the conditions before attempting to pass another vehicle. Once the decision to pass has been made, the pass should be executed quickly, with a minimum of time spent in the oncoming traffic lane.

Backing

Although backing doesn't seem difficult for most, it often results in property damage. Backing accidents account for 85 percent of the single-vehicle collisions involving ambulances. Backing accidents usually result in bent bumpers, crumpled fenders, and, occasionally, a minor injury. Although these accidents seldom result in serious personal injury, such accidents do require vehicle repair and account for a great deal of expensive "down time" for the involved vehicle.

The dangers involved in backing can be minimized with caution and an understanding of a few basic principles.

Turning Radius. When making a turn, any vehicle will let the back end track in a narrower radius than the front. The difference in radius will depend on the sharpness of the turn with the greatest difference occurring during a sharp turn. This same concept holds true for a vehicle when backing. Because the steering wheels are now the following wheels, they will move laterally some distance to pivot the leading end of the vehicle around. This effect exposes the side of the vehicle to obstacles the rear of the vehicle has missed. For this reason, the sides of the vehicle need to be monitored carefully.

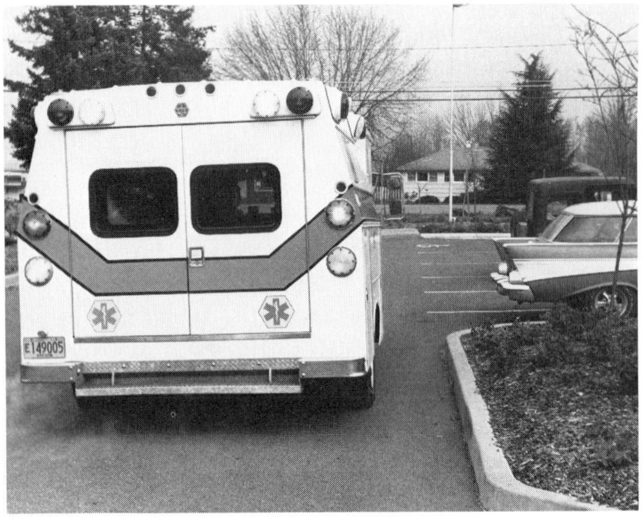

Fig. 5.5a Front wheels travel in a greater arc than the rear, especially when backing. Thus, the vehicle's side is exposed to obstacles missed by the rear.

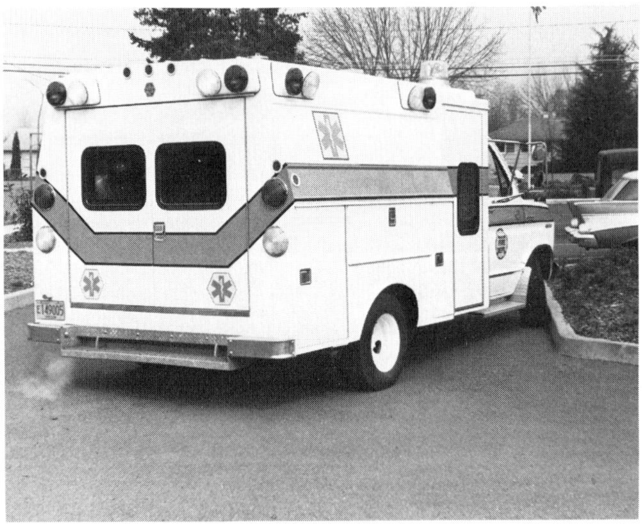

Fig. 5.5b Example of the effects of too wide a turn when backing. (Photos courtesy of **jems.**)

Pivot. The turning action of the front and rear wheels causes the vehicle to pivot varying degrees depending on the sharpness of the turn. When backing, the pivoting takes place at the rear tires, not the bumper. Although this principle sounds quite basic, it is easily forgotten when driving. The rear tires usually cannot be seen in the mirrors when the vehicle's position is observed through mirrors. The only reference the driver has to his position is the rear of the vehicle. Therefore, it is important for the driver to be familiar with the location of the rear wheels in relationship to the rear bumper. Should the driver initiate a turn as the rear bumper passes an obstacle, the rear wheels will act as the pivot point and the side of the vehicle may strike the obstacle even though the rear of the vehicle appears to be moving away from it.

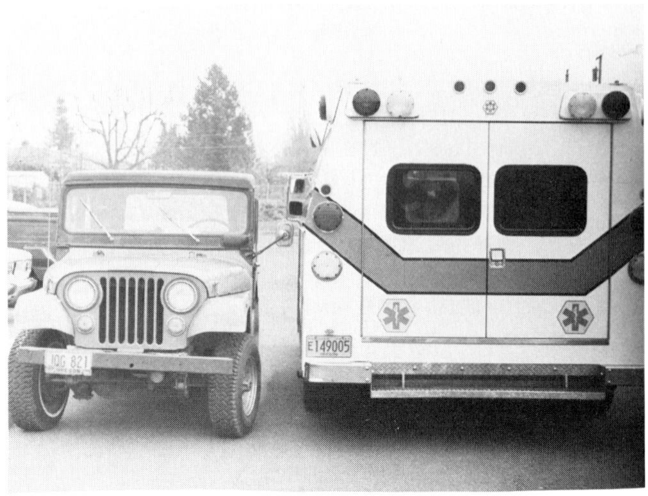

Fig. 5.6a When turning while backing, vehicles pivot on the rear tires, not the bumper.

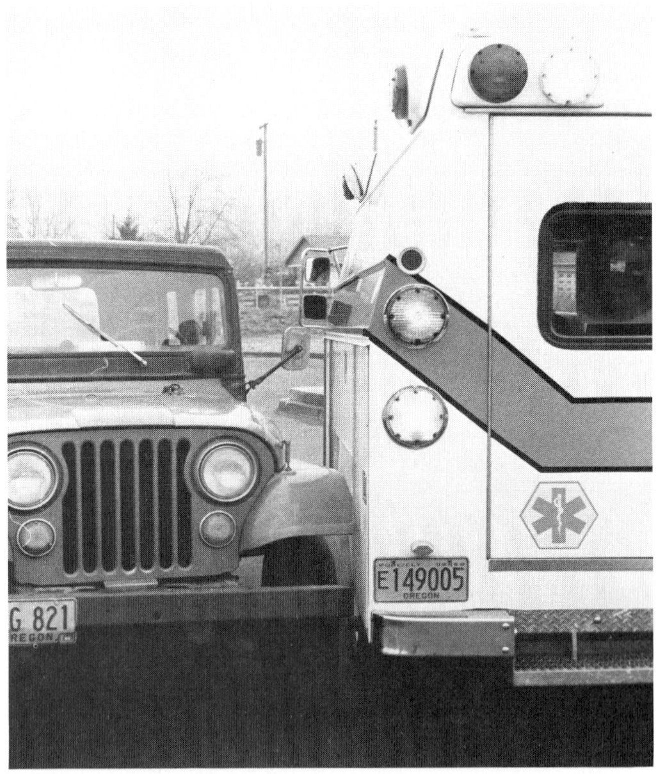

Fig. 5.6b If driver initiates a turn as rear bumper passes an obstacle, a collision may result. (Photos courtesy of **jems.**)

Plan Ahead. Because of its hazards, the driver should strive to avoid backing. Whenever possible, place the vehicle in a way that you can pull out straight ahead without having to back. It is often safer to drive around the block than to back the vehicle.

When backing is unavoidable, the driver should attempt to plan any backing maneuvers that must be made to be to the left. Left turns allow the driver to watch his most vulnerable side in his left mirror, the one with the best visibility. Since left turns are to the driver's side, he can back up using the mirrors and looking to his left side to get a better field of vision.

At an accident scene, any backing should be planned to take place immediately before or after the scene. Any backing performed within an accident scene increases the already present confusion and may result in an accident.

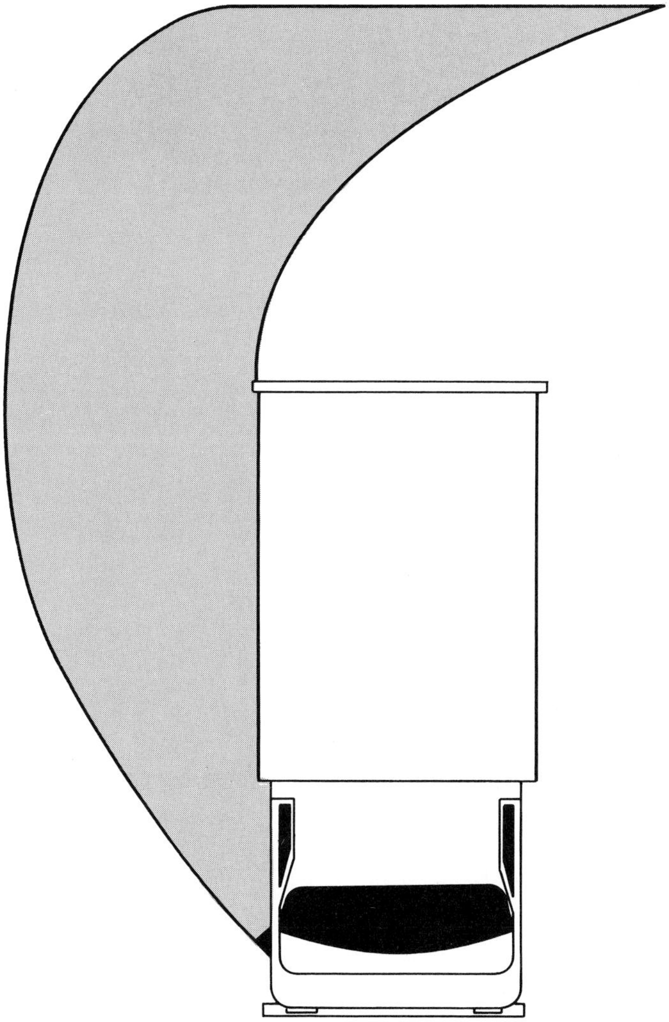

Fig. 5.7 The shaded area emphasizes the track of rear and front tires—anything in this area will be struck as ambulance turns.

Visibility. The major contributing factor to backing accidents is the lack of good visibility. One method of increasing visibility while backing a sedan is to look over the right shoulder. However, this practice usually leaves the driver steering with only one hand on the wheel. With the body turned and the driver looking out the rear window, he cannot adequately monitor what is happening with and around the front of the vehicle. This unsafe backing practice is usually the result of the vehicle being inadequately equipped with mirrors.The rear view mirrors generally found in sedans are small and inefficient and right side mirrors are frequently nonexistent.

Obviously, looking over your right shoulder while backing most ambulances won't get the job done. Even if the driver leans way out of his seat to see out the back doors, the driver still won't be able to see much out of the tiny patient compartment door windows. Visibility out of any side windows will also be very limited and of little value to the ambulance driver.

Some drivers prefer to open their left door and watch along the side of the vehicle as they back. Such a method is totally unacceptable. In this position, the driver can only monitor the left side of his vehicle. The right side is left totally blind. At the same time, this driver cannot watch the front of his vehicle. The driver himself is also placed in a precarious posture, hanging out the door and relying on a movable door for support.

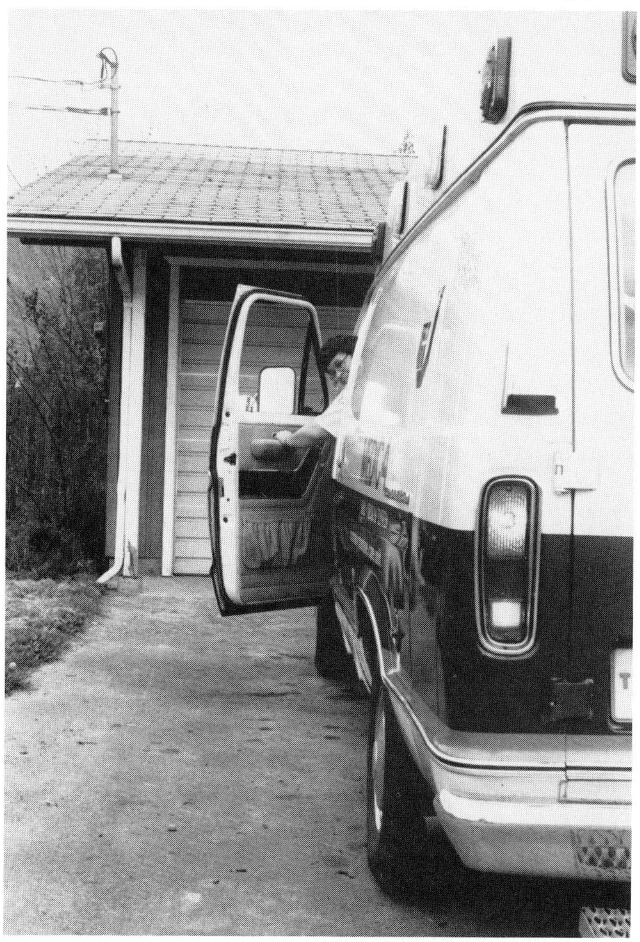

Fig. 5.8 Opening the door to watch along the side while backing is dangerous and unacceptable—only one side can be seen.

In such a position, the backing driver often becomes so intent on watching the rear of the vehicle and its interaction with the surrounding area that he may not monitor his door. It is then left free to snag on any obstruction it passes, damaging the door and pulling it from under the driver. Additionally, the driver is steering with only one hand while supporting himself on the door. One-handed driving is more likely to lead to oversteering and jerky movements.

Mirrors. Certainly the best technique for backing an ambulance is to use the mirrors mounted on both sides of the vehicle. Mirror usage allows the driver to monitor both sides and still keep his eye on the front of the vehicle. Mirror usage also allows the driver to keep both hands on the steering wheel for greater control.

Using the mirrors on any vehicle requires some getting used to. Most mirrors allow vision of only a few feet to the side at the rear of the vehicle. This limited visibility is decreased even further as the distance to the mirror is decreased. Additionally, side view mirrors only allow the driver to see as low as the rear bumper of the vehicle, often, not even that low. Also, the view in the mirror can be confusing, since the image is seen in reverse of reality. Couple these factors with the distortion caused by the angle at which the mirror must be set, and all these problems can make the use of mirrors confusing and distorted.

Rear visibility can be assisted by the use of convex or "fish eye" mirrors. These are small mirrors that allow the field of vision to be drastically widened, and make the blind spots visible. Unfortunately, such mirrors do distort depth perception tremendously. For this reason, they should not be relied on while backing. Convex mirrors should be used to check the area to make sure everything is clear before backing. Since convex mirrors are only used as secondary mirrors, they should be mounted so they don't interfere with the use of the regular mirrors.

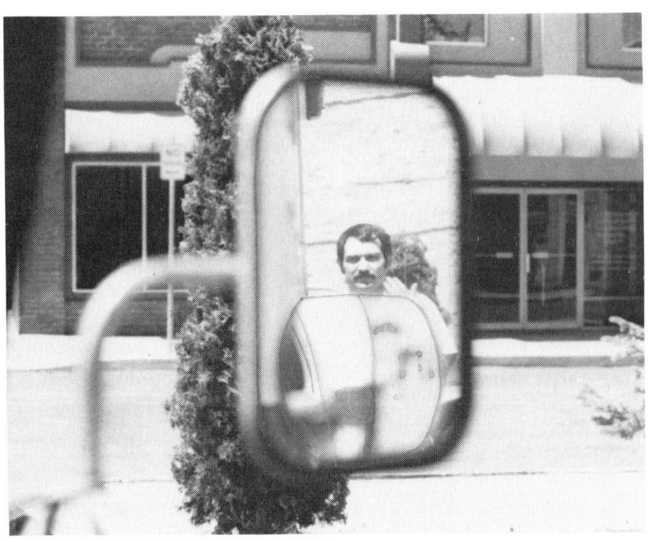

Fig. 5.9a Use of convex or "fish-eye" mirrors helps to drastically widen the field of vision.

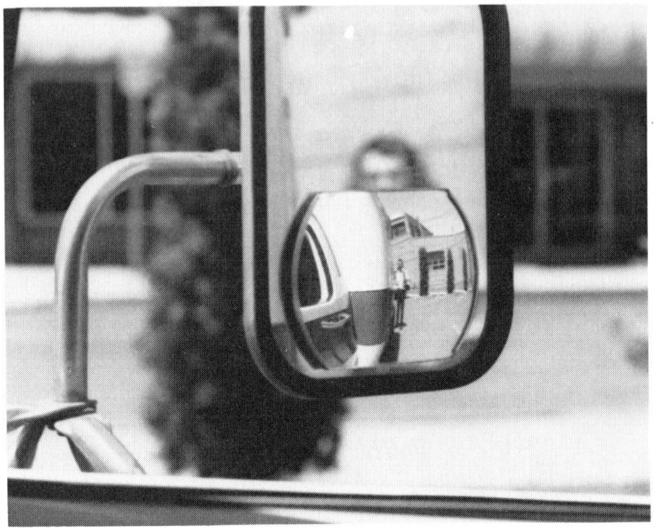

Fig. 5.9b Convex mirrors distort depth perception—should not be used for actual backing.

Another device that can increase rear visibility is a fresnel lens mounted on a rear window. A fresnel lens allows the driver to see almost directly below the back of the vehicle. It also distorts the image much the way a convex mirror does. Therefore, a fresnel lens should only be used to quickly check for hazards prior to backing the vehicle.

Act of Backing. When backing becomes unavoidable, it must be performed correctly. The driver's first act should be to personally walk the area to be covered while backing. This act allows the driver to fully understand where all of the obstacles will be in relation to his vehicle. He will also become familiar with the terrain that will be negotiated.

A spotter should always be utilized when backing a vehicle such as an ambulance. Many agencies will not allow their vehicles to be backed even along the station apron or driveway without a spotter at the rear of the vehicle. The spotter can more efficiently monitor blind spots and the vehicle relationship to its environment than the driver. The spotter is generally one of the other crew members. At the scene of a medical emergency, the other crew members may be busy with patient care, thus another spotter must be selected. When possible, utilize someone who will not be distracted by other events occurring at the

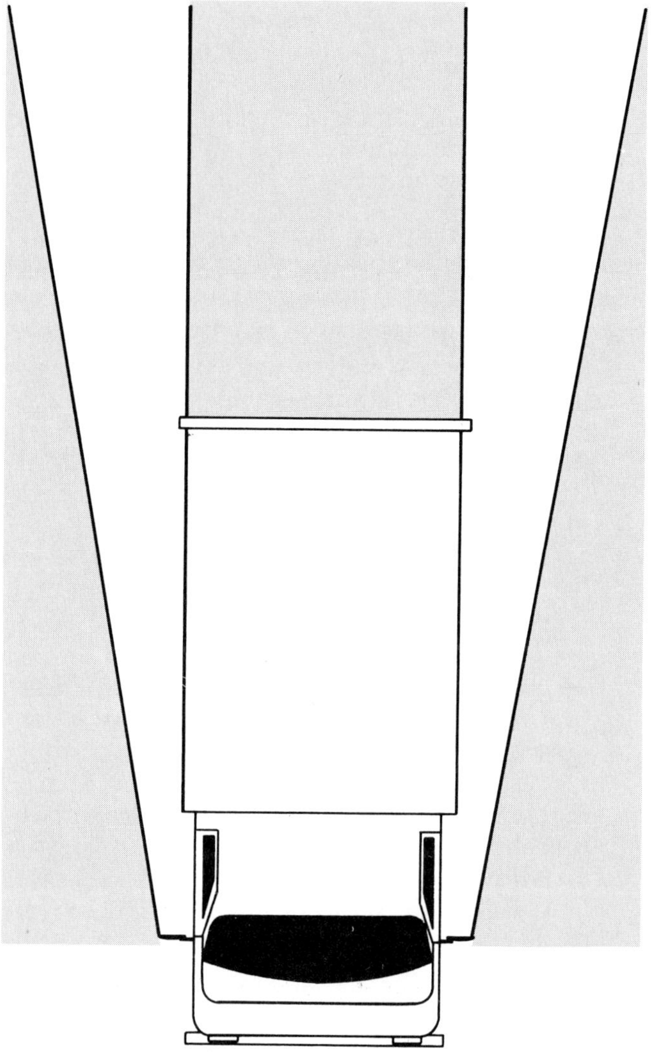

Fig. 5.10 Mirrors tend to allow only a few feet of vision to the side at the rear of the vehicle.

scene, such as a first responder, firefighter, or police officer. These people are not as likely to become distracted or walk away at a crucial moment as a bystander might. The driver should assure the spotter is positioned to be seen in the left mirror and his hand signals are deliberate and understandable. It is very important for the driver to realize that the spotter cannot monitor the right front fender of the vehicle. The driver must also keep in mind that although he is being helped by another person, he (the driver) is still responsible for the vehicle. The driver must make every effort to monitor his vehicle's progress and its relation to any hazards.

The driver must never attempt to back rapidly. Vehicles behave awkwardly and differently when driven in reverse. Because of the limited area of view in the mirrors, problems seem to arise more quickly. Judgment of distance can also become a problem when backing rapidly. No matter what the situation or patient condition, the driver must always take the time to back slowly and cautiously.

While backing, the driver must continue to use his mirrors, checking both sides as often as necessary. The driver must also make sure the front fender and the rear tire are clear of any obstructions before initiating a turn. Make the turn as wide and slow as possible. A wide turn will reduce the difference in front-to-back radius. Slow turning will be less likely to create the awkward feeling in the steering that is often encountered when driving in reverse.

There is no point in backing a vehicle any further than minimally necessary. The more backing that is done, the more likely a collision.

As you back, but before the vehicle comes to a complete stop, turn the wheels in the direction in which they will need to be to pull away. This action will decrease the strain on the steering system.

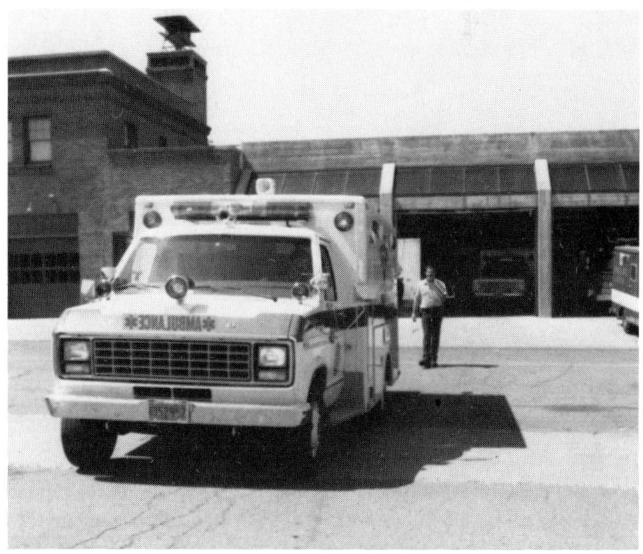

Fig. 5.11 Always use a spotter when backing an ambulance to monitor blind spots. Spotter should use deliberate hand motions.

Many ambulances are equipped with warning devices that are activated when the vehicle is being backed. It may be preferable to install a switch on the backing alarm which could allow the driver to deactivate it. The driver might elect to turn the device off when backing in a quiet neighborhood or at the hospital at three in the morning. If the device is wired through a switch, a warning light should be installed to remind the driver that the alarm is deactivated.

While these alarms enhance safety, there are some precautions worthy of mention. Backing alarms or the use of the emergency lights in no way relieves the driver of any responsibility to carefully watch where he is backing. Unfortunately, such alarms may tend to make a driver overconfident. Keep in mind that the sight of an ambulance will almost always attract children. Children may not understand the meaning of the backing alarm and dart into your path.

The professional driver realizes he has nothing to prove by backing rapidly or without the aid of a spotter. Backing is hazardous. Such a driver will do all in his power to minimize the risks involved when backing his vehicle.

Parking

Each time we drive we are faced with the problem of parking. We may be parking in our own driveway at home, in a supermarket parking lot, or at the scene of an accident. Although parking is very routine to all drivers, it can still create little problems. By gaining an understanding of what is required of a driver when parking, the task can be made much easier.

Urban Parking. Parking in the urban setting is the toughest parking problem. Typically it entails first searching for a place to park and then squeezing the vehicle into a tight space, all the while trying to keep from impeding other traffic. Urban parking usually requires the vehicle to be parked in one of three different positions.

Diagonal Parking. Parking in a diagonal space requires an approach speed of no more than 10 mph. As the vehicle approaches the space, the driver should move to the far left of his traffic lane to obtain as much space as possible between his vehicle and the line of parked cars. Typically, this space will need to be at least five or six feet. If the vehicle you are driving is large, such as an ambulance, this distance will need to be even greater. The actual side distance needed is one-third the length of the vehicle being parked.

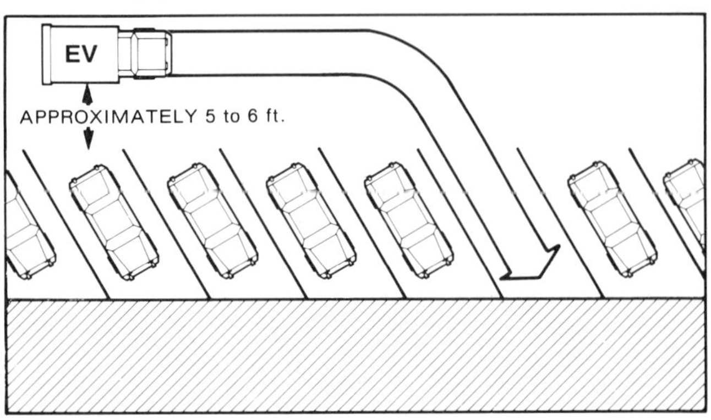

Fig. 5.12 Representation of diagonal parking

Many motorists attempt turning into diagonal parking spaces as soon as their front bumper is in line with the parked vehicle's bumper. This maneuver will often result in a collision, since the tires are the turning vehicle's pivot point.

In order to properly and safely diagonal park, the driver must wait until his front wheels come in line with the bumper of the car in the parking space before he begins to turn. As he turns the driver should visualize the track the rear tires will take. The rear wheels will track a shorter radius. The driver should estimate the path that will bring his vehicle into a parallel position with the parked vehicles.

Perpendicular Parking. Except for a much steeper angle of approach, setting up your vehicle for perpendicular parking is much the same as for diagonal parking. Perpendicular parking requires that the vehicle initiate its turn into the space from a point 7-8 feet away from the line of cars. As the turn is made, the vehicle should be straightened out (parallel to the parked vehicle) by the time it actually begins to enter the parking space. This will avoid scraping the neighboring vehicle. If the vehicle being parked is long, like an ambulance, it is often better to back into the space. Backing in allows the wheels doing the steering to trail and will pivot the vehicle into line much more quickly.

Parallel Parking. Parallel parking is usually avoided by ambulances and other emergency vehicles but it is a skill that should still be learned since it has a bearing on other maneuvers. In order to be of sufficient size, a parallel parking space must be about 25 percent longer than the vehicle that is to be parked. When parallel parking, the driver should pull his vehicle up parallel to the vehicle in front, with his rear wheels even with the rear bumper of the parked vehicle. This point is where most people get into trouble.

They often pull up further so the two vehicles are even and then attempt to pivot on their bumper instead of the rear tires. With your rear wheels even with the parked vehicle's rear bumper, you simply pivot into the parking space, guiding the rear into alignment with the vehicle parked behind. You can then straighten the wheel and pull forward to fit into the space.

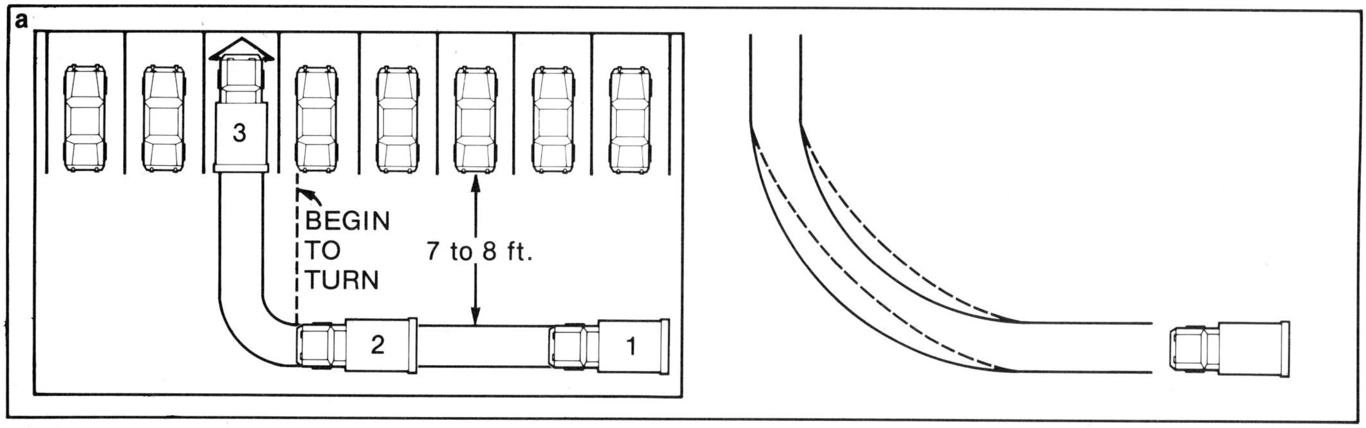

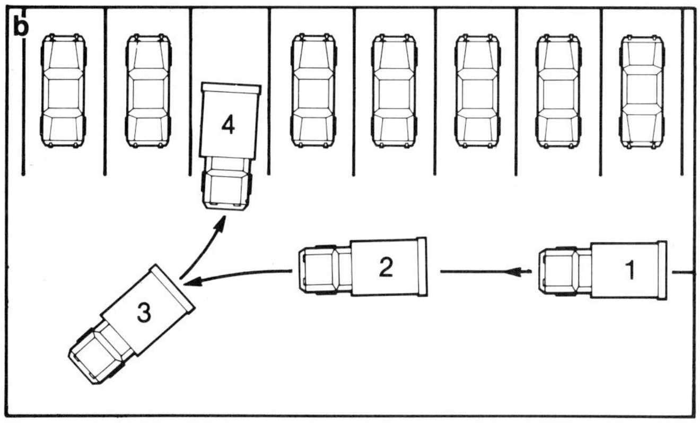

Fig. 5.13 Positioning for perpendicular parking.

While there are generally three types of designated areas for parking, many people will choose instead to park in undesignated areas, such as fire lanes, handicapped spaces, or other illegal areas. Such places are tempting to ambulance crews who are looking for a place to park. In case of a call, they offer easy access and departure.

However, nonemergency parking in such places is both illegal and inconsiderate of others. Parking in a handicapped space will certainly cause inconvenience for the paraplegic who needs the enlarged parking space to get his wheel chair out of his vehicle. Parking in fire lanes can obstruct the normal traffic flow and also create a blind spot for pedestrian traffic. Double parking will also obstruct normal traffic flow. Any of these parking indiscretions will help the public to form a negative impression of your EMS agency.

Even when parked in designated areas, because of its size the ambulance may present problems to other motorists. In diagonal and perpendicular parking spaces, the width of the ambulance may make it difficult for other drivers to get in or out of their vehicles. The ambulance parked close to a corner may also make seeing around the corner difficult for other motorists.

While still needing to park in an area with easy departure, the crew should be aware of the impact their parking site selection will have on other motorists and choose an appropriate place carefully.

Parking On a Slope. Many people don't realize that a hill or slope can make a difference in how the vehicle is parked. Cases have occurred where a vehicle's parking brakes or transmission have failed while parked on a hill. These vehicles have then careened down the hill causing collisions and often injury. Such events can be avoided if the driver places his vehicle as close to the curb as possible and then turns the wheels into the downhill curb. In the event that the vehicle should start to roll, the front wheel will be forced into the curb, and be unable to move. Where curbs are not present, turn the wheel so the vehicle will travel off the roadway should it roll downhill. This act may help avoid a multivehicle collision should the parked vehicle's brakes fail.

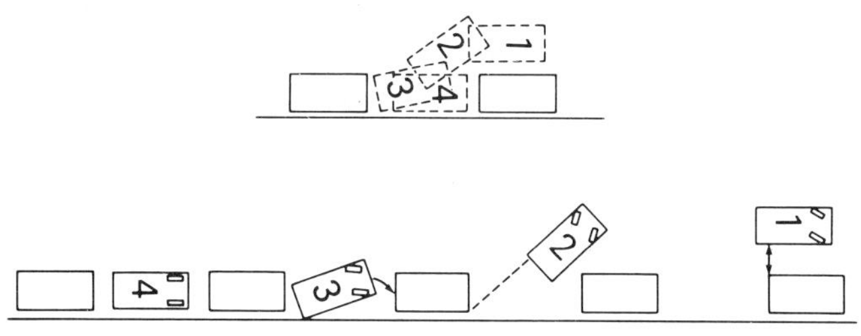

Fig. 5.14 Steps involved in parallel parking (1) line up vehicle parallel to the vehicle in front (2) pivot into parking space lining vehicle up with front of vehicle to the rear (3) turn toward curb (4) straighten out by pulling forward.

Many drivers rely only on the automatic transmission, placed in park, to keep the vehicle from rolling while parked on a hill. The pawl (locking mechanism) that holds the transmission in park was never intended for such use and cannot be guaranteed to hold on a hill. Once the vehicle is placed properly, the driver should engage the parking brake firmly *before* placing the transmission in park. This act will keep the weight of the vehicle from resting on the pawl and stressing the transmission components. One word of caution: Parking brakes will often freeze when set in extremely cold weather. This is especially true if the vehicle has recently been driven through puddles since the parking brake cables are wet. A level parking place will need to be selected to avoid the use of the parking brake during such weather conditions.

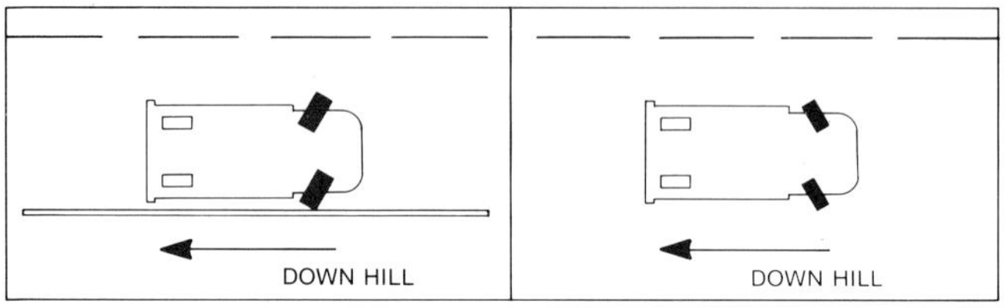

Fig. 5.15a When parking on slope, place vehicle as close to curb as possible, turning front wheels to downhill curb.

Fig. 5.15b If curbs are unavailable, turn wheels so the vehicle will travel off roadway should it roll.

Turning Around

For one reason or another, the ambulance will have to be turned around. When confronted with such a situation, drivers either drive around the block or simply pull into a driveway and back out facing the opposite direction. Some consideration must be given to these options. In many cases, the trip around the block is the best option. It is usually the safest and in some states, the only legal means of turning unless operating the vehicle in an emergency mode. There are options available for special circumstances and, grouped together, they are called turn-a-bouts. Turn-a-bouts incorporate U-turns, "two point" turns, and "three point" turns. The universal criteria for all turn-a-bout maneuvers is to pick a location that is safe. The location must have good visibility in all directions and adequate gaps in the traffic.

U-turns. U-turns are probably the safest type of turn-a-bout since they are executed in one motion without having to back up. However, U-turns require a considerable amount of space to be completed. To make a safe U-turn, the driver needs to complete it using as few lanes as possible. A turn on an expressway from the lanes going in one direction to those in the other direction, even when the median is crossed, is technically a U-turn. Such turns are rarely legal unless operating under the emergency mode.

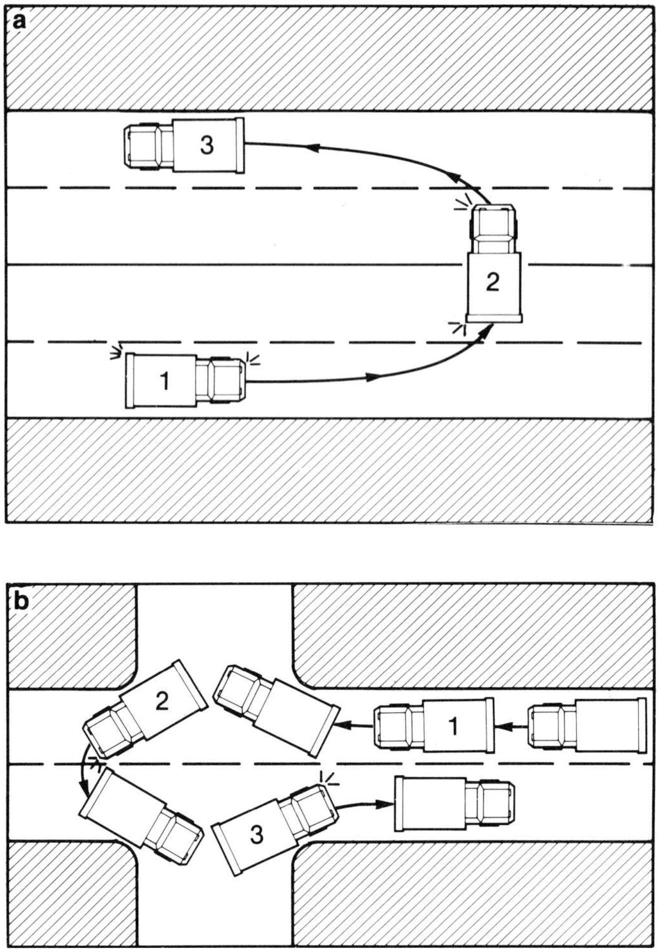

Fig. 5.16 U-turns are executed in one continuous motion and are considered the safest type of turn. But, they're usually illegal and require excessive space.

Care must be taken in selecting a turnaround site. Many median strips are nothing more than earth and are often lower in grade than the traffic lanes. Water run-off may collect in the median making it soggy and unable to support the weight of an ambulance. Once the vehicle has crossed the median strip, it will then have to blend in with the approaching traffic. To further complicate matters, the ambulance will often have to blend in with high-speed traffic while it is traveling at a reduced speed. Visibility will also be a problem for the driver since the traffic will be aproaching from his blind side.

"TWO POINT" TURNS. "Two point" turns usually incorporate a side street or driveway and forward and reverse driving.

It is far better to select a side road or alley for such a maneuver rather than a private driveway, since private driveways are often narrow and may have hidden dangers. Additionally, the driveway may not be able to support the weight

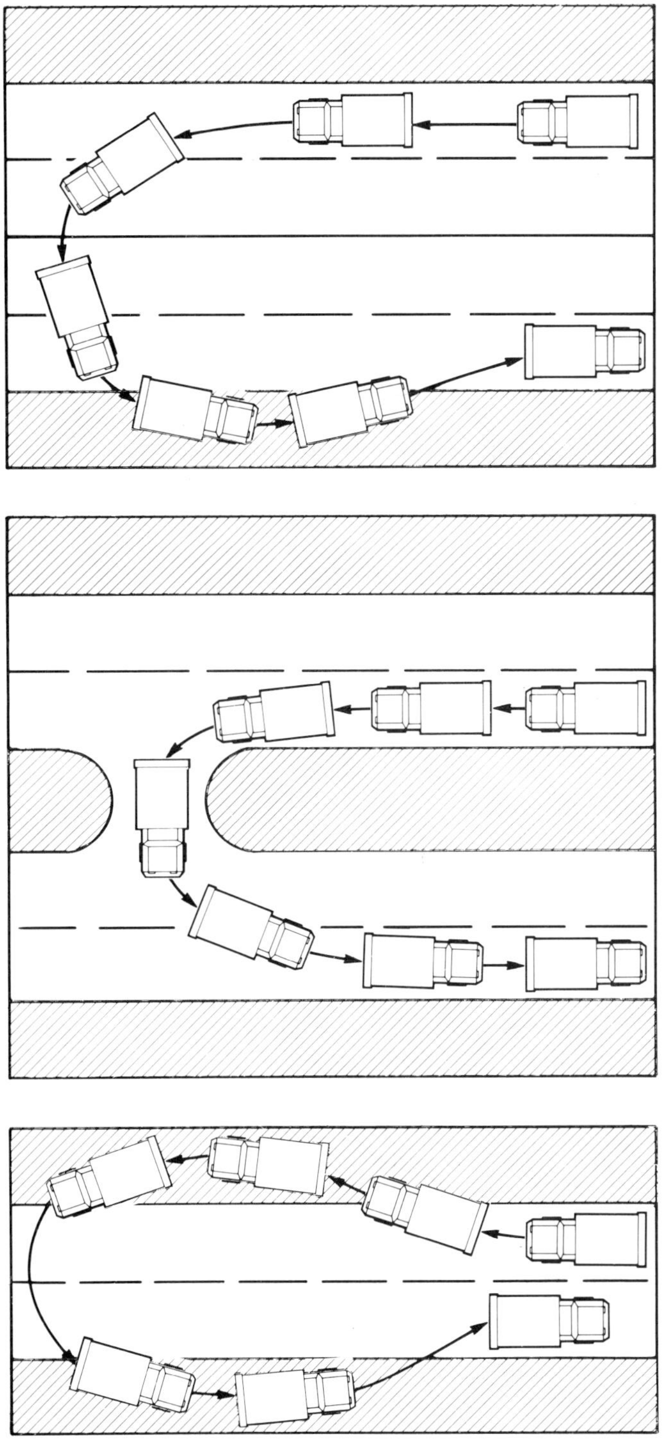

Fig. 5.17 Examples of U-turns

of the ambulance or it may have toys, shrubbery, or water stand pipes that might be damaged. There are essentially two ways to perform a "two point" turn:

Rear First Turn-about. This is the safest type of "two point" turn-about. When an alley or side road is available the driver should pull past it and then back into the road. This leaves the vehicle positioned to pull forward across the two lanes of traffic. When the alley or side road is on the same side of the street, backing is restricted to one lane of traffic and does not involve crossing traffic.

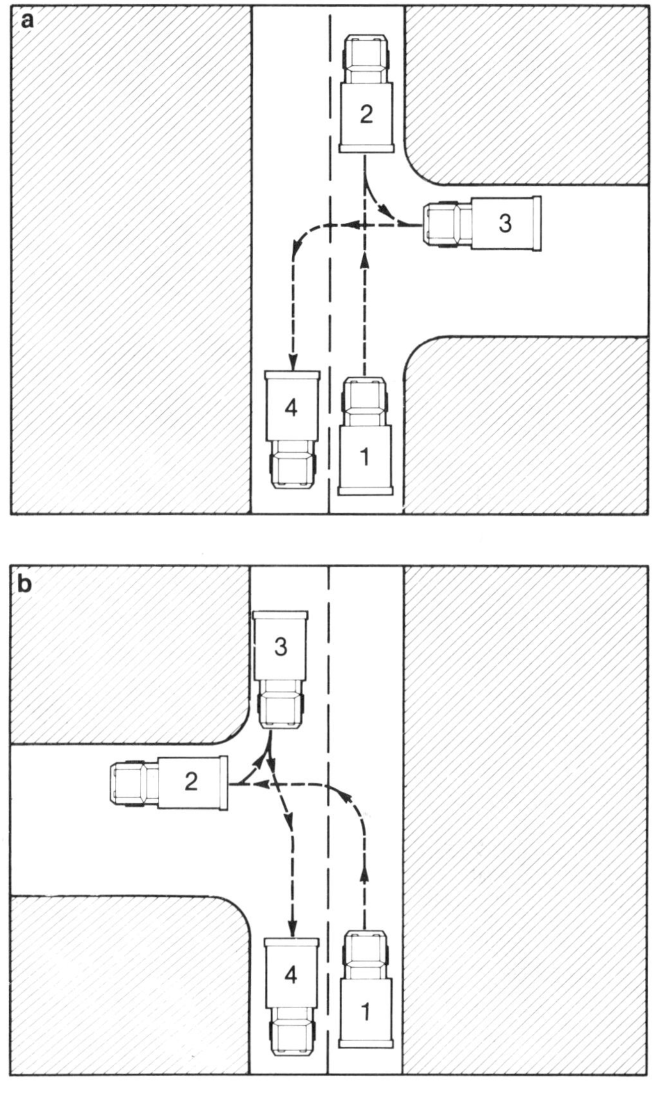

Fig. 5.18a You can use the rear-first two-point turn when an alley or side road presents on the right. Just pull past the intended side road and then back into it.

Fig. 5.18b When using the front or left side turn, the driver must back into traffic approaching on the blind side, and so this turn is not as safe as the previous type.

Front First Turn-about. This maneuver is not as safe as the rear first turn-about. It is an option when a side road on the right is not available. It involves pulling front end first into the road and then backing out. Since it forces the driver to back into traffic approaching on his blind side, it is much more hazardous to perform.

"THREE POINT" TURNS. "Three point" turns are the most hazardous turn-a-bout since they require the driver to do a great deal of maneuvering. The primary hazard of the "three point" turn is that the entire maneuver must be performed on the primary road with the potential of traffic approaching from either direction. Another hazard, backing, will also be done to the blind side. "Three point" turns should only be used as a last resort when other options are not available.

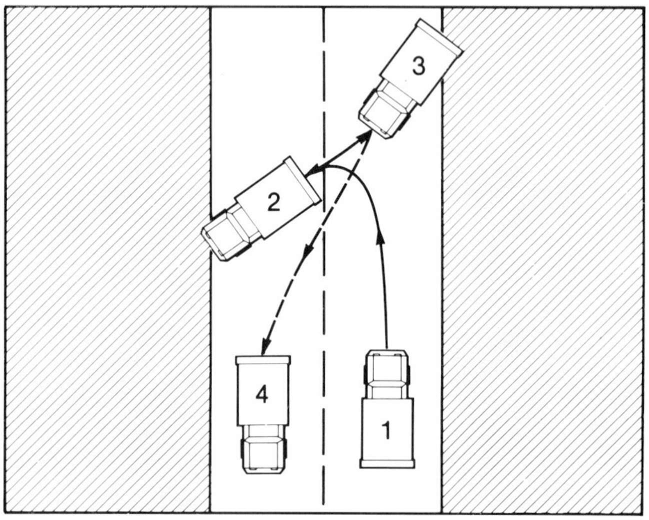

Fig. 5.19 Three point turns are considered the most hazardous since they require much maneuvering.

Y-turns. Y-turns are performed on roadways that are too narrow for the completion of a U-turn. The Y-turn requires the vehicle to cross the center line three different times before the turn-about is completed.

Urban Driving

Heavy urban driving can be one of the most challenging experiences a driver will face. In urban traffic the vehicles are surrounded by others being driven closer together than is considered safe. Traffic is constantly changing speed as it slows for stop lights, to change lanes, or to turn. Cars are merging into traffic from the curbside and out of alleys and parking lots, as well as from intersections. Such conditions can become frustrating. Drivers protecting their space within the traffic often refuse to allow others to merge. For a driver to survive in such an environment, he must drive with an aggressiveness that is often alien to his personality. Obviously, a driver must be at his peak of alertness to safely drive in heavy urban traffic.

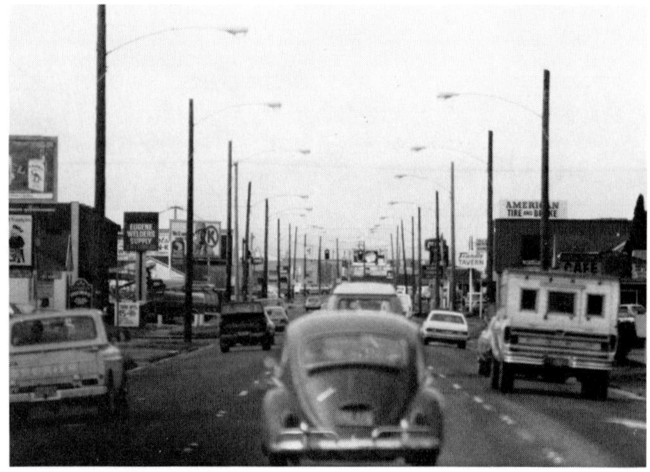

Fig. 5.20 Urban driving is one of the most challenging experiences a driver will face.

Ambulance crews encounter these same situations and must learn to handle them well. A driver must exhibit professional ability and demonstrate confidence to others. Because of his professional stature the ambulance driver might be looked to for help by other motorists trying to merge into the traffic flow. The ambulance driver should encourage others to pull into the traffic in front of him and allow room for them to do so. This type of courtesy will endear the crew and the agency they represent to the public.

In order for an ambulance driver to drive a safe emergency response in heavy urban traffic, he must first understand and be able to drive routinely in heavy traffic. Meeting the challenge of urban driving requires that the driver be observant and learn to fit well within traffic.

Observation. As in all other types of traffic, the most critical skill required of a driver in urban traffic is well-developed seeing habits.

By rapidly observing changing conditions well before they can affect him, the driver can anticipate what might happen, and can react with plenty of time so his actions won't drastically affect others on the road. The ambulance driver cannot expect others on the road to be as alert as himself. For this reason, he must allow others as much time and distance as possible in order to react ahead of danger.

The frenzy of heavy traffic can be quite confusing. Motorists often signal to make a turn, then continue straight ahead. They may have realized the street they were about to turn on was not the one they intended or was obstructed by other traffic. The situation can also be compounded if they change lanes at the same time to

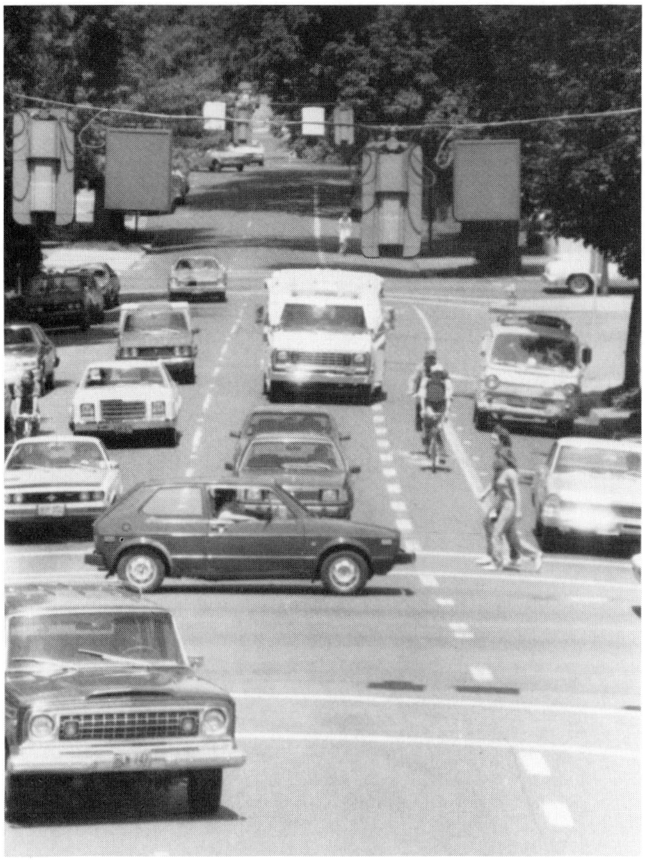

Fig. 5.21 For a driver to conduct his vehicle safely in urban traffic, he must first be able to drive routinely in heavy traffic.

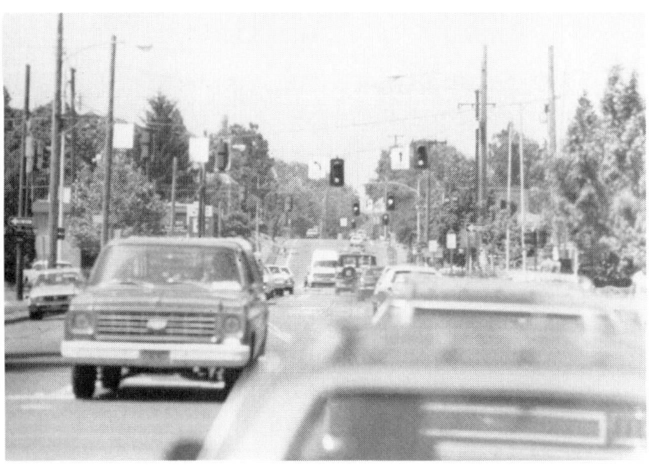

Fig. 5.22 Watching traffic and anticipating what's going to happen next enables you to adjust your position in traffic much more easily.

get out of the turn lane or into a faster moving lane. These drivers will often signal their intentions to turn off the street, but will actually turn in the opposite direction.

By carefully observing, you can frequently anticipate what these drivers are really going to do. By watching another driver's head, you can see where he is looking, a valuable clue as to his intentions. The partially turned wheel of a vehicle stopped at an intersection is a clue that the driver is going to turn. Such indicators are only clues and don't necessarily reflect what will take place. Be especially attentive to drivers doing other than what the clues indicate.

An example would be if a driver signaled to turn up a one-way street in the wrong direction, or when a driver signals to turn onto a street that is typically congested during that specific time of day. Such observations will often cause the driver to quickly change his mind and resume a position within his previous flow of traffic without signaling his intention to do so. A motorist who appears uncertain of his location or whereabouts will drive very slowly with most of his attention focused on each street he approaches. As he passes a street, he may accelerate to a point at which he can read the next street sign. These drivers give many clues to their intentions. Obviously these clues cannot be trusted since the driver himself doesn't know his intentions.

There are other clues which can help us as we drive. Cars parked along the curb become a concern when they have a driver in them and especially when exhaust can be seen. This motorist may suddenly pull out in front of your vehicle. Look at his front wheels. Are they aimed into traffic? Alleys present problems too. A motorist attempting to pull from an alley has little view of traffic until he is almost into it. Occasionally, a driver will pull from an alley directly into traffic without warning.

Safe urban driving demands that a driver have the ability to *S*earch for the hazards and clues, *I*dentify them, *P*redict how they will affect him, *D*ecide on a solution, and *E*xecute that solution (SIPDE).

Fitting Traffic. A driver must be able to fit into traffic neatly, drive at the same speed, and maintain his own lane. The driver who is constantly changing lanes seldom gets to his destination any quicker although he increases the danger and frustration for himself and everyone around him. In addition, ambulances are the object of attention by others and so their operator must drive as predictably as possible.

Urban driving seems to be a constant stop and go process. The driver who watches traffic, anticipating what is going to happen next, can often adjust his position in traffic by simply varying his foot pressure on the accelerator or by coasting with minimal use of the brake. Such careful driving will make for a smoother ride and reduce vehicle wear. It is also an indication of the driver's experience and ability.

Traffic flow can be maintained if the traffic lights fit into a timed pattern. In many communities, the lights are set so that by maintaining a certain speed a driver can make all the green lights. The driver should attempt to determine if the traffic signals are set for flow. Timed traffic lights are often equipped with a sign that states that the lights are "set" for a certain speed. If you maintain the designated speed, you should be able to pass through a series of traffic signals without having to stop.

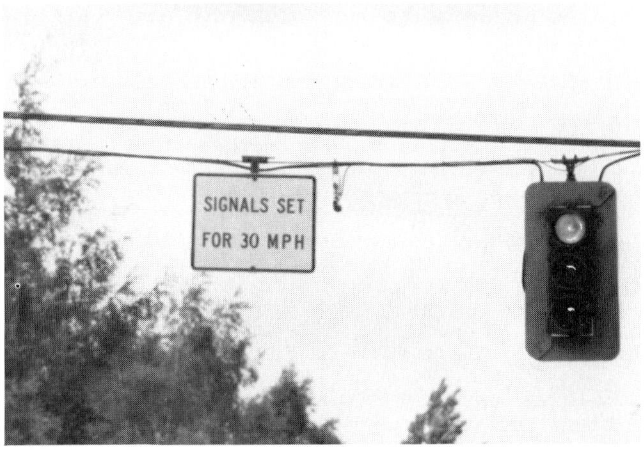

Fig. 5.23a Many communities use timed traffic lights so that a driver, maintaining a certain speed, can make all of the lights.

Another way to adjust your speed is to observe pedestrian signals. When the "WALK" light is on in your direction, you can assume the light will remain green for some time. Once the "DON'T WALK" or "WAIT" light starts to flash, the signal is about one-half way through its cycle. When the "DON'T WALK" light remains constantly illuminated, you can assume the signal will soon change. Once a driver has entered onto a street, he should decide which traffic lane he will travel in and move to it. Once in this lane the driver should not constantly need to change lanes. If he is going to remain on the street for some distance, he might initially pick a lane that is comfortable, changing to the appropriate lane well before the next turn. On multi-lane, two-way streets, the lane closest to the center of the street can be slowed with drivers waiting for oncoming traffic to pass before turning left, unless a center turn lane is available. Traffic close to the shoulder or curb will also be slowed by traffic attempting to turn right. If more than two lanes are available, those in the middle can be viewed as express lanes.

If the road has a high crown to facilitate water run-off, the left lanes may be the most comfortable lanes to drive. The right or outside lanes of a road with a high crown often gives the driver a feeling that the vehicle is pulling to the right or that it wants to fall off of the road.

By thinking several turns ahead, a driver can often determine which lane will be the one to turn from to put him in the proper lane on the next street. When doing this he must be aware that unless otherwise designated, such as with more than one turn lane, the driver is expected by law to turn into the nearest lane. Example: A left hand turn should be into the far left lane of the new street. Where two left turn lanes are pro-

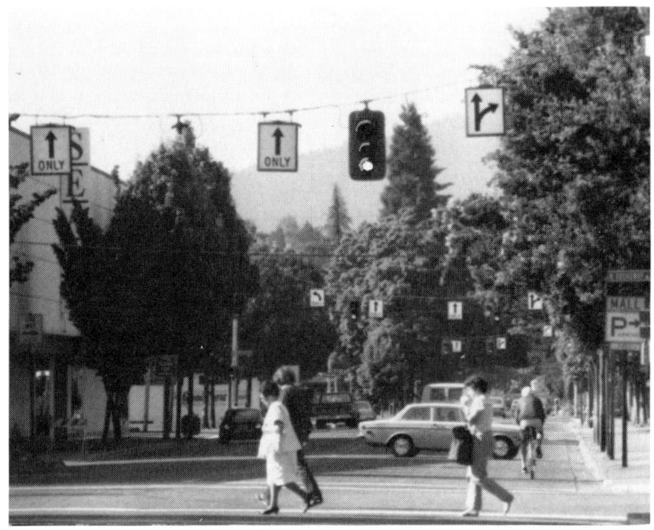

Fig. 5.23b Observe pedestrian signals to adjust your speed. Continuously lit don't walk sign means traffic signal will soon change.

vided, you may choose to turn from the second lane to better position yourself for an upcoming right turn.

Urban driving presents a variety of challenges to the driver. One who is conscientious, courteous, and observant will progress well through the traffic at a minimum of risk.

Intersections. Nearly 50 percent of all multiple-vehicle accidents occur within intersections. It is easy to understand the need for proper driving techniques and visual habits when passing through an intersection. It is at the intersection that vehicles come into direct conflict with others as each tries to cross the other's path. Poor visibility, confusing control systems, and driver error all lead to intersection accidents.

Approaching an Intersection. The driver needs to prepare himself for the intersection as he ap-

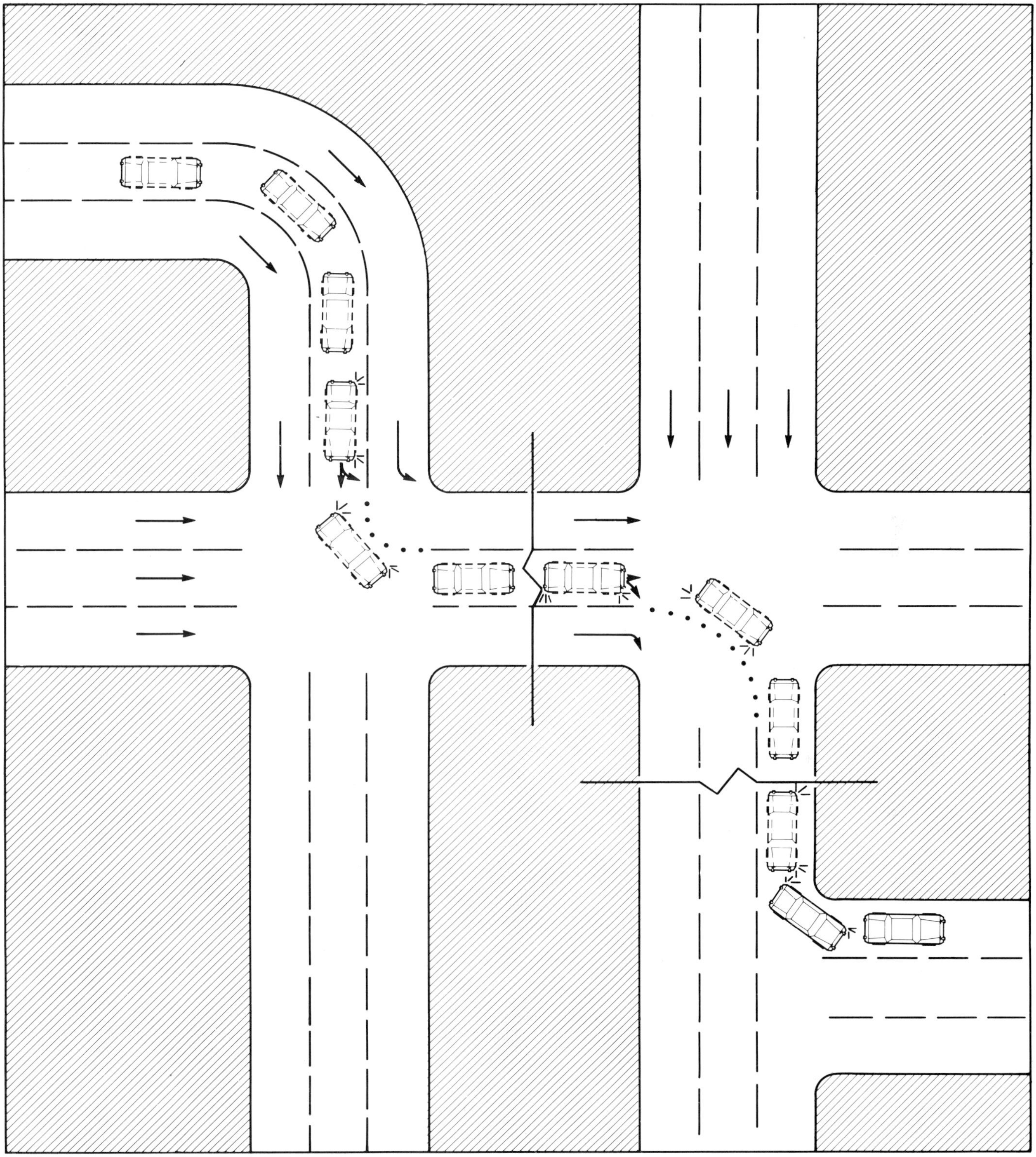

Fig. 5.24 Plan several turns ahead to determine which lane to turn from to put you in the proper lane for the next turn.

proaches it. He first needs to determine the speed at which he can safely approach. This will be determined by the traffic congestion, the type of controls at the intersection, and visibility. Signaling in advance of a turn is extremely important. It gives others a valuable clue to your intentions. All too often, a lazy driver will stick his finger out to hit the signal lever as he starts turning the wheel. Such late signaling is of no value to others. It is frequently recommended that a driver should signal his intent at least 100 feet prior to a turn. The key to where to begin signaling is time, not distance. Other drivers must be given a reasonable amount of time to see your signal and interpret your intent before a turn is initiated. Conversely, caution should be used so that a signal isn't given so early that an oncoming motorist thinks the intention is to turn before you arrive at your actual turning point.

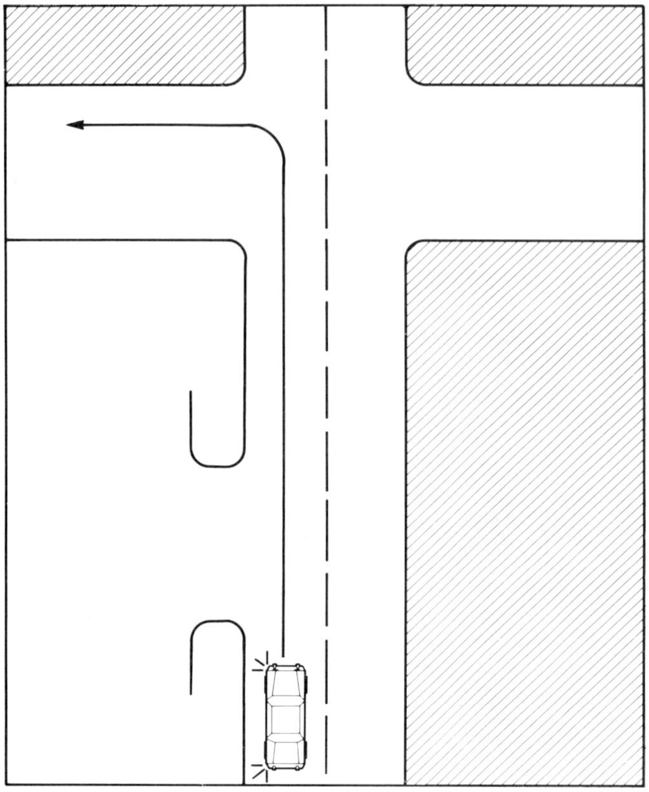

Fig. 5.25 Begin signaling at a point where other drivers cannot misinterpret your intentions.

While approaching an intersection, it is also important to allow an extra space between your vehicle and any trucks in front of you. Because of its height, a truck may block your view of overhead traffic lights so they are not visible until just before you enter an intersection. If the light changes while the truck is blocking your view, you may find yourself entering an intersection against a yellow or red light.

One of the more difficult driving decisions that motorists are faced with is whether or not to stop for a traffic signal that is changing to red. Once a signal turns yellow, you should attempt to stop before entering the intersection. If the traffic behind you is following so closely that it is likely they will not be able to stop without colliding with you, you should not attempt to stop. Another concern will be patient comfort. A hard stop may be very uncomfortable for your patient.

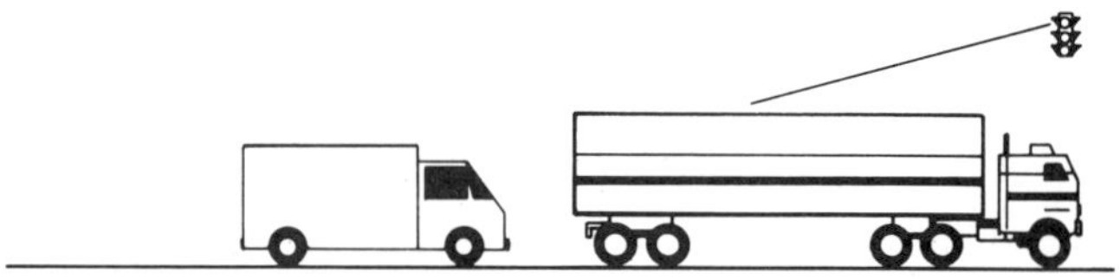

Fig. 5.26 Allow extra space between your vehicle and any trucks in front so you can see the light before entering an intersection.

Your good driving habits will reduce the need for hard braking and thus make your patient ride more comfortable.

Another common error is motorists stopping within intersections when caught in a line of stopped traffic. Stopping in the intersection is inconsiderate of cross traffic and is also illegal. If you keep your eyes aimed high and watch the traffic well in front of you, you shouldn't find yourself in the position of having to stop within intersections.

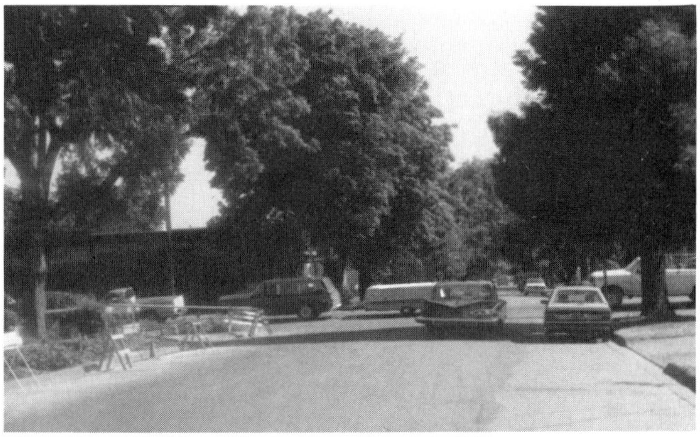

Fig. 5.27 Don't stop within intersections when caught in a line of traffic—it is both inconsiderate and illegal.

Ambulances, like most trucks, are blind to much of their right side. This condition means that any roads that meet you at an angle greater than 90° may be difficult to see down once you have stopped. By anticipating such a condition ahead of time, the driver can position his vehicle by turning it slightly towards the cross street. While this approach increases your visibility, you must be aware that you are giving false clues to other motorists as to your intentions. Proper signaling and extreme caution must be exercised when you give false intention clues.

When a traffic light turns green for you, look both ways before pulling ahead. Be aware of those who are trying to slip through on yellow lights. Always visually clear the intersection before pulling out into the intersection.

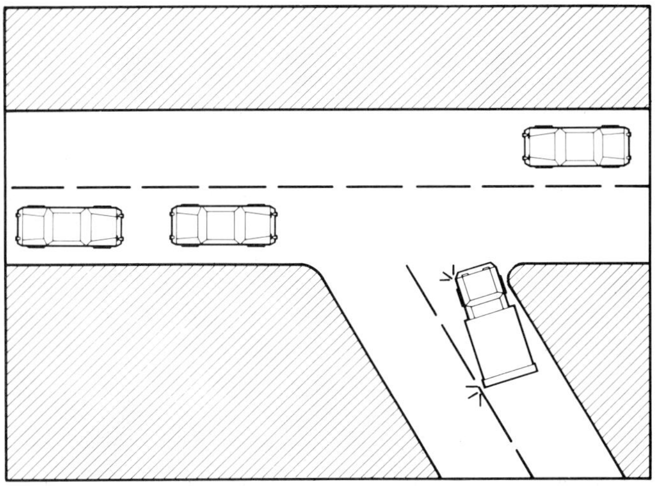

Fig. 5.28 Since ambulances are usually blind to much of their right side, roads that meet at an angle under 90 deg will be difficult to see down.

Techniques for Negotiating the Intersection. A driver must be aware of the time it takes to cross an intersection. From a standing start, it will take a minimum of four seconds to cross a two-lane street. For safety's sake, the driver should allow a margin of at least six seconds between himself and any approaching cross traffic.

Before entering into any two-way traffic intersection, the driver should first look left, since the first traffic he will cross will be coming from this direction. He should then look right to assure the traffic in this direction is also clear and back to the left again to assure that the original status has not changed. When crossing intersections with one-way traffic, first look in the direction from which the traffic is approaching, then quickly check the opposite side for wrong-way driving motorists.

As a driver prepares to turn right, he should first assure there are no bicycles or pedestrians to his right that may cross his intended path. Once a right turn is initiated, it will take about six seconds for the vehicle to turn and accelerate up to 30 mph. For this reason, a right turn should not be initiated unless the traffic approaching from the left is at least eight seconds away. This will put the turning vehicle at a safe two-second interval ahead of traffic once the turn is completed. Of course, in faster moving traffic, a larger gap will be needed. When initiating a left-hand turn, this interval must be increased by a couple of seconds since a lane of traffic will have to be crossed.

Left turns across the path of oncoming traffic present an additional safety problem. It is not uncommon for a stopped vehicle to be struck from the rear by an inattentive driver. If the vehi-

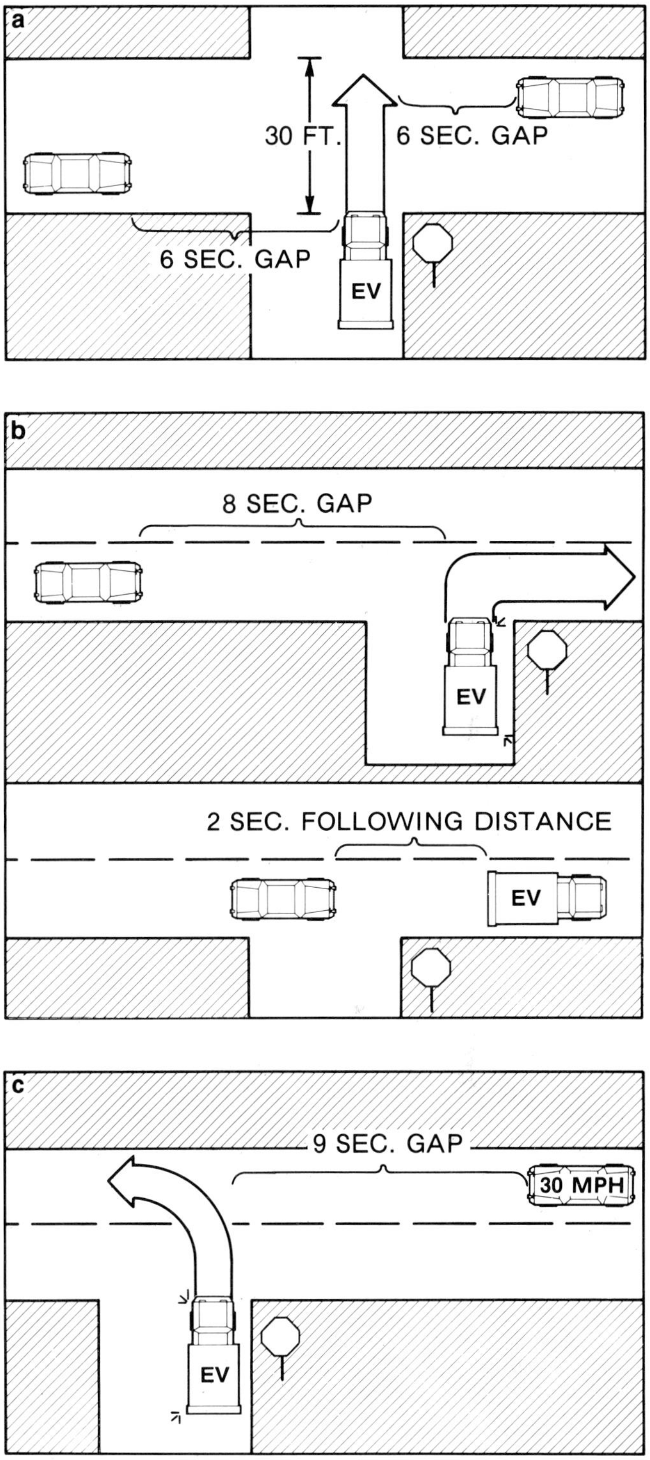

Fig. 5.29a It takes a minimum of four seconds to cross a two-lane street from a standing start; allow at least 6 seconds between yourself and approaching traffic.

Fig. 5.29b It takes six seconds to turn a right hand corner and accelerate to 30 mph. Allow eight seconds so that oncoming traffic can follow at two second intervals.

Fig. 5.29c The same time interval is needed for left hand turns, except that you'll need an extra second to cross the first lane—thus you'll need nine seconds total.

cle intending to turn left has its wheels turned in the direction of the turn when struck, it will be shoved forward, into the path of any oncoming traffic. This type of head-on collision is easily avoidable. The turning driver should not turn his wheels until he actually begins his left turn. If he is struck from behind prior to this time, he will simply be pushed forward in a straight line, avoiding the potential head-on situation.

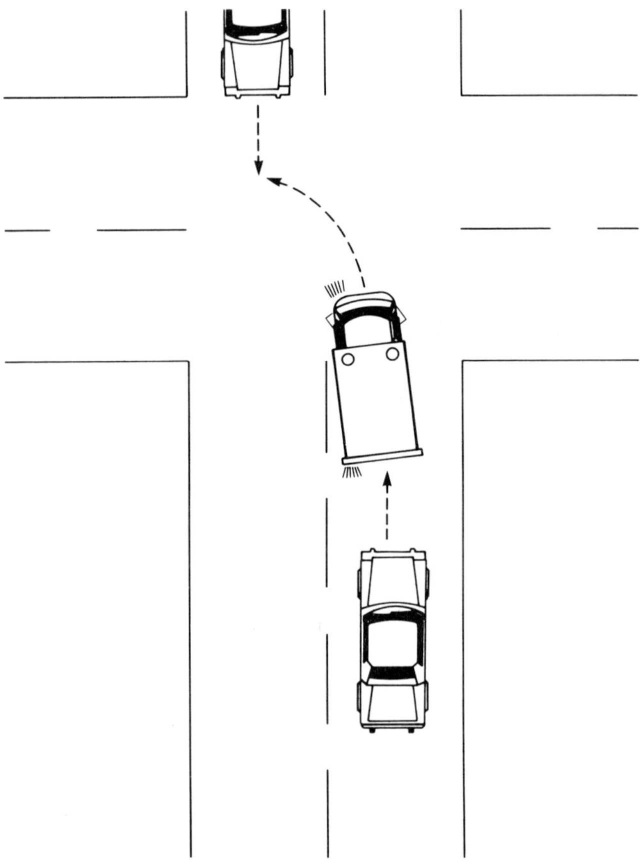

Fig. 5.30 It's not unusual for a stopped vehicle to be struck in the rear by an inattentive driver. Leave wheels pointing straight ahead when waiting to turn so that, if struck, you'll move in a straight line.

The dangers of driving through an intersection can be greatly reduced if a driver will aim high and keep in touch with the traffic around and to the rear of his vehicle. Courtesy and common sense will also help you avoid collisions. If the intentions of a driver are questionable, exercise added caution while entering an intersection. If an oncoming driver signals his intent to cross your path, it is often safer to wave him across in front of you because you can then totally understand his intent. Extreme care must be taken to insure traffic following you, perhaps in a lane to your right, is not endangered by your apparent "courtesy." Any traffic approaching the intersection on your right side will most likely be in a blind spot created by your vehicle. This type of intersection collision is very common and like most accidents, avoidable when good driving techniques are employed.

Driving On an Expressway

The term expressway describes any multi-lane, limited-access, high-speed highway. The expressway system present today in the United States started with a mandate delivered by President Eisenhower as a means of uniting America through an efficient highway network for the modern traveler. From that initial, federally subsidized system, many smaller systems have evolved uniting more areas. These expressways allow efficient travel within urban areas or are often a means of efficiently bypassing the urban area.

Properly engineered expressways are specifically designed for high speeds and traffic safety. Traffic directions are divided so the risk of a vehicle crossing a lane and creating a head-on collision are almost nonexistent. Most expressway curves are engineered to be driven comfortably at high speeds. Ramps are provided for speed changes while entering and exiting the highway so traffic can travel at a uniform speed. Expressway lighting and sign poles are usually situated well away from the edge of the road, and the poles are designed to break away if struck to reduce vehicle damage and occupant injury. Many expressways have concrete dividers between the opposing traffic lanes that are designed to guide a striking vehicle back into its own traffic lane, eliminating head-on collisions.

Due to the presence of all of these safety features, driving on an expressway may seem routine, requiring little or no decison-making. Because of this relaxed attitude, a driver can easily be lulled into a false sense of security. He may become hypnotized by road noise or by the endless center line, and so lose his awareness of what is happening around him. An expressway driver must consciously fight such conditions and remain alert.

At expressway speeds of 55 mph, it will require about 300 feet to stop the average passenger car. An ambulance will require even more distance. Therefore, it is important to continue looking far down the road beyond the vehicle in front to observe brake lights or any other signs, such as a puff of dust, that trouble looms ahead.

As traffic travels along an expressway, it will tend to develop into bunches with long spaces of open road between. These bunches of vehicles are often called wolf packs. A driver should consciously avoid these packs whenever possible. Such packs tend not to allow for proper spacing between vehicles and leave the drivers without any maneuvering room to use in case of a crisis.

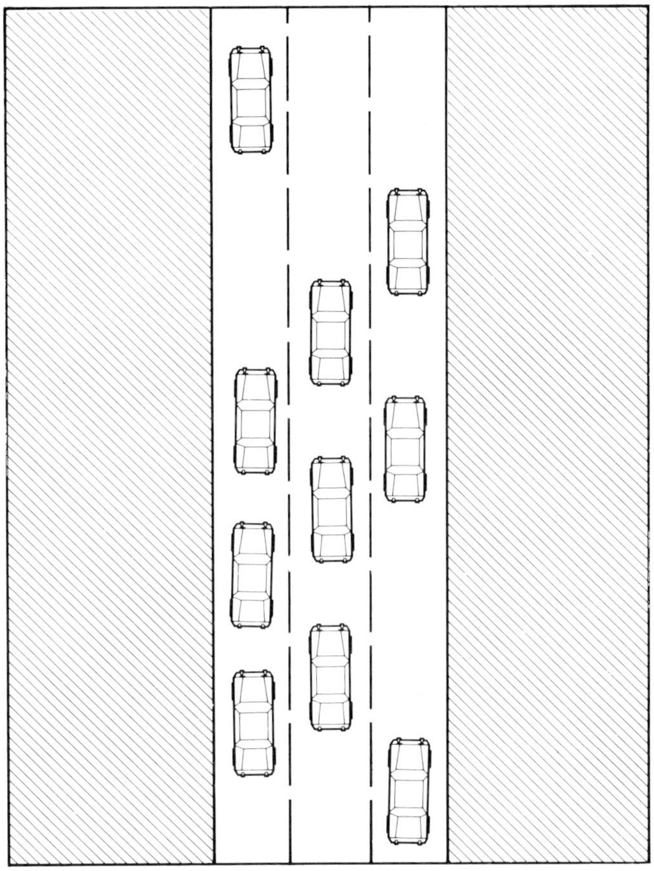

Fig. 5.31 Clusters of vehicles on expressways tend not to allow enough spacing between vehicles, thus minimizing escape "outs." Such "Wolf packs" should be avoided.

Expressway driving is safest when all traffic is moving at close to the same speed. People driving faster or slower than the rest of the traffic create new dangers. A slow-moving vehicle will startle an inattentive motorist using a cruise control. A speeding motorist will also surprise the inattentive as they rapidly pass. For these reasons, speed changes should only be done to help avoid wolf packs, and should be done with only a small change in speeds.

In some states, it is illegal to travel in the left lane of an expressway unless you are in the process of overtaking another vehicle. It can be discourteous to drive in the left lane, even when it's not illegal. The left lane is for those vehicles that are traveling faster than the rest of the traffic. It enables these drivers to safely overtake other vehicles with minimum risk. As we all know, it becomes quite frustrating to have our path blocked by two cars traveling side by side at the same speed. Such frustration often causes the driver attempting to overtake others to follow too closely. This unsafe practice can then lead to the creation of a wolf pack.

Entering an Expressway. Since expressways are built for traffic to flow at a fairly uniform speed, entrance and exit ramps are provided so speed changes can occur out of the normal traffic flow. When entering an expressway, it is important to accelerate up to the speed of the traffic with which you are merging. As the merge area is being approached, the driver should activate the appropriate turn signal and begin watching for a gap in the traffic. Once a suitable gap is observed, the driver can adjust his speed to fit into the gap. When a driver is trying to gain access onto the expressway, if traffic is light to moderate courtesy dictates that motorists move over one lane to allow access. Such a rule is only a courtesy and is not always followed. Technically, the motorists already on the expressway have the right-of-way. It is the responsibility of the driver entering traffic to merge safely. On occasion, this will require the merging driver to slow to almost a stop while looking for an adequate gap in which he can merge. Such a situation should be avoided since a stopped vehicle will require a very long gap in order to merge into the traffic safely. Should you be forced to slow down on an entrance ramp, carefully watch your mirrors. Any motorist behind you will be accelerating to merge with the traffic and may not be looking ahead as he searches for his own traffic gap. This driver is almost certainly going to hit you. To avoid such a rear-end collision, attempt to pump the brake pedal a few times in order to flash your brake lights on and off. Hopefully, this will alert the other driver and allow him time for slowing or stopping.

Exiting an Expressway. A driver should always anticipate his needs well before an exit and be in the proper lane. While most exits are to the right-hand side of the road, there are some that exit off to the left. When traveling in an unfamiliar area, the driver should always look for signs telling which lane he should be in for an exit. Be especially alert for those "exit only" signs. When the driver decides to exit, he should maintain a constant speed and activate the proper turn signal while still on the expressway. Deceleration should not begin until the vehicle is actually on the exit ramp, unless the ramp is unusually short. Safe exit speeds are typically posted at the begin-

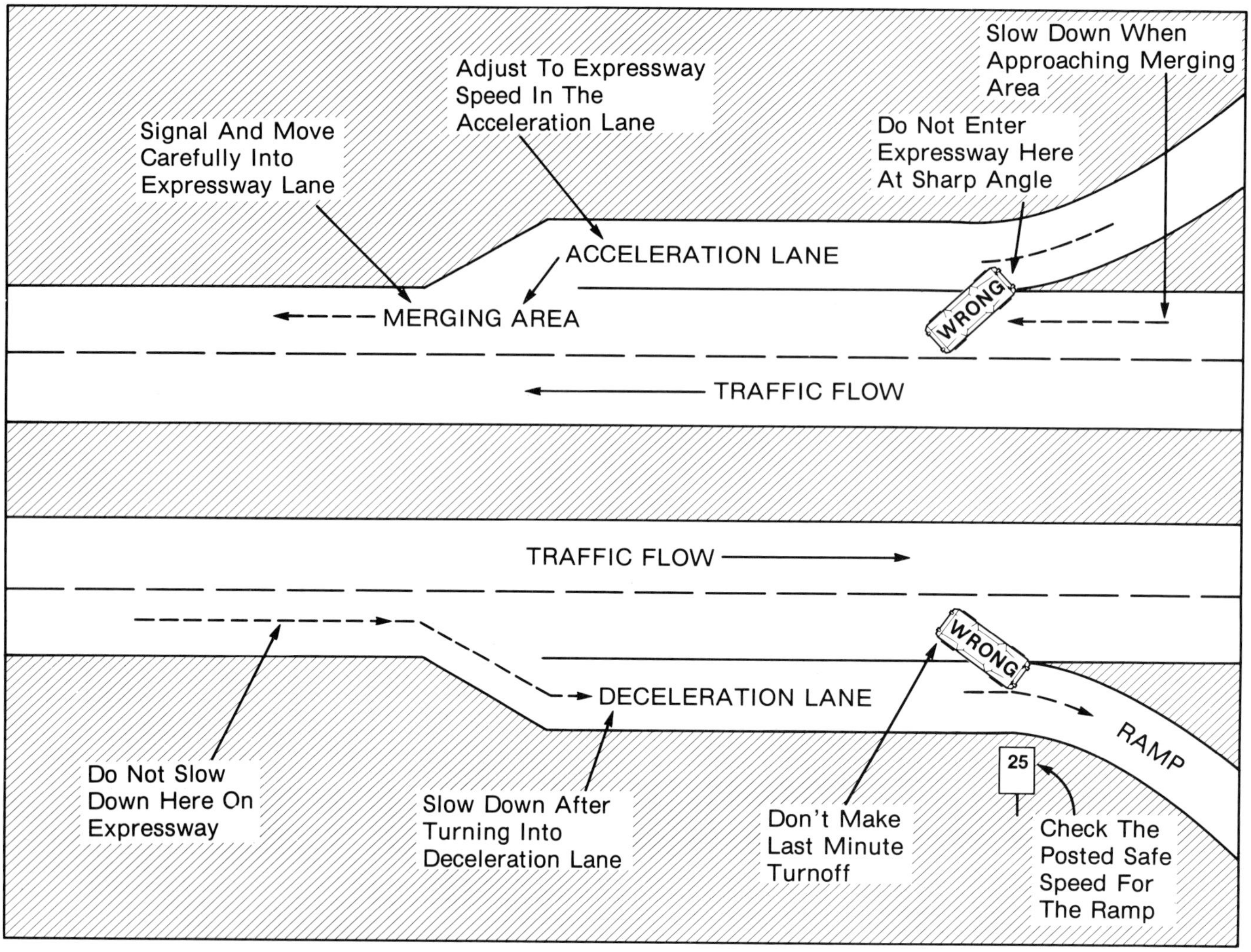

Fig. 5.32 Technique for entering and exiting an expressway.

ning of the ramp. On some exits and cloverleaves, speed may have to be adjusted before reaching the ramp. In those situations, it should be apparent to the driver well before he actually needs to slow down. The exit speeds will be posted before the ramp.

As mentioned earlier, any time a vehicle is changing lanes, or entering or exiting an expressway, it is important to signal your intent well in advance.

Cloverleaf Interchanges. Where two high-traffic-volume roadways meet, quite often there is a special cloverleaf type of intersection. Cloverleaves can present problems since traffic ends up using the same lane for both acceleration and deceleration. In addition to this, the ramp is often very short. A driver entering the expressway has to accelerate rapidly after coming through a tight curve, while the driver leaving the expressway must decelerate rapidly in anticipation of an equally tight curve. Such a situation requires each driver to be extremely alert to what the traffic around him is doing in order to merge safely.

The expressways of America are among the safest roads in the world. In order for them to remain safe, it is important for the drivers who use them to be courteous and alert.

Employing the fundamental concepts of passing, backing, and parking will help the ambulance driver reduce his chances of a collision, both on and off the job. Whether driving an emergency response vehicle or taking the family out for a Sunday drive, utilizing the principles discussed in this chapter should make your driving task much more enjoyable as well as safer.

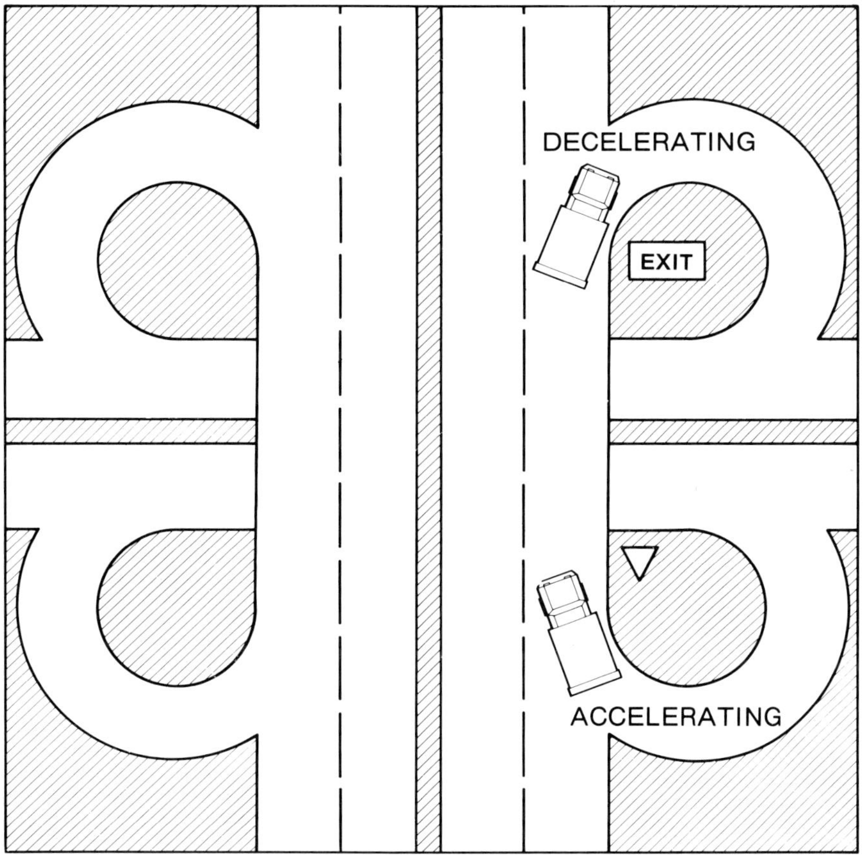

Fig. 5.33 Cloverleafs have special problems: The same lane is used for acceleration and deceleration and the ramp is too short for proper merging.

6 VEHICLE DYNAMICS

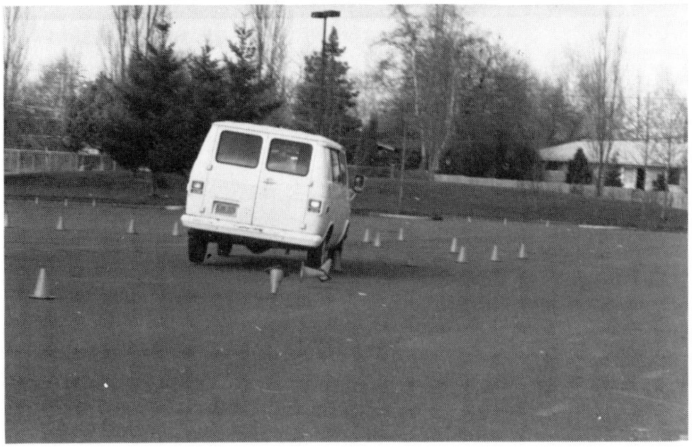

Physics! Many of us have not thought about the principles of physics and the forces that affect us since high school. Oh, we know those forces are there, but we don't really think about them. However, they do have a profound effect on us and our driving. Even small changes in vehicle control can have such an effect because of these forces.

By understanding vehicle dynamics (the study of the relationship of motion between a vehicle and an object, or two or more vehicles, and the forces effecting this motion) you can better predict how the ambulance will handle in a given situation and therefore be better able to control it. By employing physical forces, a vehicle can often be driven to avoid a collision. If the driver does not understand the dynamics that act upon the vehicle's steering and tires, he may not be able to maneuver around an obstacle and may instead end up in a collision. While a driver can routinely accelerate, decelerate, and turn corners without paying attention to those forces, he cannot exert full control without using them.

In this chapter, some of the basic principles of physics will be reviewed as they apply to the operation of a motor vehicle. The information will be presented in a simplified manner to avoid much of the confusion associated with advanced science courses.

Physics and the Vehicle

Inertia, centrifugal force, kinetic energy, the coefficient of friction, and gravity all affect the vehicle and how it handles. These influences can be a big help in controlling a vehicle. They can also hinder it. Therefore, it is important for you to understand just what these forces are and how they interact with the operation of a motor vehicle.

Gravity

Gravity is important to vehicle dynamics. It is this force that pulls us and the vehicle toward earth, resulting in weight or mass. Without weight we would have a difficult time developing traction against the road surface as a counter force to inertia.

Inertia

Inertia can be defined as the resistance of a body to change in its direction or velocity either at rest or in motion. Inertia is affected by the mass (weight) of the object. For our purposes, the object is a vehicle, and the heavier the vehicle the greater the inertial force it exerts against change. Inertia is also affected by the distribution of its mass or weight in a vehicle. But more importantly, inertia is affected by the speed or velocity of the vehicle. The faster a vehicle travels, the more inertia it has to resist change. In fact the speed has so much influence on inertia that resistance to change increases in proportion to the square root of the speed. Inertia is important to understand when driving because it affects the amount of time required to make the transition from straight ahead driving to turning.

Centrifugal Force

In actuality centrifugal force is an inertial force. This force is generated by the motion of the vehicle as it moves toward the center of

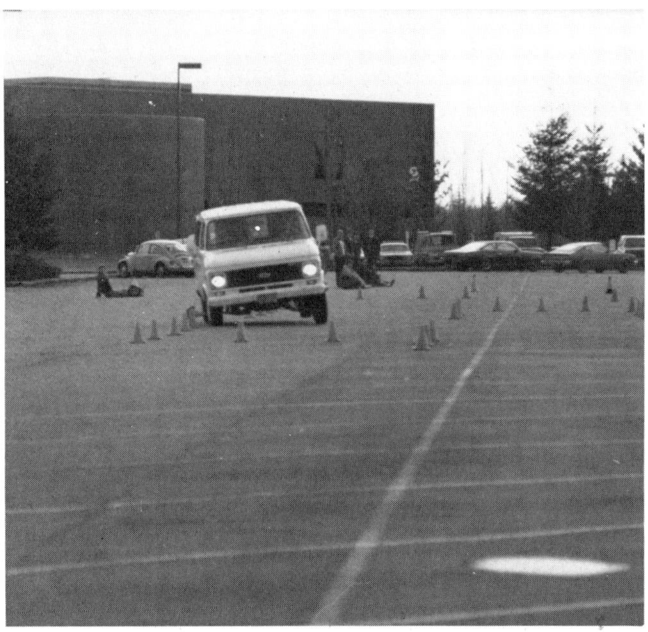

Fig. 6.1 Inertia and centrifugal force have a profound effect on steering.

the circle. The formula for centrifugal force is centrifugal force = mass multiplied by the square of velocity, divided by the radius of the turn $\left(CF = \frac{\text{mass} \times V^2}{\text{radius}}\right)$. It is centrifugal force which pushes a vehicle to the outside of a curve. Once again you can see by the formula how force increases by the square root of the speed. In addition you can see by this formula that tighter radius turns driven at a constant speed create more centrifugal force than do longer radius turns.

Coefficient of Friction

When discussing friction as it relates to control of a moving vehicle, we are usually concerned with the traction a tire can develop on a given surface. Such traction is governed by the coefficient of friction, the maximum force that can be created by a tire on a given road surface condition divided by the weight on the tire. The coefficient of friction then limits the traction available for accelerating, stopping, and cornering. The traction force that goes into the coefficient of friction depends on the tire's construction, its rubber compound and its tread pattern, as well as the road surface and weather conditions. Traction can be applied in three directions.

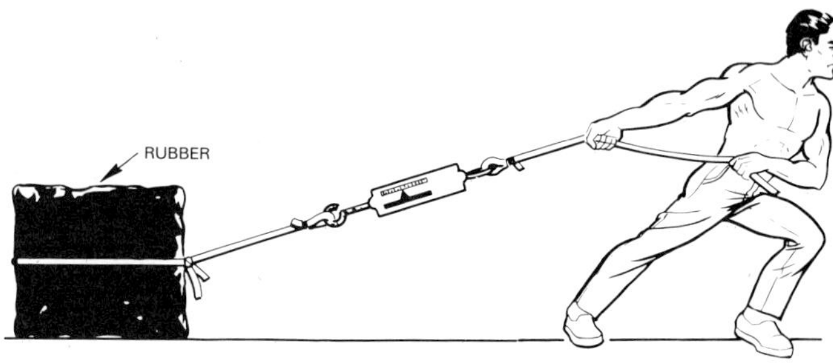

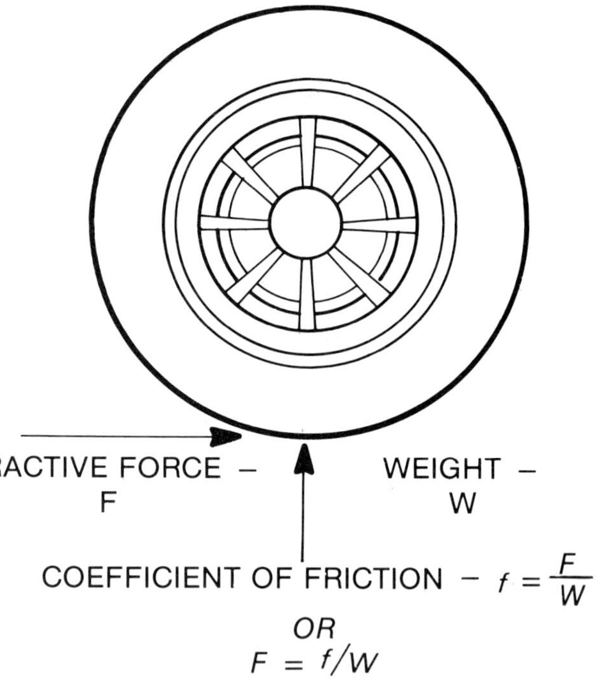

Fig. 6.2 The relationship between tire and road is measured by the term "friction coefficient"—the amount of force needed to move an object is divided by the object's weight.

Driving Traction: The force of the tire pushing against the road to make the vehicle move forward or backward.

Braking Traction: The force of the tires pushing against the road to make the vehicle slow or stop.

Cornering Traction: The side force generated by the tire pushing against the road surface allowing the vehicle to overcome centrifugal force in a turn.

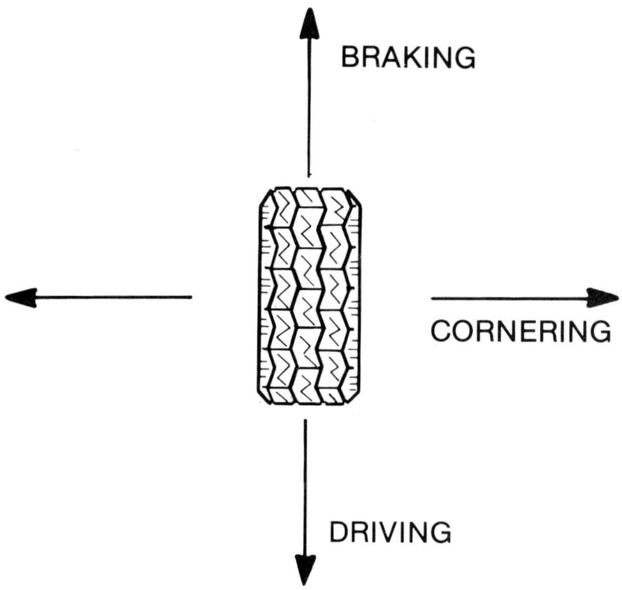

Fig. 6.3 A tire's ability to produce traction is finite and is used during braking, driving, and cornering.

Kinetic Energy

A vehicle has two forms of mechanical energy: potential energy and kinetic energy. Potential energy is the energy the vehicle possesses while stopped simply by its potential to move. Kinetic energy is the energy a vehicle has due to its mass and speed. To find kinetic energy for a vehicle in motion, the formula is kinetic energy = ½ mass (weight) multiplied by velocity (speed) squared ($KE = \frac{1}{2} \text{mass} \times V^2$). This formula tells us a great deal. Since kinetic energy is a force present in a moving vehicle, the vehicle's speed or velocity becomes an extremely important factor. Just as with inertia and centrifugal force, kinetic energy is influenced by the square root of the speed. Therefore, if the speed of the vehicle is doubled, the kinetic energy is increased four times. Even slight changes in speed can affect the kinetic energy of a vehicle. A 10,000 pound ambulance increasing its speed on the highway from 50 to 55 mph will add potentially destructive energy on top of that which was present at 50 mph equal to the energy the vehicle had at 23 mph. To take this further, if the ambulance then increases to an emergency run speed of 70 mph, the additional force added to the 55 mph force is more than the vehicle had at 43 mph. This awesome increase in energy is usually no problem for the driver. However, if the driver needs to suddenly avoid a collision, the vehicle will have to dissipate or redirect that energy quickly. To dissipate the energy it must either stop or collide with the object. Stopping at such a speed will require over 300 feet (including the driver's reaction time). In order for the vehicle to redirect its path, the vehicle must first overcome inertia.

You can easily understand that the combination of inertia and kinetic energy (each increased by the square root of the speed) become significantly more difficult to influence as speed increases.

Principles of Vehicle Control

Driving is simple, right? It only requires you to do three things: steer, accelerate, and decelerate. These acts are so simple some people do them with one hand! In reality, these acts are not simple. Let's examine each of these actions, and how they are affected by the laws of physics.

Steering

Many drivers take steering for granted. To them, steering is an automatic reflex that simply comes because one has experience in driving a car. Many feel that steering consists merely of aiming their eyes in the right direction and then turning the steering wheel right or left, and then the vehicle will follow the input. That's not the case. Steering is the most important driving control function.

Hand Position. Steering a vehicle should begin wheel rather than turn it smoothly, moving the wheel too fast to accurately control the amount of turn. This is especially noticeable when trying to avoid a collision where the wheel may be turned in panic. Using both hands on the wheel will set up a kind of counterforce between the two hands, making it easier to turn the wheel accurately. It is therefore easier to make smooth turns with two hands.

Not only should two hands be used for steering, they should also be properly placed on the wheel. For many years, experts advocated placing the hands at the ten o'clock and two o'clock positions on the steering wheel. More recently it has been determined that the nine o'clock and three o'clock hand positions are actually better for safe driving.

Often during an evasive maneuver, the driver will not have time to change hand positions as he executes the maneuver. For this rea-

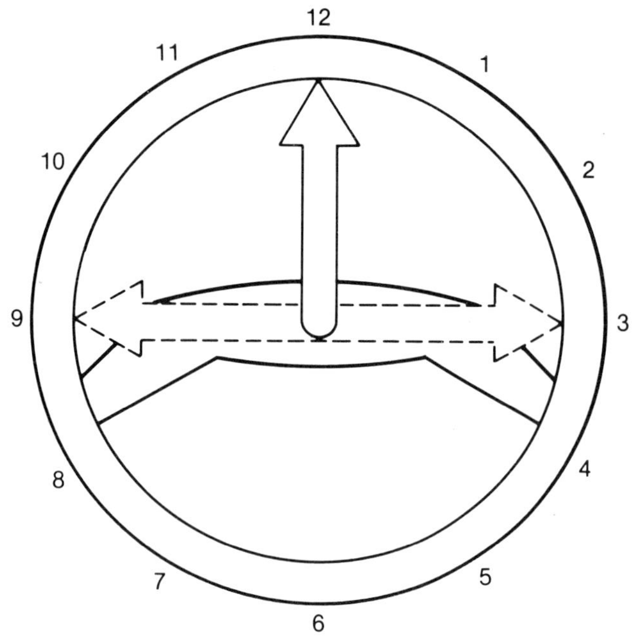

Fig. 6.4 Hands placed at nine and three on the steering wheel help achieve maximum amount of steering before hands have to be moved.

son, the driver must place his hands where they can turn the wheel the maximum amount without having to change hand position. This placement happens to be at nine and three. Additionally, the closer the hands are together the less they counter-balance one another, and so in that same evasive maneuver, steering precision is lost. By placing your hands at nine and three, they are at a maximum distance from one another and thus counter each other very well.

Driving with your hands in such a position may at first be uncomfortable and feel foreign. As you use the position, it will begin to feel natural, particularly since most modern steering wheels are designed with this position in mind. This is not to say that a driver must always hold the wheel only at the nine and three positions. After a while, any hand position becomes fatiguing and reduces efficiency. In areas of low hazard and minimal turning, the driver should vary his hand positions to some degree, but always maintaining two hands on the wheel. The hands should be apart a distance of at least one-third of the circumference of the wheel to maintain balance, with one hand placed above the midline of the steering wheel. In areas where traffic increases or curves and corners become more prevalent, the driver should slide his hands into the nine and three positions. Certainly, any time an EMT is driving in an emergency mode, hazards and risk increase, and so this position should be used. If a skid is encountered which requires more turning than is available from the nine and three position, the hands should be moved hand over hand rather than slid along the steering wheel.

The Dynamics of Steering. By turning the steering wheel we turn the tires on the road and so the vehicle turns the curve. But there's more to it than meets the eye. In order for a vehicle to turn, the tires must create a cornering force to oppose inertia. The tires do this by pushing to the side, across the road surface. This results in a counter force (centripetal force) which opposes centrifugal force and pushes the vehicle toward the center of the circle, or in the case of a curve, along its path. In order to create the required turning force, the tires must be turned to a greater angle than that of the curve being negotiated. The resulting angle of the tire in relation to the road direction is called the "drift" or "slip" angle.

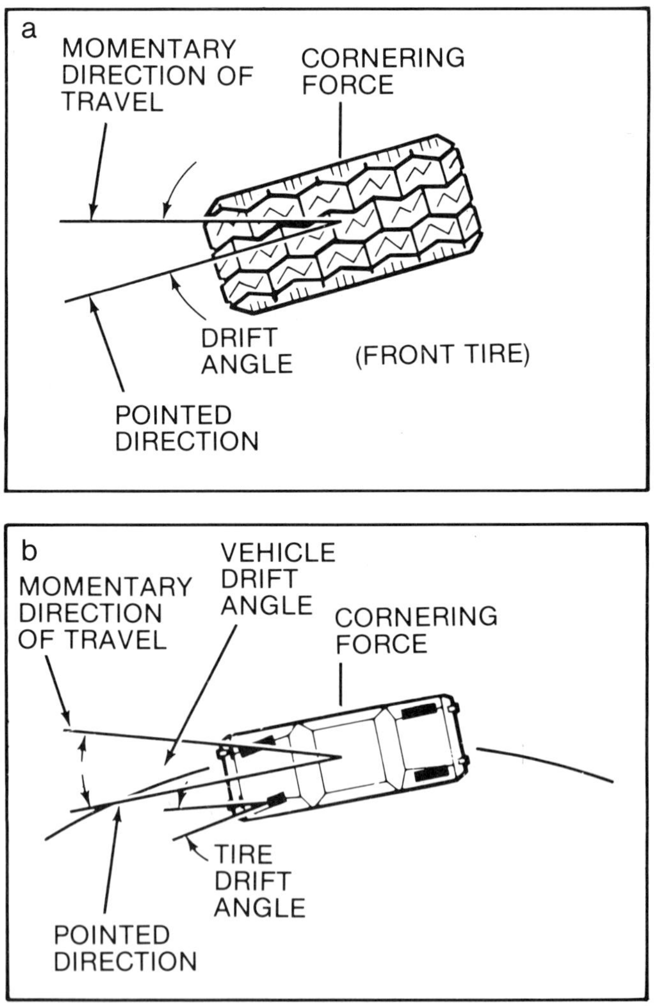

Fig. 6.5a The angle of the tire in relation to the road direction is called tire drift angle.

Fig. 6.5b The angle of the vehicle in relation to the road direction is called vehicle drift angle.

Cornering force must be developed by both the front and rear tires to successfully negotiate a curve. However, the rear tires cannot be steered, and cannot set up a drift angle. Thus, the cornering force is set up by turning the front tires and the whole vehicle, then, offsets slightly from the projected curve to be driven, developing a vehicle drift angle.

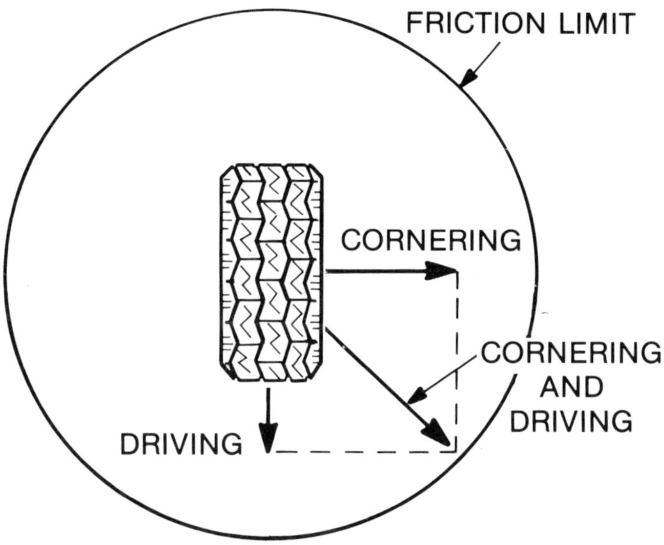

Fig. 6.6 The sum of two driving forces cannot exceed the friction limits (traction) between the tire and the road.

By increasing steering we increase the drift angle and the vehicle naturally follows. This increased drift angle in turn creates more cornering force; up to a point. Once the tires have reached a certain angle in relation to the direction of travel, maximum drift angle is achieved.

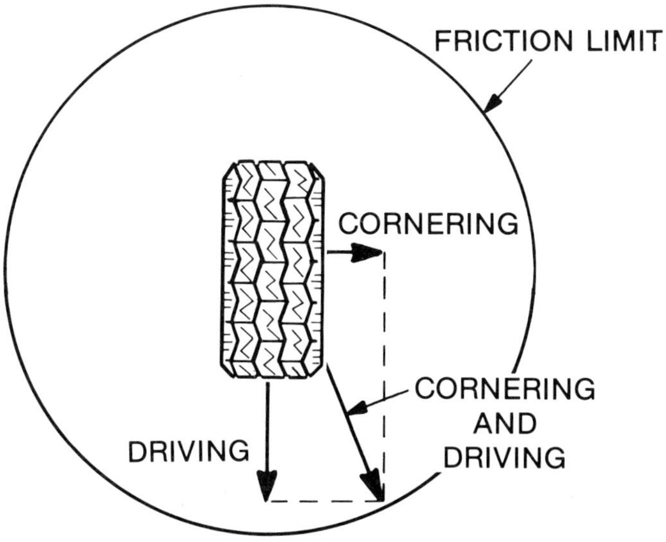

Fig. 6.7 The more driving (acceleration) or braking traction applied to the tire the less cornering traction is available.

To go beyond that most efficient angle, traction is lost rapidly, and can cause the vehicle to go out of control.

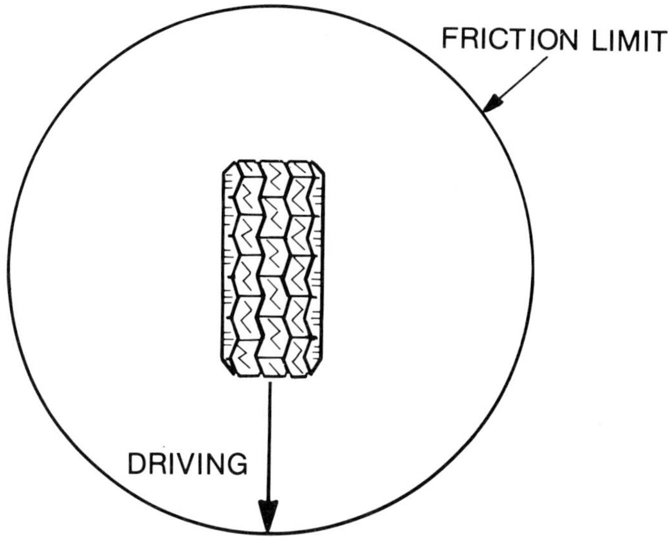

Fig. 6.8 A locked or spinning tire surpasses the tire's traction ability for speed control, thus no traction is available for cornering.

Cornering force is significantly affected by either braking or acceleration. Each of these vehicle controls require traction. However, the coefficient of friction allows only a finite amount of tire traction to prevail. If tire traction is effected by the vehicle trying to slow or accelerate, the amount of traction available for cornering will be reduced. If driving (braking or acceleration) force is applied to an extent that causes the tires to spin or wheels to lock up, traction will be greatly reduced for the desired control input. Furthermore, because all of the available tire traction is being expended by any spinning or skidding tires, absolutely no traction will be available to develop cornering force. Thus, spinning or skidding rear tires greatly reduce a vehicle's ability to turn; spinning or skidding front tires totally prohibit directional control of the vehicle.

The shorter radius a vehicle has to turn from its path the greater the centrifugal force developed for a given weight or speed. Excessive amounts of centrifugal force, combined with either a high coefficient of friction (good traction) or high vehicle center of gravity, the greater the chance that the vehicle will have of rolling over. The high center of gravity is an important factor because a vehicle's body is not directly in contact with the road and will tend to roll, or lean away from the inside of the curve. It is this roll of the body which tends to make the driver of a vehicle uncomfortable and take a corner slower or wider

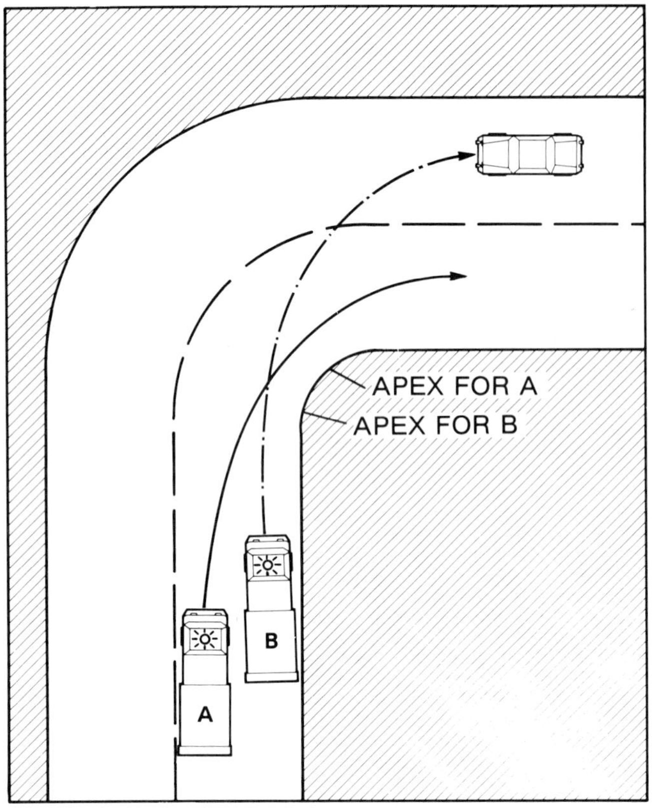

Fig. 6.9 Curve radius can be changed slightly by altering vehicle approach.

than would be the case if roll were not present. This action, when extreme, can make the ambulance feel as though it is going to roll over. In fact, some ambulances are built with higher centers of gravity and are more susceptible to a rollover situation. Usually though, the coefficient of friction (traction) is not high enough to hold the tires once such extreme maneuvering begins and the vehicle only slides, unless it is tripped.

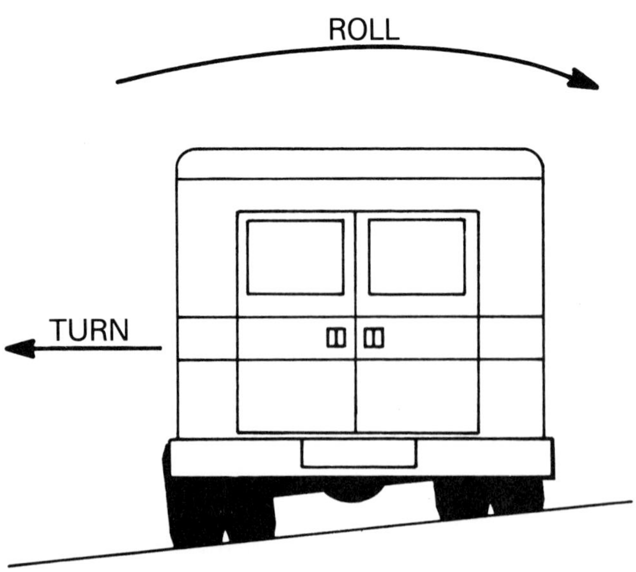

Fig. 6.10 When rounding a curve, centrifugal force pushes a vehicle into a straight line. Vehicle tends to roll or lean away from the axis of the curve.

Tripping results when a vehicle hits a curb or chuckhole, breaks a wheel, or pushes up ground with the tires. These hazards stop the tire's slide while the kinetic energy of the vehicle continues. Tripping can also result when the lateral forces against the tire are too great for the air pressure to hold the tire bead to the rim. The tire fails, allowing the rim to dig into the pavement.

Rollover is more likely to occur, especially for a top heavy ambulance, when steering is input rapidly in one direction and then in the other. As steering is imparted in one direction, let's say to the right, the springs on the right side of the vehicle begin unweighting rapidly. Those on the left begin absorbing this weight shift. This transfer in turn places the vehicle in a lean to the left as it attempts to turn right. Now as the driver turns rapidly back the other direction, weight travels from the left springs all the way back over to the right. As the springs on the left unweight from their compressed attitude, they can actually help throw weight to the right side. Since the weight is then moving to the right in an arc, this exaggerated motion can lead to a rollover or loss of control. The likelihood of such a circumstance depends on the weight of the vehicle, the height of the vehicle's center of gravity, its suspension system, the tires, the road surface, environmental conditions, and the amount and rapidity of the steering input.

When a curve is entered too fast, knowledge of vehicle dynamics can prevent an accident. Fact: centrifugal force increases by the square of the speed, creating significant problems for cornering. At the same time, the fact that the speed is squared means that a vehicle does not have to reduce its speed by half in order to reduce the centrifugal force present by half for a given curve. Additionally, the cornering force developed by the tires creates drag proportional to the drift angle. This drag is very effective at slowing the vehicle without affecting steering control, if the limits of effective drift angle aren't exceeded as the vehicle proceeds through the curve. Simply stated, a corner can often be negotiated more safely if the brakes aren't applied in the curve.

Acceleration

Acceleration is the process of increasing speed and is stated as a rate of changing speed per unit of time. In order to accelerate the vehicle must work to overcome the effects of inertia. Simplified, Newton's second law of motion states that the greater the force acting upon a vehicle the faster the speed of the vehicle will increase. It also states that the less a mass weighs the faster a given force can change that speed. Acceleration by itself is not a problem. However, if acceleration takes place during cornering, traction becomes more limited.

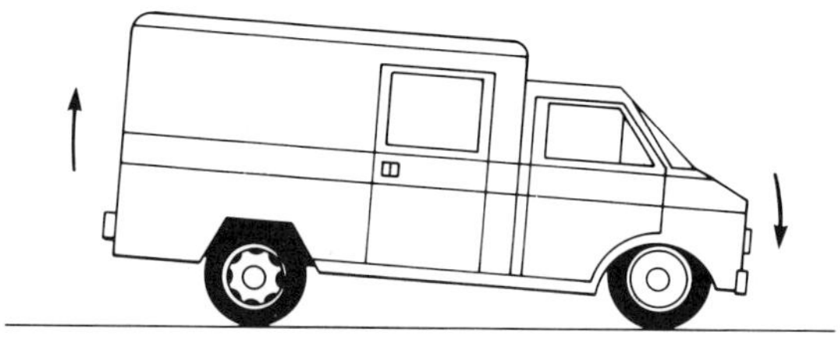

Fig. 6.11 Pitch is produced during deceleration and acceleration.

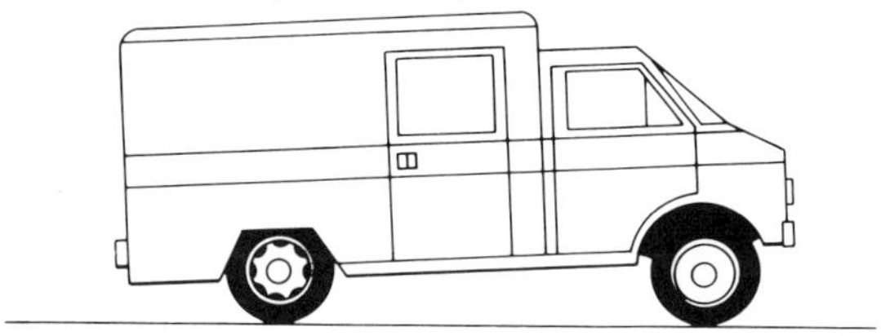

Fig. 6.12 Inertia affects acceleration—it causes vehicle to pitch to the rear as it accelerates, and weight is transferred to the rear.

Deceleration

Deceleration is simply any slowing a vehicle might undergo. Deceleration can be caused by any driver action from slightly reducing pressure on the accelerator to applying hard pressure to the brake pedal. The rule of inertia simply states that a vehicle in motion will tend to stay in motion unless acted upon by an outside force. Therefore, in order to slow a moving vehicle, a counter force must be developed. By reducing pressure on the accelerator, a counter force is developed from the friction of the atmosphere as well as the friction of the engine, drive train, and the tires. All these factors help to slow a vehicle. However, reducing accelerator pressure alone only works as a partial solution to stopping and only when there is time to coast to a stop. Otherwise, you must exert a counter force (friction) through the braking system in order to stop. And this friction develops a tremendous amount of heat at the brakes.

Because of the potential for excessive heat buildup, the brakes should be used judiciously. As was pointed out in chapter 5, "Fundamentals of Driving," whenever possible, you should drive according to traffic flow, looking ahead at all times to allow time for your vehicle to slow without using the brakes.

It can be argued that a driver using his left foot can apply the brake a fraction of a second faster since he doesn't have to first lift his foot off the accelerator. However, a driver using the left foot may have a tendency to rest his left foot lightly on the brake pedal. Such an action can cause excessive wear on the brakes, and may also cause the brakes to heat prematurely so they will not be adequate when really needed. In addition, if the driver rides the brake pedal, the brake lights will be on constantly. Such a false clue does not give the driver following a fair warning as to when braking is really taking place.

The left-foot braker may also have a tendency to apply the brake before his right foot is totally off the accelerator. This act will, in turn, exaggerate the pitching present when a vehicle decelerates.

Brake Construction

Today the braking system for most passenger cars, vans, and light trucks is a hydraulically operated combination of two different systems: drum and disc.

Drum Brakes. Drum brakes consist of an almost totally enclosed drum that has pressure exerted against its inside walls by two shoes.

Disc Brakes. Discs are more efficient than drums. In this system a disc, exposed to the air, rotates between two calipers that are squeezed against the disc when activated.

Most newer vehicles are equipped with the more efficient disc brakes in front and drum brakes in the rear. The brake system is designed

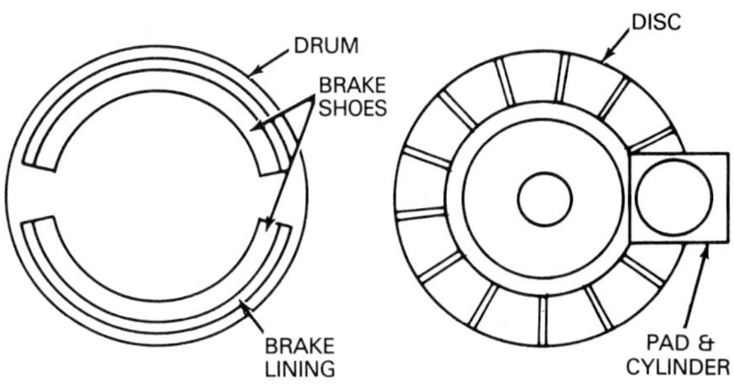

Fig. 6.13 Note the mechanical differences between drum and disc brakes.

this way in order to keep the rear brakes from locking up before the front brakes, which could cause the vehicle to spin.

Brake Fade

Brake fade occurs when the brakes become so hot that they lose their efficiency. When hard braking takes place, heat builds up rapidly. As the heat reaches approximately 700° F., the lining on the brake shoes begins to melt. As it melts, it turns to liquid, lubricating the potential space between the shoes and the drum. Such an occurrence will cause the brake drum to glaze. This extreme heat can also cause the drum itself to expand. When this happens, the brake shoes must travel further to reach the walls of the drum. The presence of these two conditions requires an increased amount of pressure to be exerted against the pedal in order for the vehicle to be slowed or stopped.

Drum brakes, having a high percentage of surface area in contact with the shoes, cause heat to build at a tremendous rate which increases the likelihood of brake fade or failure. Disc brakes, on the other hand, do not fail easily. As they become hot, the disc actually expands and braking improves somewhat. However, disc brakes with more than 50 percent of their friction pads worn away have a 300 percent higher chance of failure than a new brake pad.

Braking Efficiency

Ask a driver what is the most efficient method of braking and you might receive any one of a number of answers. Some drivers think that they can get maximum braking by jumping on the brakes for all they're worth and allowing the vehicle to skid to a stop. As you have learned earlier, a tire can exert the most force against the road surface by continuing to rotate or by constantly putting down a new segment of rubber. Allowing the wheels to lock up and the tires to skid reduces traction. At this point, directional control of the vehicle will be sacrificed since a cornering force cannot be generated. The driver will not be able to steer and the vehicle may slide into any object in its path.

Some drivers feel they can stop faster by pumping the brakes. Often this technique is used when the road surface is slick. By using this technique a driver might actually be inviting trouble. Intent on the pumping action, the driver may not be able to sense when the brakes are locking up, thus actually becoming more likely to skid the tires. When this occurs the driver spends alternating moments of braking inefficiently by skidding and then moments of coasting toward the obstacle he is trying to avoid. Such practice can increase stopping distances significantly.

Wheel lockup is also more likely when pumping the brakes, especially disc brakes, on slick roads because the brake does not release immediately when the pedal is released. By immediately pumping the brake pedal back down the driver can actually induce brake lockup.

Many motorists pump the brake with the idea that they can keep the brakes cooled down and therefore keep efficiency high. Brake heat is produced at such a tremendous rate that the heat dissipated in that second the brake is released is so insignificant as to be nonexistent. This is especially true of drum brakes since the drum has very little exposure to air which helps to convect the heat away.

The best way to stop a vehicle is to squeeze the brake pedal to the point just before wheel lockup occurs, so as much braking force as possible is exerted but not so much that a skid is induced. This can be a difficult skill to master. Faced with a panic situation the inclination for many drivers is to hit the brake hard and fast. Using this approach, the panicked driver may suddenly find himself locking up the brakes and skidding. This is especially true since brake lockup can occur simply because braking conditions change from moment to moment. Weight transfer of the vehicle, composition and surface temperature of the road, or any foreign matter such as water or gravel can change braking conditions. By squeezing the brake pedal, the driver can feel when lockup is about to occur. However, the driver must also be able to quickly recognize skidding when it occurs. He must then back off the brakes until tire traction is regained and then squeeze down again. Backing off the brakes in a conflict situation can be very difficult. Instinct says to stay on the brakes but the pedal *must* be released enough to allow the tires to regain traction.

Braking on Hills and Curves. Brake fade or failure rarely occurs under short-term braking conditions, such as are experienced when trying to rapidly stop the vehicle to avoid a collision. This statement is, of course, only valid as long as the driver has used his brakes judiciously prior to the incident. Brake fade or failure might develop when the brakes are continuously applied while coming down a hill. For this reason, many long hills have emergency escape ramps for trucks.

Because trucks have more momentum (due to mass), more braking energy is required to control their speed on a long hill. More energy increases brake heat so the driver may soon find himself in a condition of brake fade, with loss of braking control on the hill.

Again, many drivers advocate the method of pumping the brakes to avoid such a situation. As stated earlier, the time spent coasting will not sufficiently cool the brakes. Additionally, the vehicle's speed will increase, thus more force will be required to bring the speed back down again. When descending a hill, it requires less braking force to hold a vehicle at a given speed than it does to slow the vehicle from a higher speed to a lower speed. Therefore, constant pressure on the brake pedal is more efficent when descending a hill.

Start your descent with cool brakes and place the transmission in a lower gear. A lower gear will allow the engine compression to assist in the slowing of the vehicle. Even shifting an automatic transmission down one gear can help keep your speed under control. However, if this is done once speed has built up and if the road surface is slick, it can result in a skid. When braking is needed, apply a constant pressure on the pedal. Not allowing the vehicle to accelerate beyond the desired speed will reduce the possibility of brake fade or failure.

Brake fade can also develop when the brakes are applied intermittently but hard, as might happen when driving through numerous curves. In such a situation the driver uses the brakes to slow for a curve, then accelerates out of the curve, and then must brake again to slow for the next curve. Such action may cause heat to build up over a period of time and eventually, the brakes begin to fade. A wise driver will recognize that such a condition can occur and will adjust his speed so less braking is required for each curve.

Tires

Tires play an extremely important role in how the vehicle handles. After all, control of the vehicle is exerted through the tires and their contact with the road surface. In order to better understand how the tires exert their control, we first need to examine their construction.

Tire Construction

Tires are constructed differently for each driving application by each manufacturer. In general though, when looking at a cross section of a tire each will have certain common components.

Casing. The casing of the tire is made up of layers of rubber coated cords called plies that are bonded together and run from bead to bead. A protective cover called the side wall runs from the bead to the tread. Often the inside of the tire will have a rubber liner bonded to it called an inner liner. This inner liner takes the place of a tube in tubeless tires, retaining the air pressure inside the tire. The manner in which the casing is constructed can have significant effect on the tire's performance. Basically there are three types of construction.

Conventional Bias Construction. This uses two, four, or more plies laid on top of each other in an alternating bias or diagonally from bead to bead. Bias ply construction provides a very stiff tire side wall.

Belted-Bias Construction. Tires constructed in this manner will have cord bodies laid in the same fashion as a bias ply tire. In addition they will have two or more belts laid, one on top of the other, circling the tire.

Radial Play Construction. Radial construction utilizes one or more plies of cord running perpendicular to the bead from side to side. This type of construction requires two or more stabilizing belts to be placed between the plies and the tread.

Belts. Strong layers of inextensible cord or steel often circle a tire just under the tread. These are known as stabilizer belts. They actually restrict the pliability of the casing, stabilizing the tread and making it resistant to compression.

Tread. This is the portion of the tire that comes in contact with the road surface. The rubber used in making the tread is compounded from various materials to provide optimum traction and wear for the specific purpose of the tire. The tread is made up of ribs; the raised portion that actually comes in contact with the road surface; grooves, the cut away area between the ribs; and in many cases sipes, tiny slots cut into the ribs.

Tire Performance

The tire exerts its force through its contact with the road. The more rubber in contact with the road the better traction the tire will have. With this in mind, you might question the need for tread since it actually reduces the amount of rubber on the road surface. In fact, many racing tires have minimal or no tread. A "slick" tire used

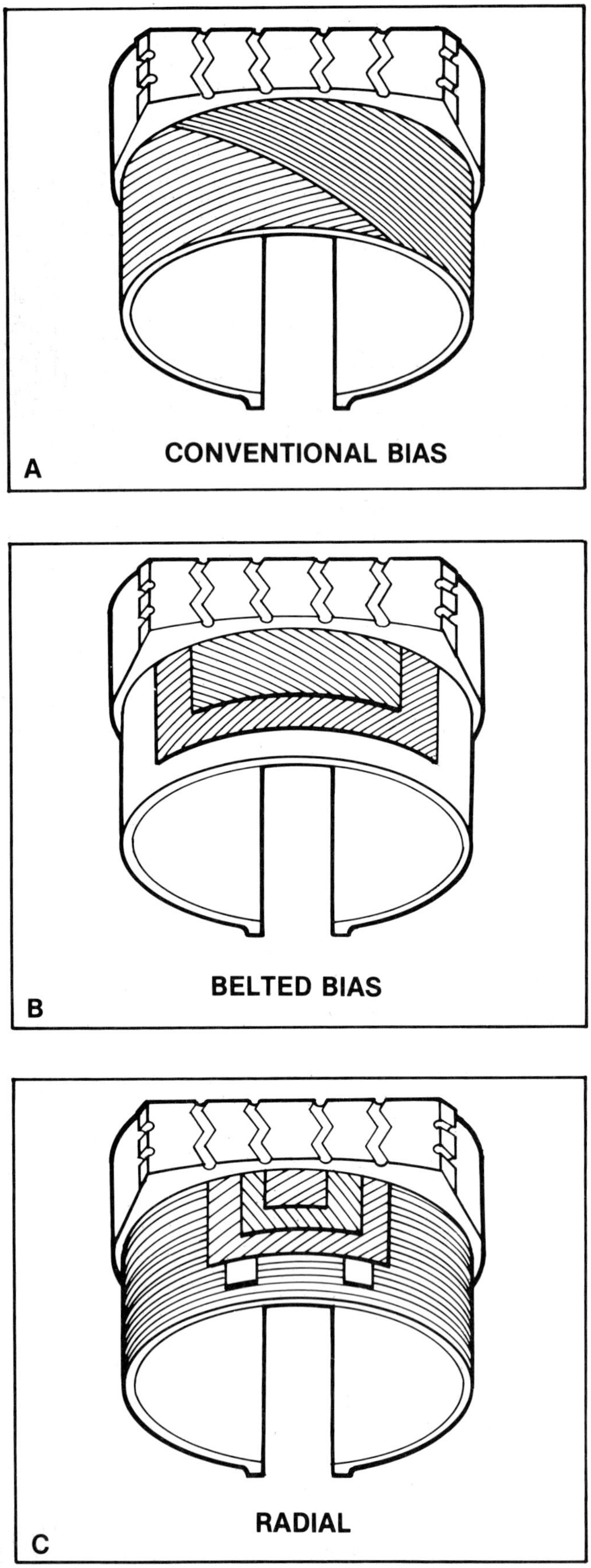

Fig. 6.14 The three types of tire construction illustrating the plies, stabilizing belts, and tread.

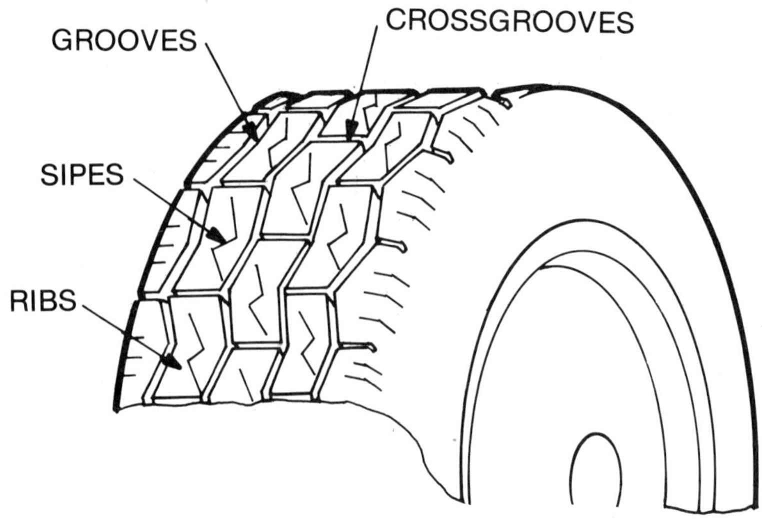

Fig. 6.15 Tread is made up of ribs, grooves, and sipes.

for drag racing has no tread, so the full surface of the tire will meet the road. Tires designed for circle track racing have little more than many sipes for a tread so that the maximum possible amount of rubber meets the race track while the sipes provide many edges for the tire to grip with.

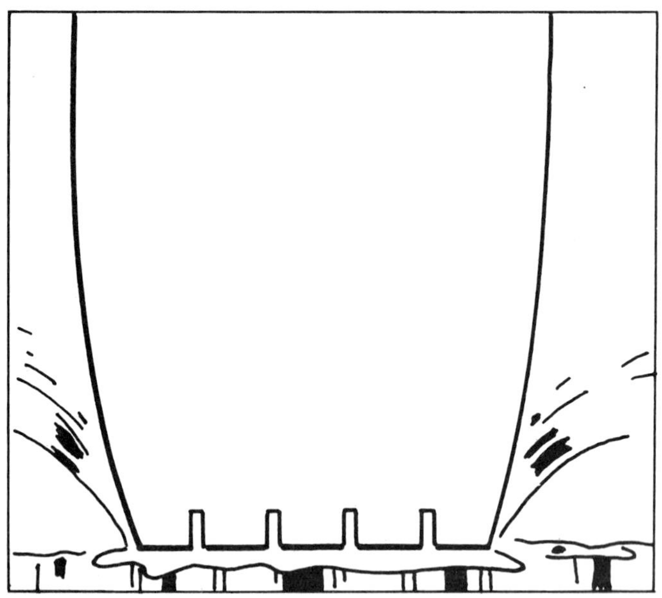

Fig. 6.16 The main purpose of tread on highway tires is to dissipate water; tires with good tread will not hydroplane easily.

Tires designed for the highway have a tread to give cornering ability and traction when encountering rain, snow, dirt, and other surface variables. The main purpose for the tread pattern is to remove foreign matter such as water from under the ribs. Example: As a tire rolls over a wet street, water is trapped between the road and the tire. Water resists this trap by spraying out in front of the tire, thus building up a wedge of water. As vehicle speed increases, the water may not be adequately displaced, and the tire rides up on to the wedge of water. This condition is called hydroplaning. When it occurs, the driver will experience reduced or total loss of steering. That is where the tread comes into function. The ribs can effectively cut through the water to get down to the pavement. The grooves of the tire can channel the water out from under the tire to the rear. The sipes further channel the water from under the ribs toward the grooves. The greater the tread depth the less likely the vehicle is to hydroplane. Generally speaking, as long as tread depth is greater than water depth a vehicle will not hydroplane *except* at higher speeds.

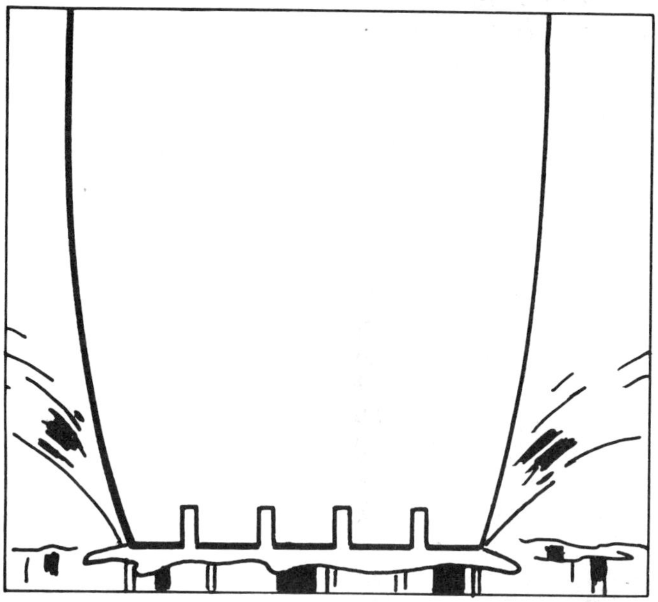

Fig. 6.17 As tires roll over wet streets, water trapped between the road and tire sprays out to the sides and front of the tire, creating a wave.

When mounted on the vehicle a tire is not perfectly round since it must absorb the weight of the vehicle. For conventional bias ply tires this weight is absorbed at the "contact patch," that area where the tread actually comes in contact with the road. As the tire rolls, the contact patch is pushed upward toward the center of the wheel. This action pulls the ribs toward the center of the tread causing them to slide laterally over the road surface a slight amount. As the tire continues to rotate and the section is freed from the pressure, it expands out beyond its normal width slightly before resuming its normal shape. This lateral movement of the tread is called "squirm." Squirm is the cause of much of the wear a bias ply tire receives and creates tire heat. Squirm also reduces the traction of the tire since the tire is constantly skidding a tiny bit. In addition squirm

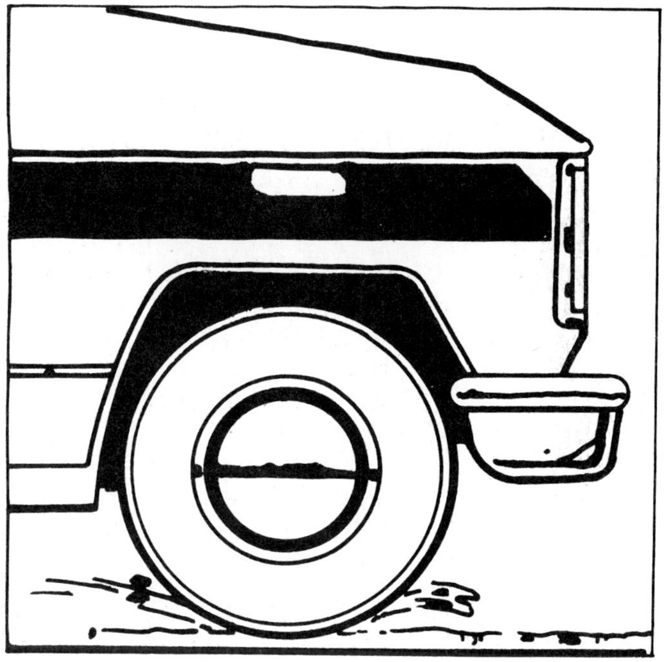

Fig. 6.18 As vehicle speed increases, water cannot be dissipated adequately and tire begins to "surf."

narrows the tread grooves at the contact patch reducing its ability to dissipate water. Belted-bias tires also exhibit squirm but not in as great an amount as a conventional bias ply tire since the belts help stabilize the tread and resist compression.

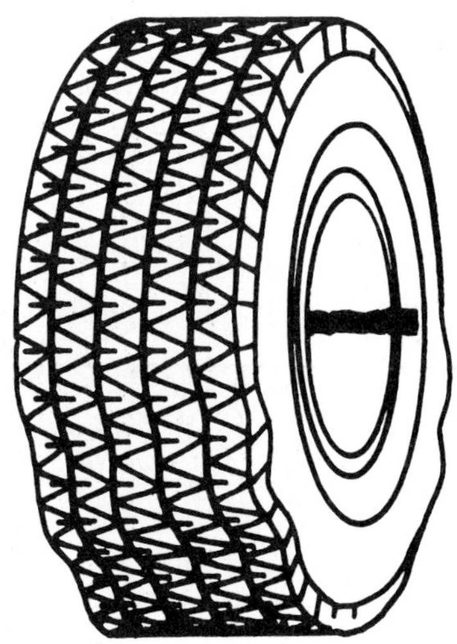

Fig. 6.19 Vehicle weight tends to deflect or flatten the area in contact with the ground and thus the area immediately in front of and behind this area. Increasing speeds cause tires to ripple in these areas.

A radial ply tire has a more pliable sidewall which flexes more easily and has the benefit of the belts to stabilize the tread. Because of these characteristics, radial ply tires exhibit little or no squirm. Thus traction is increased. A radial ply

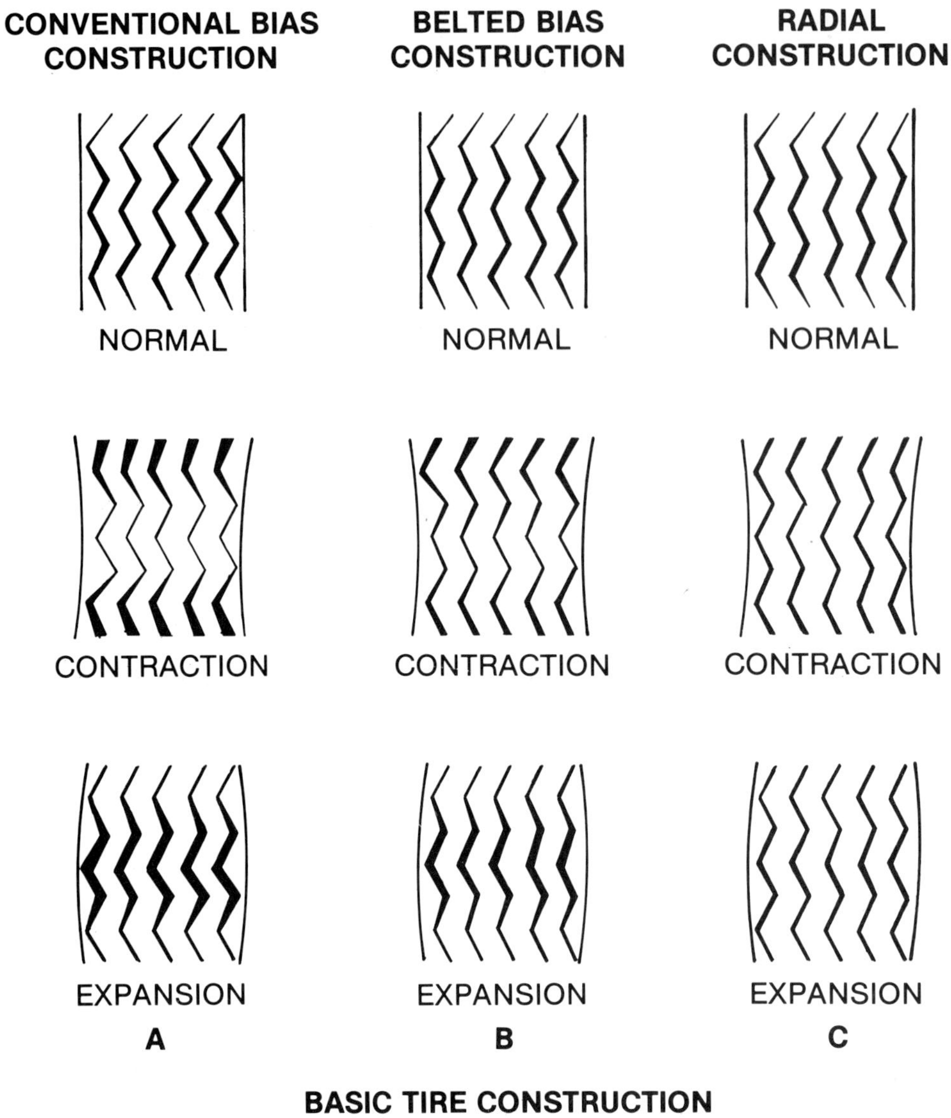

Fig. 6.20a With conventional bias construction the contact patch of the tire is pushed upward, pulling the ribs together, and then, as the tire rolls, causing the ribs to expand out.

Fig. 6.20b With belted bias construction the belts reduce the amount of squirm at the contact patch.

Fig. 6.20c With radial construction squirm is almost nonexistent when the tire rolls.

tire will develop cornering force much quicker than a conventional tire and at a lower drift angle since the tire is not skidding at the contact patch. That means the tire will stay locked into a corner much as if on a rail until the limits of traction are reached. Since a radial ply tire has little or no squirm, tire life generally increases. Fuel mileage also improves since the tread does not deform as much, thus producing less rolling resistance. Radial tires also run much cooler and thus are safer at higher speeds for longer periods of time than bias ply tires.

Tires used on ambulances are usually designed for load carrying capability. They are not designed for high speed driving. High speeds increase squirm which will build heat in the tire through the constant flexing of the tire material. With excessive heat a tire is more likely to fail. This is because tires are constructed under a heat process and will come apart when exposed to the same extreme heat used in their manufacture. For this reason, ambulances should not be driven for long periods at speeds higher than 70 mph.

Tire Inflation

Proper tire inflation is critical to vehicle performance. A tire that is under-inflated will produce more squirm. In a corner the under-inflated tire will tend to roll under the vehicle as it reacts to centrifugal force and the tire creates its centripetal force. These properties combine to in-

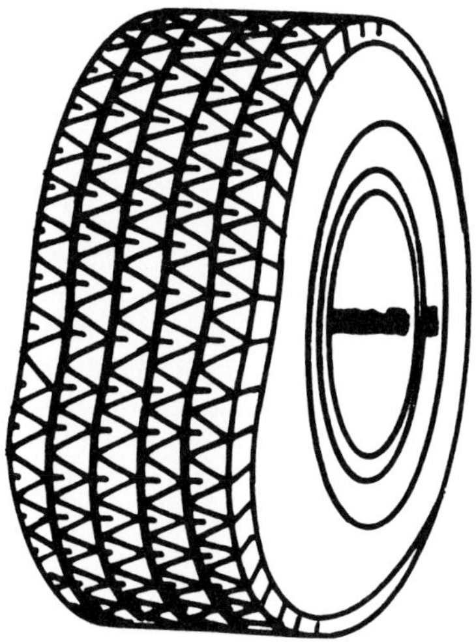

Fig. 6.21 High speeds also increase the potential for tire failure—high speed turns generate excessive lateral pressure on tire.

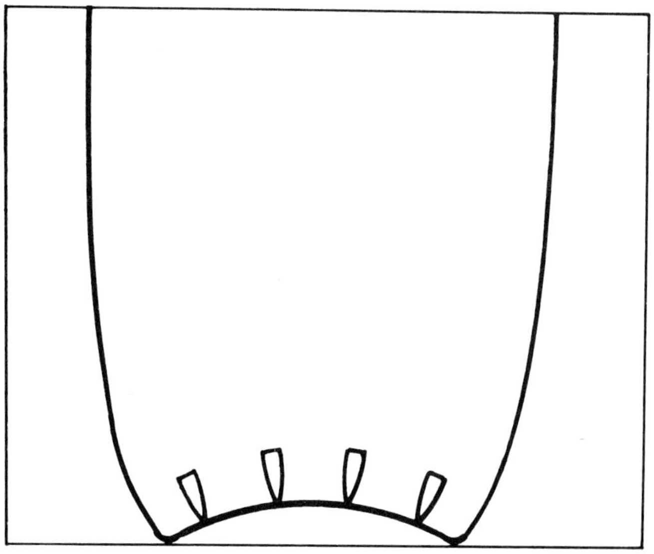

Fig. 6.22 Underinflated tires tend to cup in the middle, closing off tread pattern and causing hydroplaning.

crease the steering angle required to negotiate the curve. As a result, this combination lowers the speed at which the curve can be safely taken. Low pressure and tight cornering can also cause the tire bead to pull away from the rim. If this happens with a tubeless tire, it can fail instantly. The increased squirm caused by underinflation of tires will cause a tire to wear much faster. The reduction in pressure will cause the tire to cup in the middle of the tread, creating even more wear at the tread edges. This also closes off the tread grooves making the tire more likely to hydroplane.

Heavy loads over the rear axle can cause the vehicle to handle radically. Increasing the air pressure in the rear tires when carrying a heavy load will help stabilize driving. However, tire pressure should never exceed the amount recommended by the manufacturer.

To increase vehicle performance and reduce tire wear, you should keep your tires inflated to the higher end of the recommended pressure limits provided on the tire sidewall and in the vehicle owner's manual. Tire pressure should be checked when the tires are cold and only with a reliable gauge.

Tires for Inclement Weather

A tire works on wet pavement by channeling the water out from under it so the ribs can gain traction against the road surface. This principle is also true on ice as the water layer often found on ice (warmed by passing tires) is penetrated. However, traction on snow has little to do with friction between the tire and the surface. Instead, the tire gains traction by building soft snow up into firm ridges and then pushing against them.

The two most important abilities needed for a tire to perform well on snow are that it is able to penetrate into the snow and that the tire has many edges that can build, and push against, snow ridges. In order to penetrate the snow the tire needs to have deep tread. It must also have a profile generally narrower than a highway tire to allow it to sink into deep snow rather than float on top. The tread ribs should also be far enough apart to allow the tread to clean itself as it rotates, throwing out the snow. Otherwise the snow will accumulate in the grooves and won't allow the tire to penetrate the snow in its path.

Standard snow tires are narrow and have large voids between the ribs. However, these types of tires are most efficient only in deep new snow. On the other hand, the snow we encounter most of the time is compacted or deep slush. Under these conditions, the standard snow tire will not be able to build the many edges needed for pushing.

Probably the best tire for any inclement weather other than virgin snow over four inches deep is an all season radial tire which is offered by most tire manufacturers. An "all season" tire offers many zig-zag edges for pushing that are still far enough apart for self cleaning and also have the ability to move water from under the ribs because the individual ribs are narrower than on a standard snow tire and usually have sipes cut into them. All season radial tires also work well on ice because they cut through the water film. In addition they retain their elasticity better than snow tires because of their special rubber compounding. For highway driving they offer almost as much rubber to the road surface as a conventional highway tire.

Tire Mixing

It is not unusual for vehicles to have tires of different construction mounted at the front and rear. However, this practice is discouraged, especially on an ambulance. Because bias ply tires and radial ply tires perform so differently, combining them on the vehicle can dramatically alter the handling characteristics of the vehicle. To be sure, tires of different cord construction should never be mounted on the same axle.

Just as tires of the same cord/ply construction should be used on all four corners so should those tires all be designed for the same purpose, preferably of the same make and model. It is not unusual to see an ambulance with snow tires on the rear drive wheels and conventional highway tires on the front. This practice apparently is to provide as much traction as possible to the drive wheels. However, the mix of tires can cause a significant change in the vehicle's handling characteristics, either on dry or wet pavement or snow and ice. If moving the vehicle requires help from special tires so does steering and stopping it.

Skidding

Skidding is usually the result of attempting to change the speed or direction of the vehicle too abruptly for road surface and tire conditions. Such situations can be extremely frightening for the driver of the vehicle as he experiences sudden loss of vehicle control. It does not matter whether a vehicle is front or rear wheel drive. Each type of vehicle will react in the same manner. However, the front wheel drive vehicles may respond a little quicker to steering input due to a tighter steering gear ratio, or suspension system, which is more responsive than some rear wheel drive vehicles. In either case, it is important when skidding occurs to bring the vehicle back under control as quickly as possible. By understanding what causes a skid you can understand what needs to be done to correct it.

There are six types of skids that can affect an ambulance:

Front Wheel Skid. Front wheel skids occur when the front wheels are locked up and quit turning. It can be caused by poor brake maintenance or because the road surface has a lower coefficient of traction because of water, snow, or ice. Any time the front wheels are locked they will slide. As has been stated earlier, controlling the vehicle's direction in a skid becomes impossible since a cornering force cannot be set up by the tires. Thus, the vehicle will continue in a straight line as a result of inertia.

To correct a front wheel skid it is important to reduce the brake pressure. By doing so steering can be regained as the tires begin rolling again. Generally, the steering wheel should be in a center steer position to help regain control from a front wheel skid.

Rear Wheel Skid. The rear brakes can lock for the same reason that the front brakes lock. When this happens the rear tires lose traction and therefore cornering force. A rear wheel skid can be avoided by controlled braking. Also, it is important for the driver to recognize that inclement weather can reduce the coefficient of friction and cause a rear wheel skid. This is often encountered when a driver downshifts on slick pavement, adding a brake-like force to the drive wheels. Occasionally when rear wheel skid occurs, the rear of the vehicle will attempt to overtake the front. When this occurs, the skid should be handled in the same manner as a spinout skid.

All Wheel Skid. The all wheel skid is one of the most common types of skid. Once again it is caused by overbraking. In this case, all wheels lose traction and begin to slide. All wheel skid is corrected in the same way as the front or rear wheel skid. Get off the brakes quickly and steer in the direction of your intended path.

Power Skid. Skids are not only caused by overbraking. Applying more power to the drive wheels than can be utilized by the vehicle will cause the rear wheels to begin spinning. This type of skid is not as common for ambulances as for passenger vehicles since so much power is required to move heavier vehicles. However, it is more likely to occur for all vehicles in inclement weather. To correct a power skid the driver needs to ease off the accelerator until the tires regain traction and then begin applying throttle again at a lesser pressure.

Spinout Skid. A spinout occurs when negotiating a curve. In a spinout skid, the rear tires do not develop the cornering force needed, thus the rear of the vehicle begins to skid as a result of physical forces and inadequate traction. This type of skid is often the most frightening for the driver as the vehicle starts to move laterally. Recovery from such a skid is dependant on the driver regaining steering control. Drivers are often taught to turn in the direction of the skid. As they perceive the rear of the vehicle to be moving in one direction and the front to be moving in the opposite direction, they can become confused as to which direction the skid is actually going. The object is to keep the front tires pointed in the direction the driver wants the front of the vehicle to travel. By looking at the situation in this manner, the driver can more easily understand which direction to turn and how much.

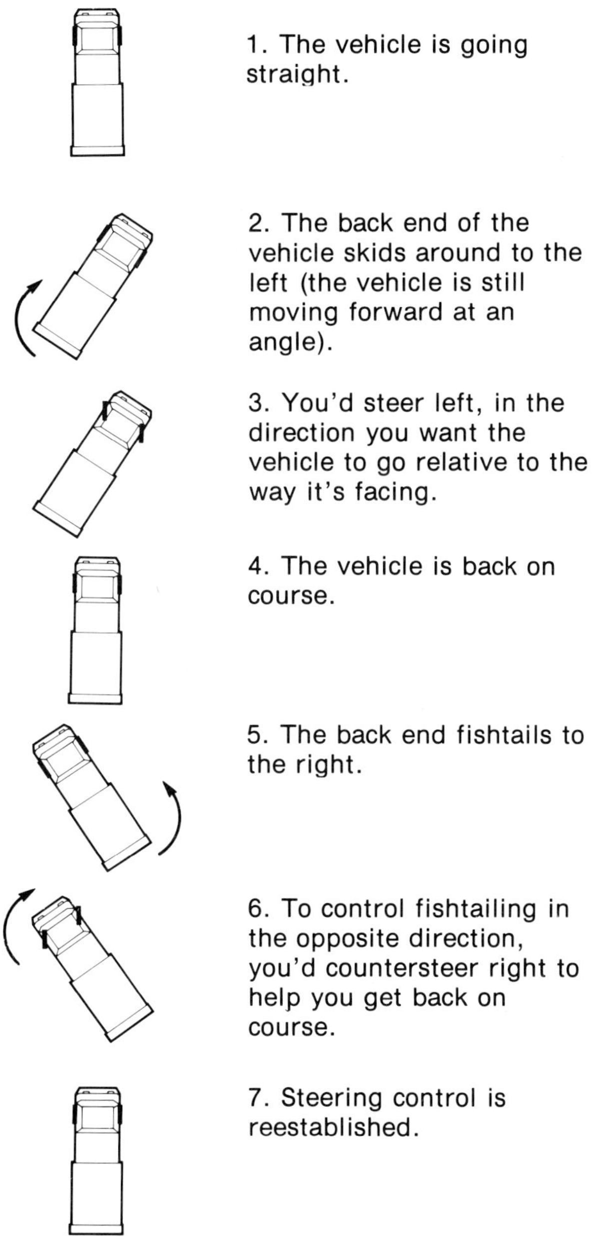

Fig. 6.23 Steering in a skid is intended to keep front wheels pointed in the direction you want to travel.

The driver also needs to be aware that as he corrects for the skid, the rear of the vehicle may actually swing beyond the desired direction or path, skidding in the opposite direction. This action, which is called fishtailing, is often the result of applying too much steering input. The driver must be prepared for such a situation and continue to attempt to keep the front wheels lined up with the direction which you desire the vehicle to travel.

Sometimes the rapid steering required to regain control from a skid can cause the driver to lose awareness of where the wheels are pointed in relation to the road. It helps if the driver knows how many revolutions of the wheel are required to turn the wheel from its center position to maximum steering input in each direction. Armed with this knowledge and by actually counting the revolutions of the wheel as they are put in and taken out, the driver is better able to remain aware of his capability to affect the situation. Also, the driver will improve his tendency to apply the proper amount of steering in the proper direction if he continues to look in the direction of intended travel. Even if the vehicle is in danger of hitting the guardrail, the driver can best regain control by *continuing to look down the road.*

It is not uncommon in spinouts for the driver to immediately hit the brakes. Such an impulse should be avoided. Since traction is already reduced significantly for the rear wheels, use of the brakes will only serve to exacerbate the situation. By braking, the rear wheels will readily lock and the tires will skid until the brakes are released or the vehicle stops.

Hydroplaning. When discussing tires we discussed what causes hydroplaning. Water buildup under the front tires reduces traction, and so cornering force is reduced to the front tires. To compound the situation, the front tires may have removed enough water from the tracks to allow the rear tires to maintain driving traction so the vehicle is continually pushed in this state of hydroplane. This same situation can be experienced without actually hydroplaning when a driver attempting to negotiate a curve does not have enough corner traction to overcome inertia. Such a skid might occur if a patch of ice is encountered.

The instinctive reactions to combat such a skid are to continue to turn the wheel further and to hit the brake. Both these responses are likely only to get the driver into deeper trouble. Once cornering force is lost, no amount of steering will allow the vehicle to take the corner. However, if a patch of ice or puddle of water helped initiate the skid, once the hazard has been crossed and if steering continues to be input, the vehicle may steer violently as cornering traction is regained.

Often in hydroplaning situations the front wheels stop turning altogether. Even slight application of the brakes will lock the wheels and the wheels will remain locked up even after they might otherwise have regained traction. To regain control in such a skid the driver must back off the accelerator and allow the vehicle to slow to a point that the wheels start turning again and regain traction.

Although it is easy to discuss what happens in a skid and how to control it, good driving skills do not come about easily unless a driver has had adequate chance to practice under the supervision of a highly trained driving instructor.

For this and other obvious safety reasons, learning to control skids should only be done under direct supervision of a qualified advanced driving instructor on an adequately prepared driving range.

7 ROAD CONSTRUCTION AND ENGINEERING

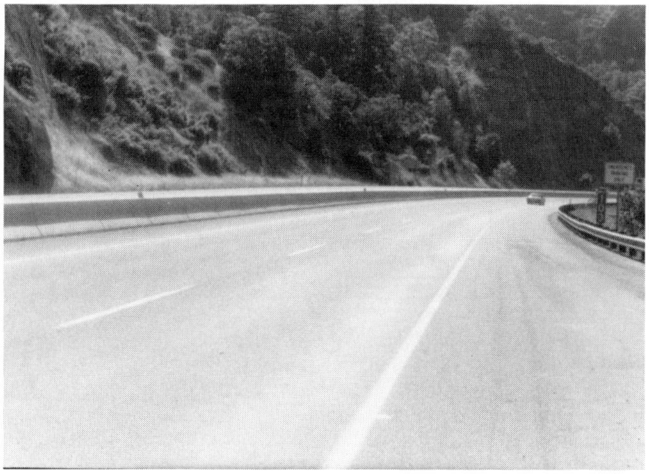

We travel the roads and highways every day. How often have you thought about them, their construction, their engineering problems, and how they affect your driving? On numerous occasions, you have driven over sections of sagging road, or through corners that were less than ideally banked.

The average motorist may view these conditions as little more than a nuisance. On the other hand, the ambulance driver must be aware of the many types of road conditions and adjust his driving accordingly to offer his patient the most comfortable ride possible. Only by knowing each road well can the EMT offer the patient the best ride. As weather changes, so too will many road conditions. If you know a particular road well, you can predict where standing water might exist after a heavy rain. If the road freezes, you can expect it to have fractures that will create a rougher ride. Knowing that the bridge ahead has a sharp bump on each side should cause you to adjust your speed prior to hitting the bump.

Any number of conditions can come into play which will cause the ambulance driver to adjust his driving or route. Understanding some basics of road construction and engineering can help you predict conditions, even on an unfamiliar road.

Road Surfaces

Many different materials are used to make up road surfaces. Anything from the dirt on a path down to a favorite fishing hole to the concrete of a modern expressway may be used. Different surfaces have different characteristics. Each surface will be affected differently by such variables as weather, traffic load, underlying road bed, and terrain. The result of these effects will have considerable bearing on driving. Let's examine the common road surfaces found in the United States and the influence these variables will have on them.

Asphalt and macadam (oil mat) surfaces are probably the two most commonly used materials on today's roads. Both offer good friction coefficients with less expense and complexity than some of the other materials used. Asphalt is not as durable as some of the other common surfaces. This means that the road will require repair more often. Asphalt repair is often accomplished by patching the surface with more asphalt or with tar to fill in cracks. These patches then create bumps in the road. When wet, tar can create slick spots. Asphalt also has a propensity to leach the oils used to make it, thereby reducing the friction coefficient of the surface. Such leaching occurs during hot spells as the road surface heats. Its adverse effects are then noticed when the next rain comes, mixing with the oil on the surface.

The composition of an asphalt road also makes the surface subject to compression. As traffic continually drives over it, typically the compression will result in two ruts in each lane where the tires of the traffic ride. These ruts can be dangerous as they inhibit water drainage. Water buildup on the road will contribute to vehicle hydroplaning.

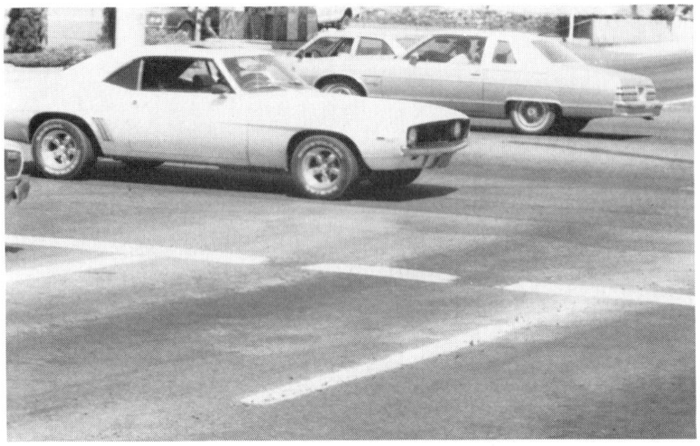

Fig. 7.1 Asphalt road composition makes the surface subject to compression: usually, two ruts will develop in each lane where the tires of traffic ride.

An asphalt road is to some degree pliable. This pliability allows the road surface to conform to changes in the road bed. Road bed changes occur as the underlying bed continues to settle after the road has been built. The road bed also changes in cold weather when the water in the ground freezes, expands, and then thaws. This action allows the road to settle even further. Settling can also occur where new asphalt is laid to cover construction for underground power lines, sanitary sewers, or drainage lines.

Freezing temperatures can also cause the need for many other road surface repairs. Water will infiltrate the tiny cracks between the gravel which makes up an asphalt surface. As this moisture freezes, it expands and loosens the asphalt composition. Where new surfaces have been laid over old, or where the surface is thin, whole sections of the surface can break away, creating chuckholes literally overnight. A driver needs to be especially observant for new chuckholes right after a freeze and when the ground begins to thaw.

A large volume of truck traffic will also contribute to the rapid decay of the asphalt roads. The asphalt surface will compress and bend under such weight. Tree roots lifting the bed under the asphalt can also create fractures.

Concrete is more durable than asphalt or macadam, but it also is more expensive. Concrete, too, is influenced by heat and cold, expanding and contracting accordingly. However, concrete cannot compress as easily as asphalt. Therefore, when concrete is laid down, expansion joints must be provided between slabs to allow them to expand and contract.

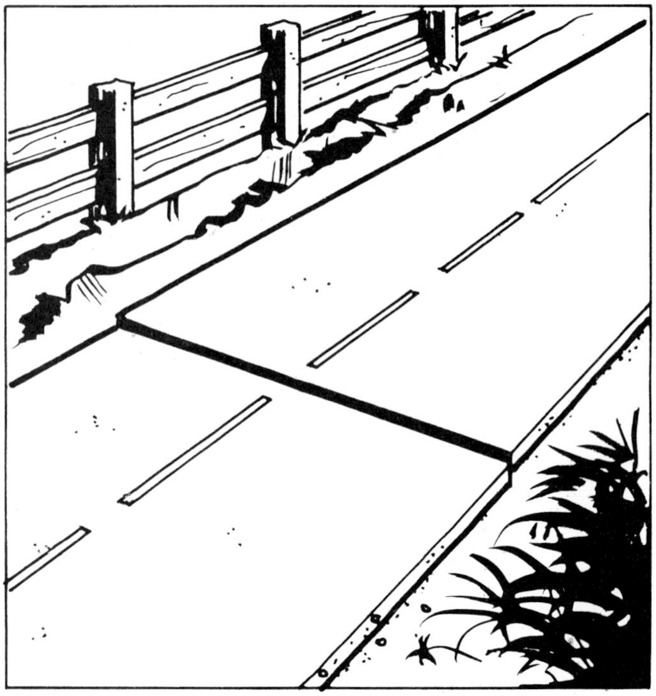

Fig. 7.2 Concrete roads won't conform to the settling of the road bed but develop differences in elevation from one slab to another.

It is these joints that cause many of the problems encountered with a concrete road. If the slabs are laid too far apart the road will create a rhythmic bumping that can be aggravating to vehicle occupants. Such a situation can also occur because of the road bed settling. A concrete road will not conform to the settling of the road bed the same way as asphalt. Instead, concrete will develop differences in the elevation of the two adjoining slabs. This minute difference in elevation can produce the same type of rhythmic bumping of the vehicle that wide expansion joints can produce. Road bed settling can also cause the individual slabs to crack which will accelerate their deterioration.

Although infrequently used for new construction, bricks can be used to surface a road. Brick roads are more commonly encountered in the Midwest and in downtown areas, especially those that have undergone recent restoration. Bricks do not have the friction coefficient of asphalt and concrete, thus they can be very slippery even when dry. Due to the multitude of joints between the bricks, tire vibration is very common on such a surface. Bricks will conform to the underlying road bed much the same as asphalt. Due to the small size of the individual bricks and their relative independence, brick roads can become very rough since each brick can project the shape of the road bed underneath. Additionally, individual bricks can easily become dislodged, which can lead to the rapid creation of chuckholes. Underlying tree roots can uplift bricks which can create solid obstructions and raise havoc with front-end alignment.

A few coastal areas have large quantities of sea shell fragments in their road surfaces. Such surfaces have a tendency to become very slick with just a hint of moisture.

Certainly, the road surfaces that have been around the longest are dirt and gravel. As the depth and compression of the dirt and gravel varies from place to place, so too does the friction coefficient. A buildup of gravel in one location will totally change the handling characteristics of the vehicle. Such a buildup can pull the steering wheel from a driver's hand. Flying rocks and dust can damage the vehicle. Dust can also block a driver's vision. The washboard effect caused by the irregularity of the road can, in short order, do severe damage to the vehicle's suspension system. For these reasons, travel on dirt and gravel roads should be kept to a minimum. If you must drive on these types of road surfaces, reduce your speed accordingly.

Most road surfaces used today have a good friction coefficient when they are first installed. After a period of time though, this friction coefficient will begin to wear down. Continual traffic will begin to polish the road surface, smoothing it out. Foreign bodies such as gravel will actually help this process, grinding the road down even further. In areas where studded snow tires are used, the studs will increase road surface wear tremendously. On some roads, this constant grinding and polishing may actually create ruts in the road. Add to this the oil and grease left behind from cars on the road and it becomes apparent that the friction coefficient can be significantly reduced on some highways.

Bridges and Ramps

Today most bridges are constructed of reinforced concrete beds suspended between con-

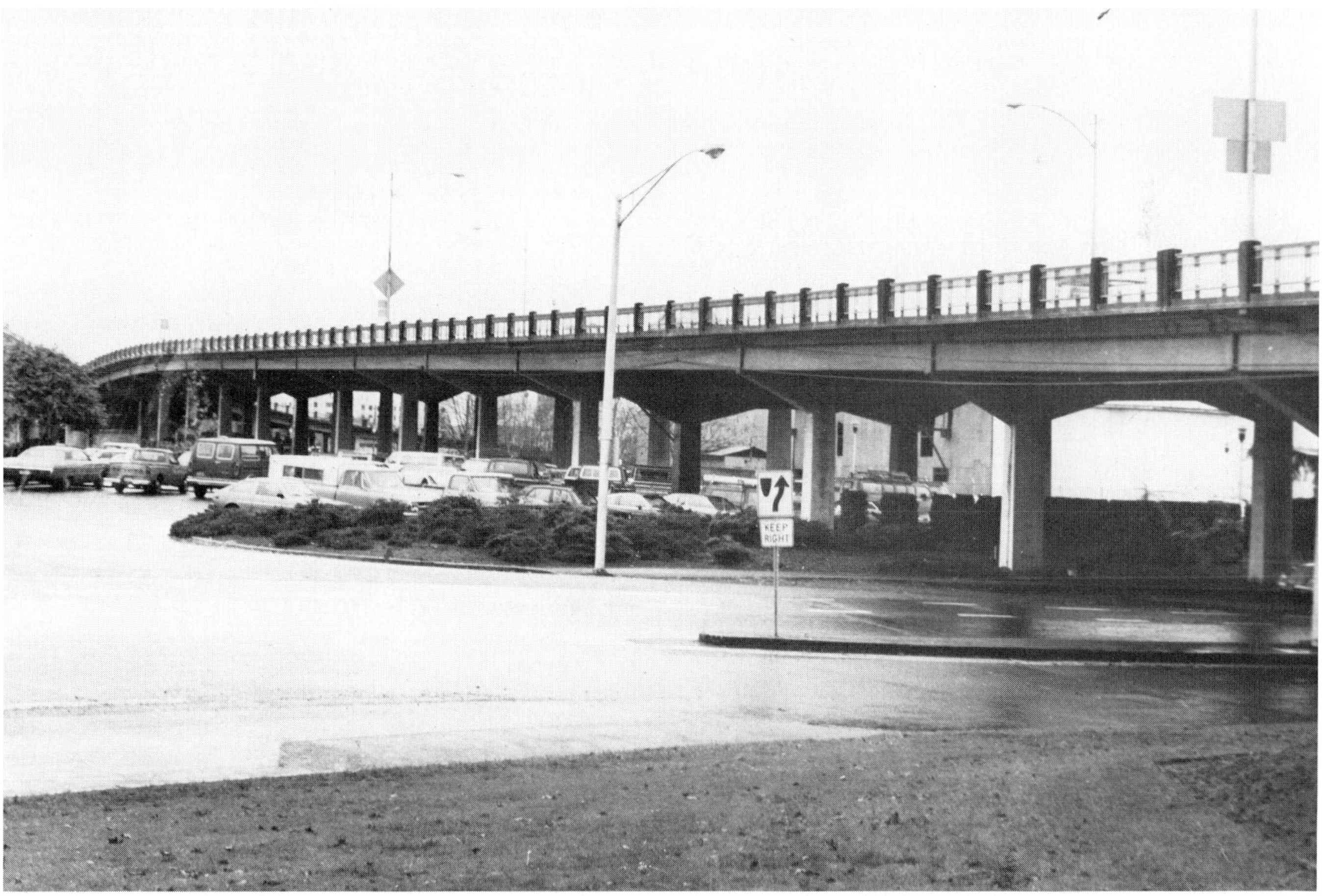

Fig. 7.3a Most bridges are built of reinforced, concrete beds suspended between concrete pillars. (Photo courtesy of jems.)

crete pillars. Since these individual sections or spans must be allowed to expand and contract, joints will occur over the supporting pillars. The individual spans are also built with some crown which will level out as traffic weight is introduced to the bridge. These bridge components (expansion joints and crown) can produce a rough, bumpy ride as a vehicle passes over each joint. Speed reduction may be indicated to keep from adversely affecting your patient or causing excessive wear on suspension components.

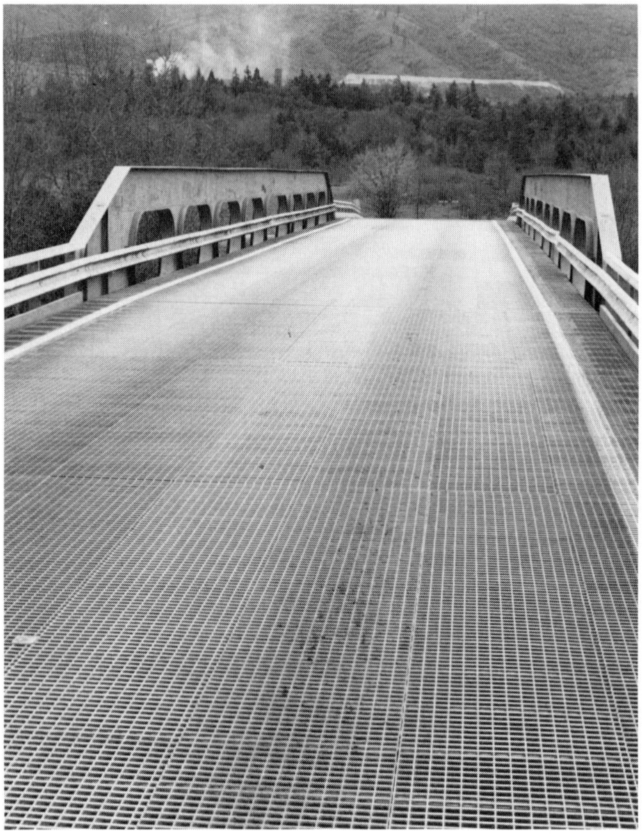

Fig. 7.3b Sometimes, you'll find bridge surfaces that are mainly metal grating, making for a slick surface and uncomfortable vibration.

Occasionally, you will encounter bridge surfaces that are mainly metal grating. Commonly, drawbridges and elevator type bridges use the metal grating in order to reduce the weight of the structure. Metal grating always seems to be slick, so added caution is indicated. Additionally, the metal grating will create an extreme vibration which will be felt by the patient at any speed. If you have an option of bridges you can travel upon, it may be better to avoid metal-surface bridges when possible.

As we drive, we will encounter several different road surfaces. Some streets may be primarily surfaced with concrete, others may use asphalt. It is common for these two materials to be used together to form one road surface, as is typical on expressways. The primary traffic lanes may be concrete, while the side aprons or emergency lanes will be paved with asphalt. It is where these two materials join that some vehicle handling problems may be encountered.

Where the two surfaces meet, there is usually a slight difference in elevation. Asphalt, as we've discussed, tends to compress under heavy traffic loads so that it is reduced in height or grade. This action is particularly noticeable in areas that actually receive the tires of the traffic. Since the concrete does not compress, a slight difference in elevation develops. To combat this action engineers will often have the area of the joint built up with extra asphalt. The end result is still a bump where the two surfaces meet.

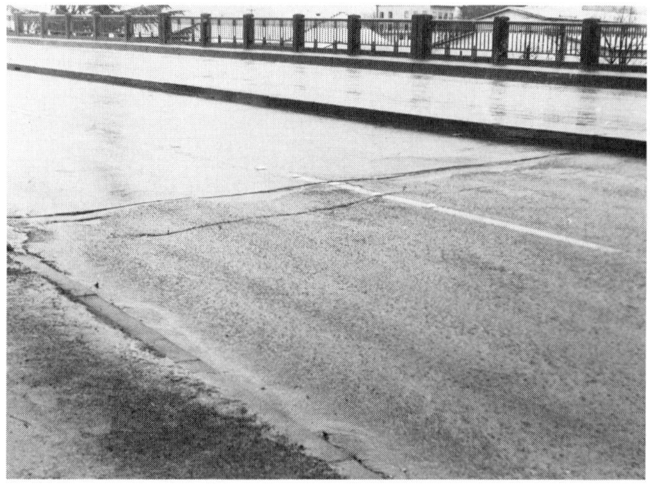

Fig. 7.4 Where two different surfaces meet, there's usually a slight difference in elevation resulting in bumps. (Photo courtesy of **jems.**)

The areas where such bumps are most often encountered include where an asphalt road meets a concrete bridge, railroad crossings, and where an asphalt entrance or exit ramp merges with a concrete expressway. Asphalt entrance ramps can create a particular problem for the unwary driver. Since the entrance ramp meets the expressway at an oblique angle, the ridge resulting from the elevation difference will resist the tires. The tires will attempt to ride over this ridge with their side walls instead of the actual tread. As a result, the vehicle will continue to travel a short distance in a straight line. At some unknown point, the tires will climb the ridge of concrete and the vehicle, with its added steering input, will then tend to lunge into the next lane. Even steering pressure and a slightly steeper angle of approach to the traffic lane can reduce much of this type of problem. Merging with the next lane at a point before or after the area most traffic utilizes will help the driver avoid the larger depressions in the asphalt.

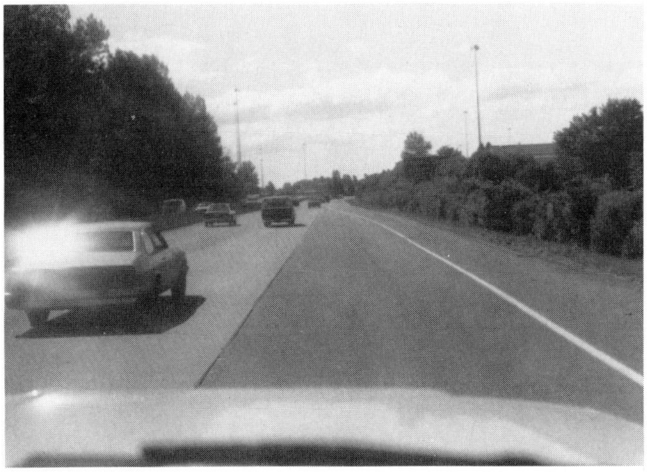

Fig. 7.5 Asphalt entrance ramps to concrete expressways create particular problems due to the resulting elevation differences resisting the tires.

Corners

Typically, low speed corners are engineered so that they maintain a constant radius around the whole turn. That is to say, the corner scribes a continuous arc that neither gets wider nor tighter through its duration. Such low speed (usually under 40 mph) engineered corners are fairly safe to drive since drivers are able to tell how much steering input will be needed at the beginning of the turn and not have to make any input changes while in the turn. If a turn becomes sharper or more acute part way through the curve, it will require additional steering input and less speed in order for it to be negotiated safely.

Unfortunately, constant radius curves are not always encountered. Many of America's roads were built before society took notice of the number of people killed on the highways and set out to correct road design problems. In fact, many of our roads date back to the horse-and-buggy days. During that era, curves couldn't be taken fast enough to really matter how they were built. Obviously, these roads were not engineered for maximum driving efficiency. Instead, their path was chosen for ease of construction. The same right-of-way may be in use today, but with higher power vehicles and impatient drivers rushing about as its traffic. Today, there is much emphasis on highway engineering and safety. An example of newer highway design is the "spiral curve." Spiral curves are engineered into the road for high speed driving comfort. A spiral curve begins slightly and increases in its sharpness and then decreases its angle slowly back to a straight line. The banking (super elevation) of the curve will also gradually increase and then decrease. This allows for a smooth continuous input and withdrawal of steering while turning as the driver negotiates the curve. New roads are being built with these concerns in mind. At the same time, many existing roads are being upgraded to make them safer. Unfortunately, many of the lesser traveled roads will probably never be upgraded. Since we do not always have the option of which of the roads we will drive upon, we need to be aware of the compound radius curve as well as the positive and negative camber curves.

A compound curve is one which, unlike the constant radius curve, becomes sharper the further into the curve the vehicle progresses. The hazards of such a curve become obvious. A driver enters a corner at a speed judged by how sharp the curve first appears. As the curve suddenly becomes sharper, the driver may discover that he is traveling at too high a speed to successfully complete the turn. Heavy braking in this condition can lead to a vehicle spin.

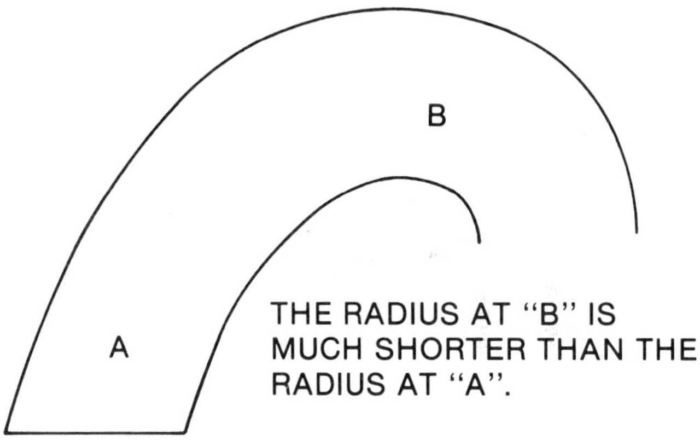

COMPOUND RADIUS CURVE

Fig. 7.6a Reducing radius curves are ones which become sharper the further the vehicle progresses.

In addition to a constant turning radius, the curve should also be properly banked. If a vehicle could be made to lean into a curve it would be able to negotiate the curve much faster and smoother. A properly engineered road will, to some extent, do this for you. The curve will be banked so the vehicle actually leans into the curve. As mentioned earlier, many of our roads were built before there was such a concern for proper engineering. Some older roads will actually have curves that are not banked or actually lean in the wrong direction. Such a curve will allow the vehicle to roll even more than natural while being negotiated. In a negatively banked curve, the vehicle will have to travel at a substantially reduced speed to keep this negative roll influence from pulling the vehicle out of the curve.

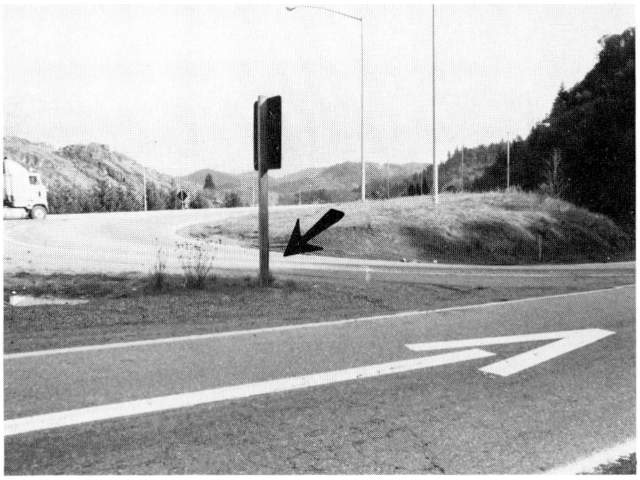

Fig. 7.6b Vehicles on this turn will accelerate to match the speed of expressway traffic upon reaching the radius reduction—a very dangerous situation.

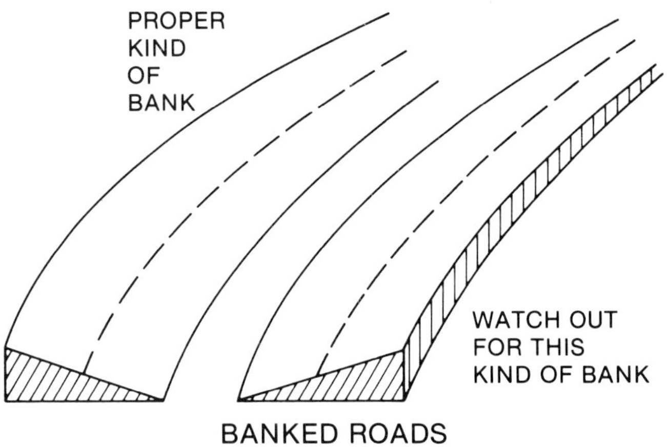

Fig. 7.7a Curves that are properly banked will allow vehicles to lean into the turn.

Most roads are built with a varying degree of crown. Road crown is where the center of the road surface is higher than the shoulders. An unbanked left curve on a road with significant crown will have the same effect as a negatively banked curve, it will force the vehicle to exaggerate its negative lean. Although very dangerous, these curves do exist and must be interpreted by the driver and negotiated at greatly reduced speeds.

Corners are usually marked with signs indicating the speed with which they can be comfortably maneuvered. These signs are placed ahead of the curve as a warning to the driver, and these curves can often be safely traversed at speeds as much as 15 mph faster than posted. Those curves marked at 25 mph or less should be

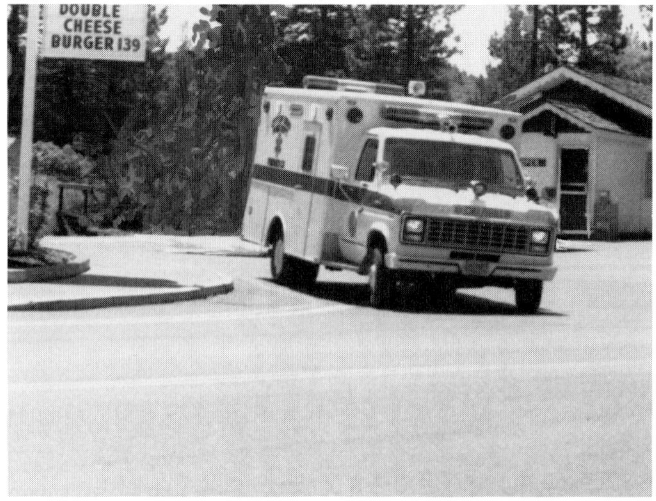

Fig. 7.7b Example of the amount of roll resulting when a vehicle takes a negative banked curve.

taken at the posted speed, as this indicates a very tight corner. When a patient is on board the ambulance, corners should be driven no faster than the posted speed.

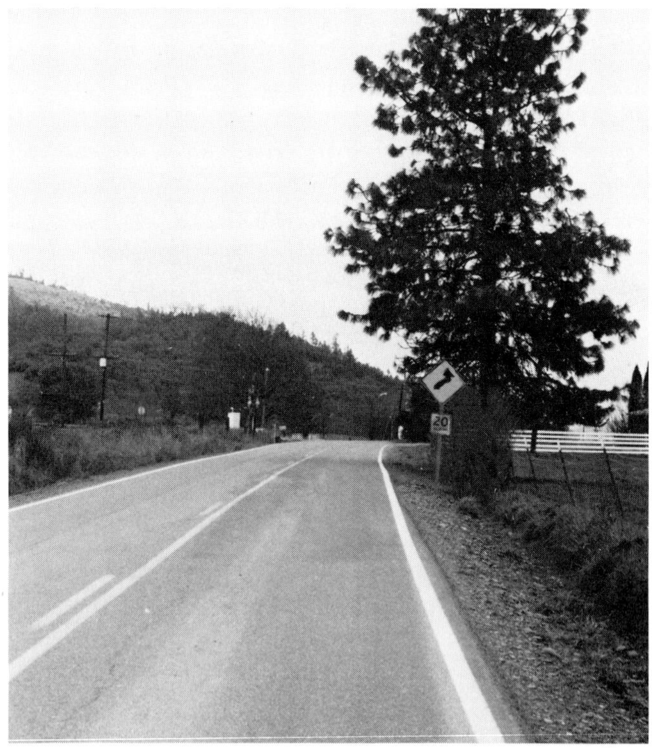

Fig. 7.8 Corners are usually marked with signs showing the speed at which they can be negotiated.

The habit of watching the speedometer to determine vehicle speed as it enters a corner is not recommended. The driver must learn to gauge the proper speed by observing road surface conditions, curve radius, personal ability, and vehicle capability ahead of time. Traveling on unfamiliar roads of fair or poor construction should be done with caution.

Water Drainage

Road crown is essential for road safety. Road crown allows water to drain quickly from the travel surface during rainy periods. The danger of hydroplaning is of course reduced when water drains from the road surface. Some concrete roads accomplish drainage by cutting many grooves into the road surface forming channels for the water to drain. This surface is then made safer for travel during heavy rainstorms. Unfortunately, some negative impact results under dry pavement conditions.

Fig. 7.9 Some concrete roads accomplish drainage through use of many grooves in the road surface.

Since a great deal of the road surface has actually been cut away, the tires come in less contact with the pavement. Less road surface area in contact with the tire surface will change the friction coefficient, thus skidding and sliding potential may be increased. These road surfaces are usually well-posted and should be respected whether it is wet or dry.

Once the water has drained off of the road surface, where does it go? This is a question you should ask yourself during and just after heavy downpours. Even when adequate drainage is constructed, an obstructed drain hole or mud slide can create instant lakes. If water is not adequately drained from the bottom of a curve, problems can be encountered by motorists traveling on the inside or bottom lane.

In some areas, the drainage runs along the road shoulders or curbs. Above-ground drainage can create large puddles at intersections. These puddles are formed by the natural damming effect where the two road crowns intersect. Slow, cautious travel is always indicated in flooded areas. Unseen hazards such as huge chuckholes may be lurking under the water.

Roadside Engineering

Most roadsides are cluttered with power poles, road signs, billboards, and other objects that can be struck by vehicles leaving the roadway. Any of these objects can be considered a hazard since they will increase vehicle damage and potentially injure vehicle occupants. Until recent years, little attention had been given to the construction and placement of these potential hazards. A few examples of increased roadside safety improvements follow.

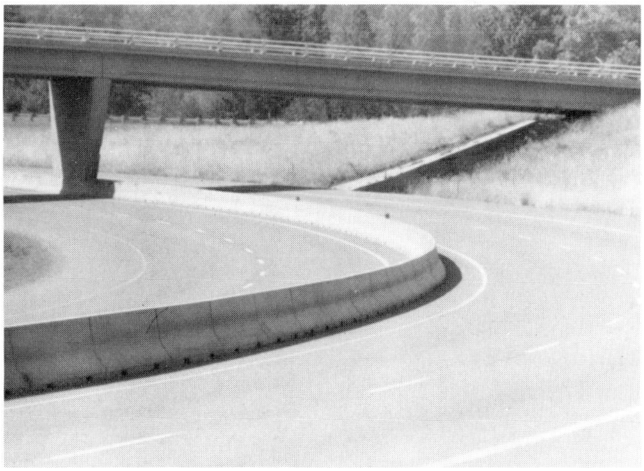

Fig. 7.10a Some barriers are designed to redirect vehicles back into their normal traffic lanes rather than stop them abruptly.

Modern sign and light standards are designed to break away when struck, usually at ground level. Such action reduces the deceleration force of the collision and avoids the horror story of the signpost passing through the windshield and the vehicle's occupants. These standards are also placed much further off the roadway than they were just a few years ago.

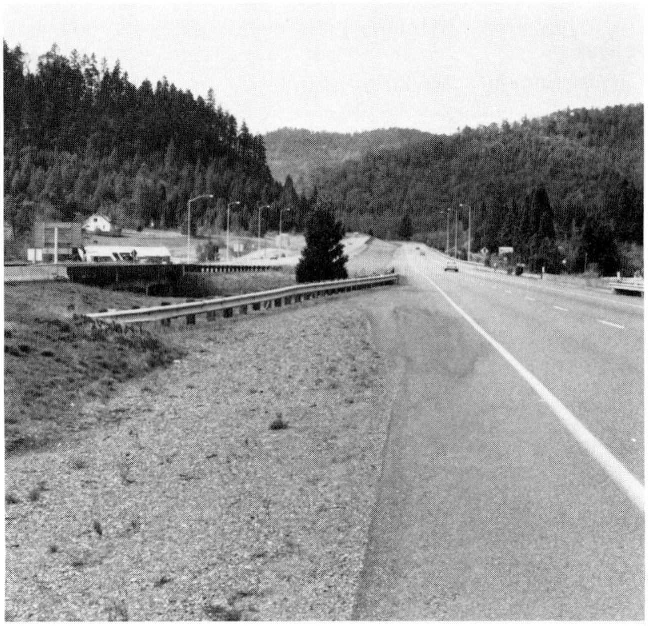

Fig. 7.10b The leading edge of guardrails is often buried so it won't protrude where it can be rammed easily.

Guardrails have been improved tremendously over the last decade. They are being placed on many more of the hazardous locations found on our roadways. These barriers are frequently designed to redirect vehicles back into their normal traffic lane rather than to abruptly stop them in their tracks. The ends of the guardrails are now somewhat protected from head-on collisions. Mounds of sod or various types of energy-absorbing barricades are found on the leading edge of guardrails and some light standards. These energy-absorbing devices will reduce the collision impact, often reducing the severity of occupant injury.

Such roadside safety engineering changes are certainly not complete. It will be many years before all of our highway systems can be brought into line with today's standards.

While highway engineering is making our roads safer for us today, the ambulance driver must be familiar with any road hazards within his coverage area. With this knowledge of construction and potential hazards, he can adjust his driving to reduce vehicle wear and increase passenger comfort and safety.

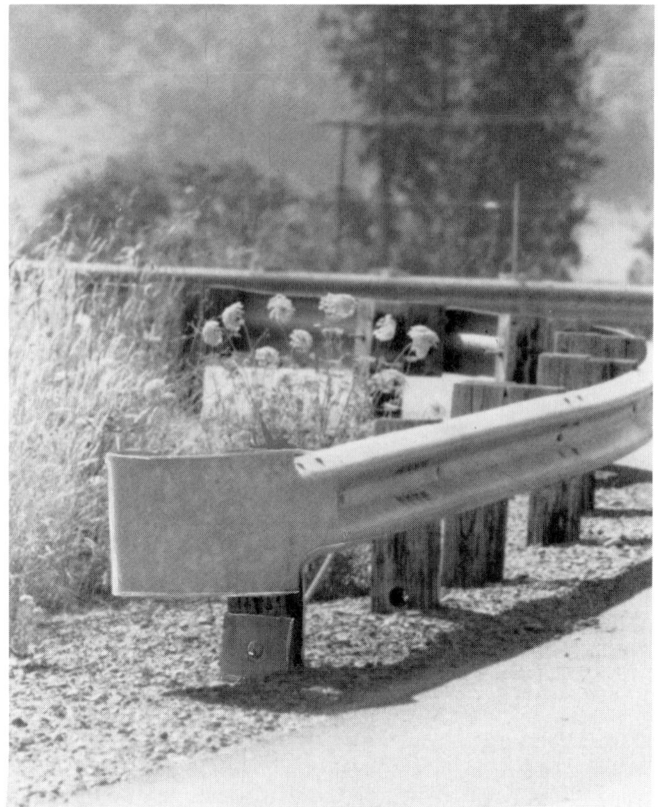

Fig. 7.10c Some guardrails have protective caps to prevent the guardrail point from being driven into striking vehicles.

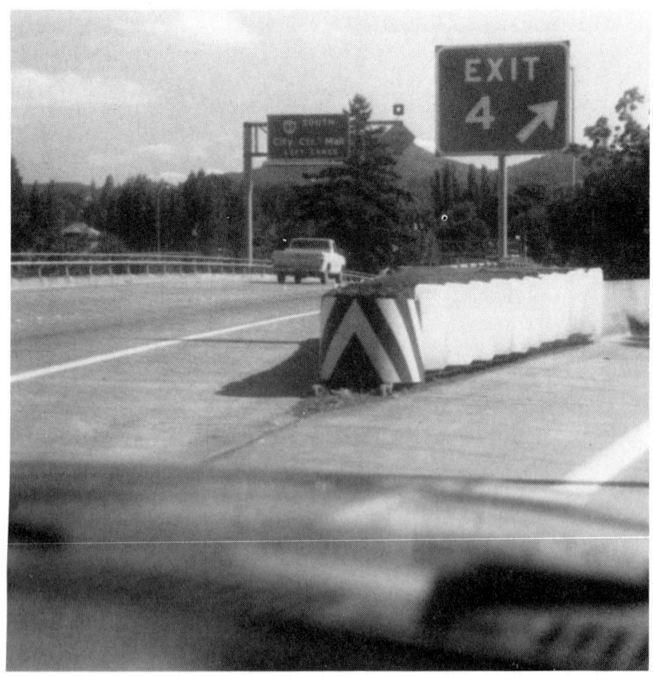

Fig. 7.10d Another type of impact-absorbing structure in use.

8 PATIENT RIDE

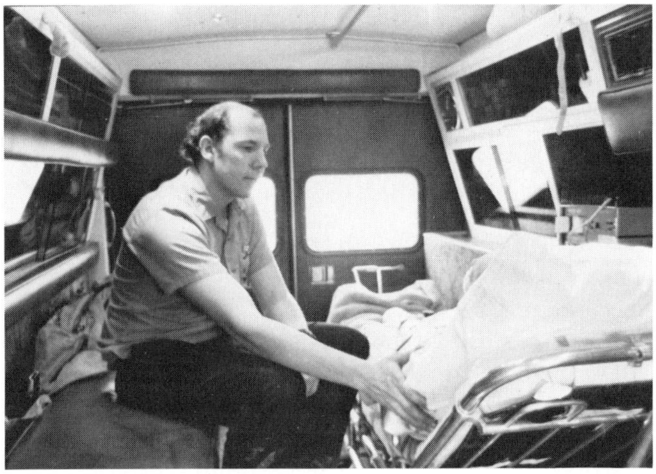

The big difference between driving an ambulance and any other type of emergency vehicle is that the ambulance transports sick and injured people. For this reason, an ambulance driver must possess a different driving philosophy than that of other emergency vehicle operators. Certainly all emergency vehicle operators strive to respond to the emergency scene urgently while operating their vehicle in a safe and sane manner. The difference becomes apparent when the ambulance is transporting a patient. The EMT ambulance operator should think of his patient as an employer, not simply cargo. The ambulance driver should think of himself as a chauffeur striving to give his employer a smooth ride. If given a smooth ride, the employer's coffee won't be spilled and his notes won't be sloppy. The patient who does not receive a smooth ride will experience additional discomfort and his condition may deteriorate. A nauseated patient may vomit, a patient with a fracture may be jostled about and have increased tissue damage, all as a result of a poor quality ride to the hospital.

It is unreasonable to expect an ambulance driver to respond to the scene utilizing one style of driving and a few minutes later for him to adopt a totally different driving style. Instead the principles of patient ride must be employed at all times the ambulance is being driven. Always driving the ambulance with the attitude that there is a patient on board will help insure the smoothest possible ride when a patient is actually present.

Adverse Effects On the Patient

Many different effects must be considered when transporting a patient. Frequently, the patient will be nauseated. Nausea is experienced both by ill and trauma patients. Any movement these people experience will increase the likelihood of the nausea progressing to vomiting. Obviously, the presence of emesis in the airway will increase the chances of aspiration and total airway occlusion. Even healthy people are susceptible to motion sickness. Place the patient on the stretcher, load him headfirst in an ambulance, and soon you will have an ill patient as he travels backwards down the road. Obviously, anyone already experiencing nausea will deteriorate if exposed to these conditions. The EMT must keep a constant vigil on every patient's airway as he is being transported. Reduced speeds may help alleviate some of this type of patient discomfort.

Should you be forced to suspend one or more patients in hanging litters, be especially vigilant for vomiting as they are very likely to experience nausea associated with motion sickness and claustrophobia.

Since most of the patients will be transported in a supine or semi-Fowler's position, their bodies are spread out in a horizontal position. Any bumps encountered will be felt through their entire bodies.

The severity of feeling the road bumps will be magnified since the patient's litter is located over the rear axle. It is at this point that the greatest deflection of a bump is experienced. If the patient could be located more towards the center point between the front and rear axles, the bumps would tend to be smoothed out as the front and rear suspension systems work. Of course, such positioning cannot be accomplished. The driver must keep this fact in mind since he will not feel the same severity of a bump as someone in the patient compartment. Even in the cab of Types II and III ambulances (van and van cabs), the bumps are not felt to be as severe since the front end of the ambulance is generally much heavier than the rear. This additional weight has a tendency to smooth out the bumps.

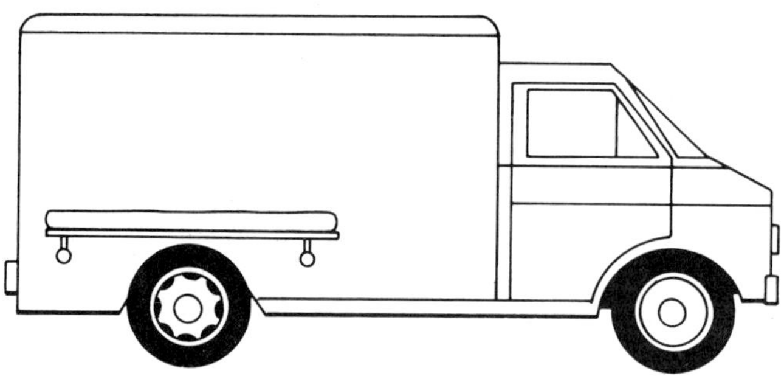

Fig. 8.1 Patient litter is situated typically over the rear axle, location of the most vehicle body motion.

Road bumps are not the only cause of these types of patient discomfort. The pitching back and forth of the vehicle as it accelerates and brakes can have the same effect.

Sudden braking to avoid a bump or to stop for a traffic light will certainly increase nausea. Hard deceleration may cause the patient to feel as though he is being stood on his head. Hard braking will also cause the muscles to contract, pulling on any broken bones.

If the ambulance enters a curve at an excess speed, centrifugal force will cause the patient to stiffen against the feeling that he is about to roll off the stretcher. This same force will have a tendency to laterally displace any fractures that are present.

Sudden changes in grade, such as those that are found at bridge entrances and road dips, have a tremendous impact on patient comfort. A sudden feeling of weightlessness can cause the patient to stiffen.

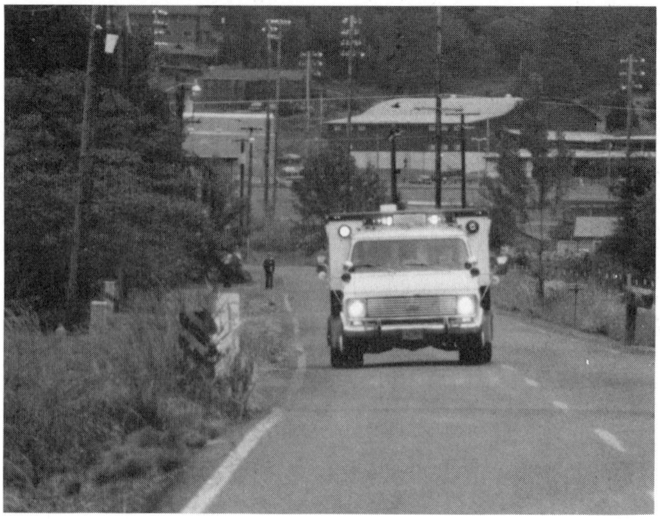

Fig. 8.2 Sudden changes in grade (such as at bridges) tremendously affect patient comfort.

Vibrations felt through the chassis will also cause patient discomfort. As speed is increased, vibrations may also increase. Even a patient with relatively minor injuries will become less comfortable if road vibrations are felt.

Along with the physical discomfort a patient might feel, the ambulance driver must also be concerned with the patient's anxiety. Anxiety increases cardiac load. Such an increase will be detrimental to most patients. The use of the emergency warning equipment can cause anxiety. The sound of the siren instantly frightens the patient as he fears the worst for himself.

Even the use of the emergency lights without the use of the siren can frighten the patient. It is not difficult for the patient to see the lights reflecting off of buildings or following traffic, especially at night. The patient will also "feel" the urgency of his condition as the ambulance makes its way through traffic. Rarely is such urgency indicated in patient transportation, especially when the negative effects of a poor quality patient ride are considered.

One way for an EMT to determine if his patient's ride is comfortable and relatively free from anxiety is to observe the patient's hands. If the patient has a death grip on the stretcher side rails and his knuckles are turning white, you can be assured that he isn't comfortable. Such an observation should be passed on to the driver so he might make an appropriate adjustment in his driving style.

Adverse Effects On the Patient's Care. Patient care cannot continue if the EMT attending the patient has to hold on to survive. Still, the way many drivers handle an ambulance causes just such a reaction. The EMT's job is to care for the sick and injured. Patient care must continue uninterrupted while en route to the hospital. The smooth ride required by the patient is also required for the EMT rendering care.

Several basic and advance life support skills are difficult or nearly impossible to perform in a moving ambulance. These skills include IV catheter insertion, endotracheal intubation, and obtaining a blood pressure by auscultation. Should these skills be attempted in a moving ambulance, it is imperative that the driver give the smoothest ride possible. Another basic skill which is greatly affected by a moving ambulance is cardiopulmonary resuscitation. Many studies have demonstrated that CPR when performed in a moving ambulance is best performed when the vehicle is traveling at speeds below 25 mph and not being driven in the emergency mode. Although such speeds may seem inappropriate, it must be strongly recommended that the vehicle not be driven in an emergency status to the hospital while CPR is in progress. It is also strongly recommended that all EMTs and EMT-Paramedics perform CPR on a recording manikin in a moving ambulance. Such practice will help sharpen the technician's CPR skills and also demonstrate how vehicle motion can adversely affect the performance of CPR.

Good patient ride directly translates into good patient care. The ambulance driver should keep this in mind at all times he is driving the ambulance. The way the ambulance is operated can affect the patient's outcome.

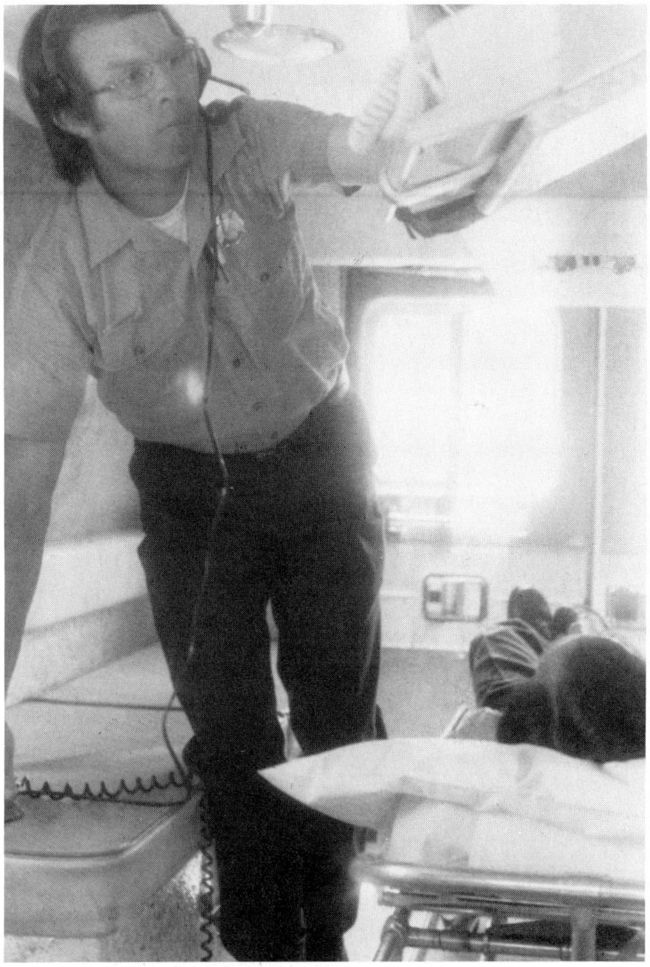

Fig. 8.3 The ambulance ride directly influences patient care. A smooth ride is required if the attending EMT is to render effective care.

Ride Influences

Generally, the quality of patient ride is influenced by four factors: road hazards, cornering, speed, and speed changes. Let's examine each of these factors and determine how to minimize their effects.

Road Hazards. Road hazards can take on many forms, some of which were discussed in Chapter 7, "Road Construction." Besides the blemishes that develop as a road slowly deteriorates, such things as speed bumps, railroad grade crossings, and general terrain can also affect the patient ride. As stated earlier, many of these hazards go essentially unnoticed by the majority of the motoring public. Such inattention cannot be tolerated in the professional ambulance driver.

Finding those normally insignificant bumps in the road is not always easy. Employing good seeing habits will often help a driver to notice those bumps not seen by others. Additionally, the ambulance driver needs to develop a "seat of the pants" feeling for them. Obviously, learning where the bumps are is only half the battle. The driver also needs to learn how to avoid them or drive over them.

In order to minimize its adverse effects, each bump must be driven differently. Once a specific bump has been identified, the bump should be approached from different angles and speeds to determine the best approach for that bump. This type of experimentation can occur while the crew is familiarizing themselves with the coverage area or when they are returning to quarters.

As a general rule, where asphalt and concrete or any other incompressible materials meet, it is best to approach the joint slightly off center of the traffic lane. The ambulance tires will then be able to track on the high points between the ruts caused by traffic. At this point, the asphalt will not have been as compressed, thus it is closer to the elevation of the concrete.

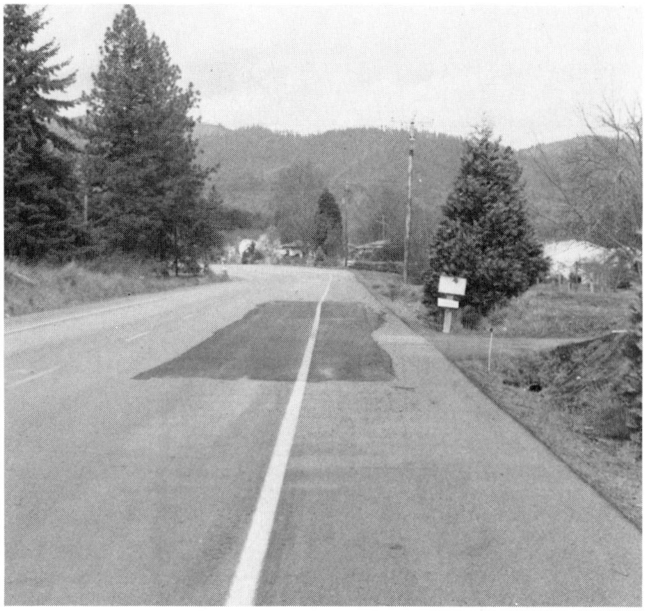

Fig. 8.4a Road repair or deterioration, usually unnoticed, can cause severe discomfort to the patient.

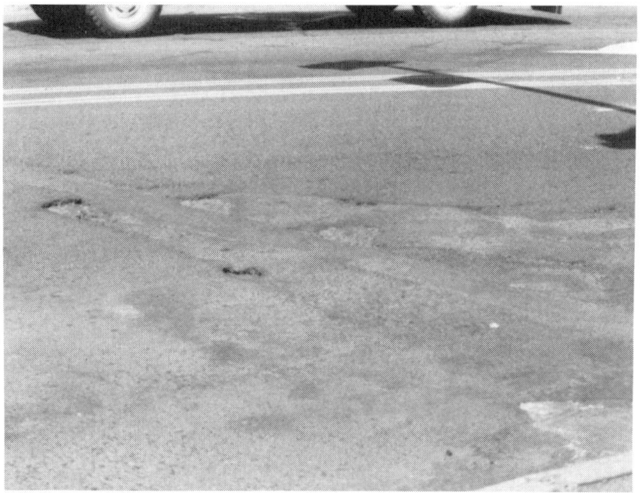

Fig. 8.4b Another example of the unevenness of road repairs.

This technique may not work as well on expressway entrance ramps where the two surfaces meet at an oblique angle. In these situations, it may be better to enter the expressway at the very beginning of the merge lane or near the end of the ramp. This will have your vehicle traveling on asphalt out of the normal traffic flow. This same technique holds true when leaving the expressway. Either way, the exact point that is best for a smooth ride won't be found without some experimentation.

Interestingly, while most road hazards will require the ambulance to slow to negotiate them properly, a few will require the vehicle to maintain speed. Railroad tracks are an example. When encountered, most railroad tracks create severe vibrations and bouncing and must be taken slowly. Others only create vibration at slower speeds and are barely noticeable when taken at the posted speed limit. Certainly, any railroad crossing should be taken at reduced speeds until proven comfortable and safe for higher speeds.

All speed changes should occur prior to negotiating bumps. For example, if braking continues right up to the point where the bump is encountered, the weight of the vehicle will not be properly distributed over each axle. This will not only cause undue wear on the suspension system but will also magnify the intensity of the bump felt by the patient.

Nothing seems to destabilize a patient so much as when the ambulance travels rapidly over the crest of a hill. Going up the hill, the springs compress, as they are fighting gravity. As the crest is passed, the springs rapidly extend. During this action, the patient may experience a momentary feeling of weightlessness which will cause changes in his hemodynamic state and frequently precipitate spontaneous vomiting.

When traveling on a road with a significant crown, it is usually better for the patient comfort if the ambulance is driven as close to the center as possible. Driving in the outside lanes, or close to the shoulder, will give the patient the feeling of being rolled off the stretcher. They will fight this sensation by tensing muscles. The adverse effects of this action have already been discussed.

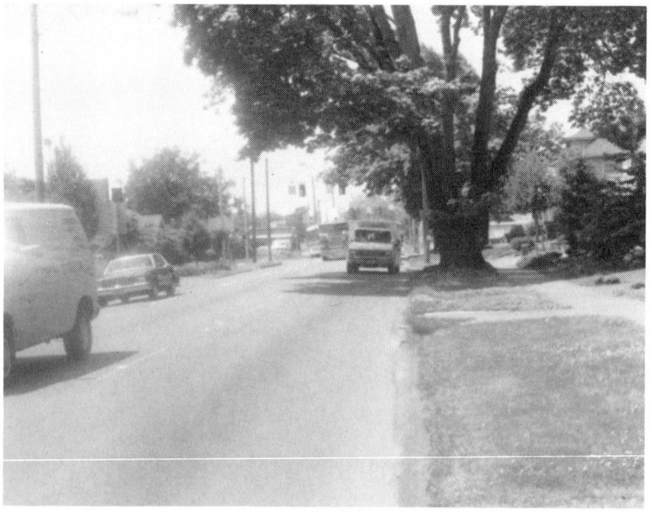

Fig. 8.5 Driving in outside lanes or close to shoulder gives patients feeling of being rolled from the stretcher.

Concrete bridges usually must be negotiated at slower speeds. The roller coaster ride that often develops on bridges is somehow ignored by the general public but is rarely overlooked by the ill or injured patient.

Cornering. Earlier we discussed how a vehicle will roll in corners as a result of centrifugal force. This roll is proportional to the amount of direction and the time involved in making that change. Since we can't affect the amount of change (turning angle) involved, we can only influence how much time it takes to make the change. Therefore, the slower the corner is driven, the less roll will be encountered. Slowing must take place before the vehicle enters the corner. This early deceleration will help to reduce the vehicle pitch which would tend to magnify the roll of the vehicle. The corner itself is then driven at a steady speed. Acceleration does not occur until the corner has been completely negotiated. By reducing the influences of excess roll and pitch, the patient's ride will be greatly enhanced.

Overall Speed. With all of this discussion on factors that influence ride, it must appear that ambulances are expected to be driven slowly. That is exactly what is expected! Not only does speed increase the effects of bumps, corners and hills, it also increases vehicle vibrations. For these reasons, travel to the hospital should routinely be at speeds at least five miles below the posted speed limit. Keep in mind that the ambulance is transporting a delicate cargo and must be driven accordingly.

Emergency driving with the patient on board is something that should be conscientiously considered rather than just being a reaction or the routine. Experts agree that less than five percent of the patients transported to the hospital warrant an emergency trip.

Emergency transportation to the hospital is only indicated in those cases where the patient's chance of survival will be greatly reduced if excess time is spent in the field. A few examples of patients who require rapid transportation include those with gunshot wounds to the head and chest, prolapsed umbilical cords, acute abdomens, and perhaps a severe head injury with rapidly reduced level of consciousness. These patients require care that is not available in the field and can deteriorate rapidly.

A point that is often forgotten, the mode of travel can be changed if the patient's condition changes. It seems much more difficult to change from an emergency mode of travel to nonemergency when the patient stabilizes or improves, but it must be considered. Traveling on a country road with little traffic may dictate that you proceed nonemergency even with a critical patient. The higher speeds and rougher ride may not be well-tolerated by the patient even though your path is clear. Always drive for the patient. Undue risks may not only further aggravate his condition but may also lead to a collision which could result in property loss, injury and litigation—if you survive.

Speed Change. Changing speed affects the weight changes of the vehicle and therefore will cause it to pitch back and forth. How fast the speed change takes place affects how much the vehicle will pitch. Drivers seldom realize that every time they move their foot from the accelerator and place it on the brake pedal, the vehicle tends to pitch. To minimize such effect, the driver must learn to drive without relying on the brakes.

Unfortunately, most drivers have been conditioned to rely on their foot being on one pedal or another at all times. Somehow, they feel uncomfortable or out of control without their foot applying pressure to either the brake or accelerator. For this reason, whenever it is time to slow, they immediately switch their foot to the brake pedal and apply pressure. Such a habit must be corrected.

Through the incorporation of proper seeing habits, the perceptual driver can observe changes in traffic speed well ahead of the time he would be required to brake. By simply adjusting the pressure on the accelerator, he can often slow sufficiently not to require the use of the brake. Such practices increase patient comfort and reduce vehicle wear.

When using the foot pedals, a driver should treat them as he would a trigger of a gun. When shooting at a target, the best results are obtained when the trigger is squeezed. The same holds true for the accelerator and the brake. They must be squeezed. When the vehicle needs to be stopped, the driver should slowly and evenly reduce the pressure on the accelerator to allow a minimum of weight transfer or pitch. Then there should be a short transition period where the vehicle is coasting, as the foot is brought to the brake. At this point, the brake is then slowly and evenly squeezed down. As the vehicle nears a stop, the pressure required on the brake pedal becomes less. If the same pressure continues to be applied, the vehicle will give a final pitch just before it stops. This final pitch can be reduced by slowly releasing the brake pedal pressure as the vehicle slows to a stop.

The driver needs not only to be concerned about slowing the vehicle but also with acceleration. When the time comes to leave the stop, the pressure on the brake pedal must be released in the same way—slowly. Vehicles equipped with an automatic transmission will tend to move in gear when the brake is not applied. If the brake is released rapidly, the vehicle will have a tendency to pitch back. This pitching is increased if the driver quickly releases the brake pedal and then abruptly transfers his foot to the accelerator. Instead, the driver must release the brake and squeeze the accelerator in the same fashion recommended for smooth stopping. The driver should slowly release pressure on the brake, allow a short transition while the foot is brought to the accelerator, and then squeeze the accelerator with a slow even pressure. This style of stopping and starting will greatly increase the patient's comfort as he rides with you.

Kicking the transmission into passing gear will also create a pitching that is uncomfortable for the patient. Such a procedure is rarely justified when transporting a patient and should be avoided.

The Drive Train

The vehicle's drive train can also affect the patient ride. A vehicle with an automatic transmission will want to travel forward when engaged in drive and back when engaged in reverse. This tendency will be felt by the patient each time the transmission is changed, even with the brake applied. To minimize the pitch encountered when the transmission gear is selected, first apply the brake firmly, then move the selector from one gear to the neutral position, hold it there for a moment and then move the selector to the opposite gear selection. This action will reduce some of the jarring experienced from quick gear changes.

Suspension System

Obviously, the vehicle's suspension system has a great impact on patient ride characteristics. Not too many years ago, most ambulances were built on luxury car chassis and gave the ride of a limousine. Today with our need for more room for patient care and equipment carrying capability, these coach type ambulances have been replaced, for the most part, by vans and trucks. Certainly, the truck chassis used today do not give the ride of the earlier limousine chassis.

Some of the ambulance chassis in use today have had their stock suspension system softened, thus delivering a more cushioned ride. Others still ride like a truck. Either way, it's up to the professional ambulance driver to provide the patient with the smoothest, most comfortable ride possible.

The effects of pitch and roll, and certainly braking and acceleration, will vary from vehicle to vehicle. It is therefore important for the driver to be familiar with the vehicle to which he is assigned and insure that he can respond properly in any situation.

The Family

While discussing patient ride, it also seems appropriate to discuss the family since they often accompany the patient to the hospital. Certainly the family should be encouraged to accompany the patient or be present at the hospital soon after the patient arrives. Preferably, the family members should travel to the hospital in another vehicle. This will allow them the mobility to leave the hospital, perhaps even taking their loved ones home after diagnosis and treatment.

There are of course times when you will want the family to ride in the ambulance or they will choose to do so. Usually it is better, because of the room available and patient safety, to allow only one member to travel in the ambulance. This passenger should be securely belted into the front seat and not allowed in the patient compartment. Even a stable patient may deteriorate. The EMT with the patient will have enough to do without having to work around an extra person or worry he will panic. Keep in mind that when transporting children, or patients suffering a psychological crisis, a family member may be a calming influence when allowed to ride in the back. If you allow the family member in the patient compartment, assign him a place to sit that will not hinder any care your partner may render. He should be sure to explain his intentions prior to performing any function that might be unsettling to the family member.

While you are transporting a family member, you may have an opportunity to discuss the functions of your EMS system. Perhaps you experienced a difficult time locating their street address. At this time, the driver could diplomatically explain the need for adequate address posting or why the dispatcher requires so much information. You may also take the time to reassure the family member by explaining to him that the emergency is now over since the care being rendered by your partner has stabilized the patient. This quality of care now allows for nonemergency driving and its direct benefit to the patient—a smooth ride. Taking such action is beneficial to the family member and your EMS agency as it reduces stress while increasing his knowledge of your system.

If a family member is distraught, don't allow him to drive. Instead, insist he ride with the ambulance or, better yet, arrange for him to ride with someone else.

If the family is not going to ride in the ambulance to the hospital, briefly explain where the patient will be transported, and why you will or will not be using your emergency warning devices. It only takes a moment to do so and can do much to relieve their anxiety. If you choose to transport in an emergency mode, be sure to direct the family NOT to attempt to follow the ambulance. Insure that they understand that they can do nothing to assist the patient while he is in your care. Direct the family to obey all traffic laws. Again, this only takes a few moments and can save someone's life.

If the family is not familiar with the area or hospital location it may be necessary for them to follow the ambulance. This should only be done if the ambulance will be traveling nonemergency. In this case, the ambulance driver should attempt to identify the family's vehicle and make sure they are following when he leaves the scene. While en route, he should also attempt to keep the family within sight. When making a turn, signal well in advance. Avoid unnecessary lane changes. All lane changes should be made well in advance of the next turn. Attempt to time traffic lights for both vehicles. If the family must stop at a light or loses sight of you because of traffic buildup between the two vehicles, pull over to the curb and wait until they come back into view.

These simple actions will help to reduce the family's anxiety and will carry over in reducing a conscious patient's concerns as well. Such courtesy will do much to improve the patient's ride and his mental status.

9 THE ROUTE

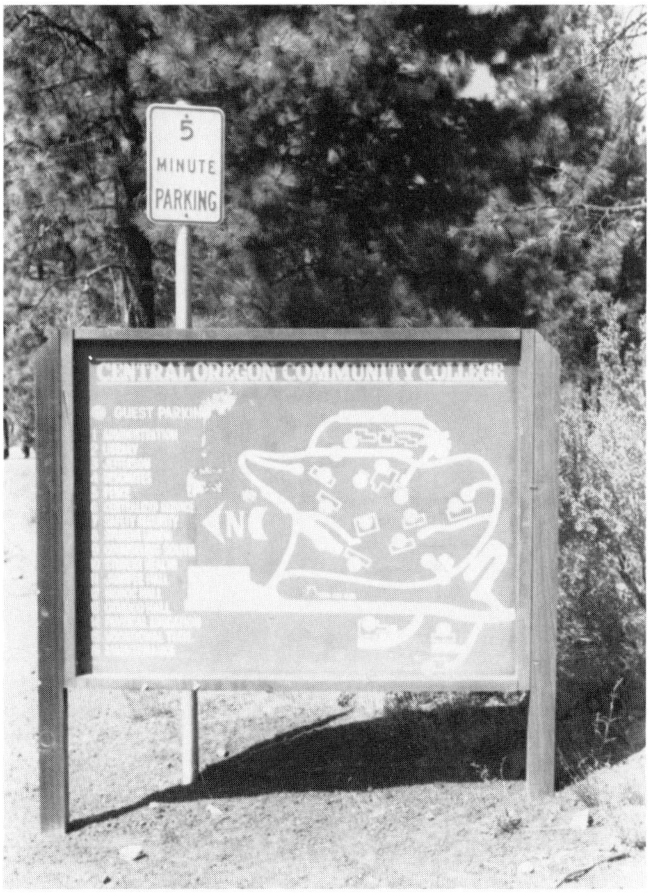

It is interesting to learn how most people navigate even within their own neighborhoods. Even after spending much of their life in one area, many people cannot tell you specifically where many of their community's streets lie. Instead, they drive by landmarks. In order to get to their dentist, they will only recall that they must turn at the Texaco station, or that their child's school is on the street three blocks past the Safeway. If really pressed, most would be able to find a specific street because they are familiar with its general location. The familiarity would allow them to drive a major thoroughfare until they come upon it. This layman form of navigation does not require drivers to memorize street names or their sequences. Obviously, ambulance crews cannot afford such a luxury. In order to swiftly arrive at the patient's side, crews must learn the street names, their sequence, and their individual characteristics.

Additionally, the ambulance crew must learn how to plan a route of travel and why. The mission of the crew is to get to the patient rapidly and safely, stabilize the patient, and then to safely transport the patient to the hospital. This can be done more efficiently when the many alternatives available for getting from Point A to Point B are utilized. By making efficient use of the road system the driver can minimize the travel time, and make the trip safer by using routes that will present the least traffic exposure. When proper route planning techniques are used, the driver can devote more of his attention to driving, secure in his knowledge of where the next turn will be and what lane to be in to prepare for it.

Rules of Route Planning

Many agencies set up standard routes of travel from one sector to another. These routes may vary for any given time of day. This predetermined route system is ideal. It gives the driver more time to concentrate on his driving while not having to heavily consider the route. Such a system must also have guidelines to follow when the preplanned routes are not appropriate. Such guidelines will help the driver to modify his route and yet remain in compliance with his agency's policies.

The first rule for shortening travel time is to keep backtracking to a minimum. Any travel time in the opposite direction doubles as the distance is then doubled. As simple as this sounds, you must always be thinking about backtracking. It is often less time consuming to stop and park, look at a map, and then proceed in a more direct route than to hastily charge off in an emergency status in the wrong direction. This statement obviously excludes various road conditions (construction, lack of cross streets, etc.) which make backtracking unavoidable.

Another factor to consider is a route that minimizes stops and turns. Each of these requires time. As you slow and stop, or make a turn, time is again doubled since the vehicle must be brought back up to speed.

The fastest route of travel will also serve to minimize accident exposure. Most accidents occur at intersections, particularly those without traffic controls or have only a Yield sign. Blind intersections, those where neither driver can see the other, can be particularly dangerous. Negotiating a blind intersection may force a driver to take evasive actions when he observes a motorist that has cut the corner, or missed the Stop sign. Typically, there is little room for an escape route in blind intersections.

Residential streets present real hazards. You must constantly be alert for pets, children, cars backing from driveways, and the fact that most residents are unaccustomed to emergency traffic in their neighborhood. Typically, these streets are narrow, limiting visibility as well as any escape route that might be required.

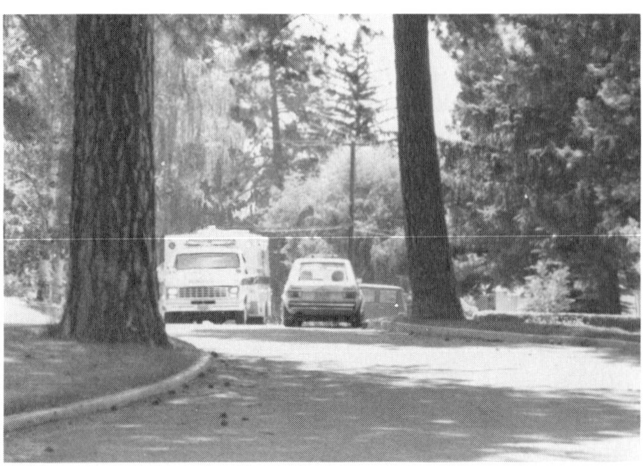

Fig. 9.1 The hazards of residential streets include the fact that they are narrow with limited visibility and escape routes.

Ambulances should, whenever possible, avoid railroad crossings, even if it requires doubling back a short distance. If used, railroad crossings will eventually catch up with you as you wait for a slow train to pass.

Opticom® Systems. Many communities have installed electronic traffic light systems that are capable of being changed by approaching emergency vehicles. The Opticom systems have come about due to the unusually high number of emergency vehicle accidents which occur at intersections. Although these systems are expensive to install they have saved many dollars in property loss and human suffering.

This system is easily understood. The emergency vehicles (usually fire suppression and EMS) are equipped with a high frequency strobe light which is faced forward on the vehicle. These strobe lights require a tremendous amount of electrical energy and should only be used as designed. Most of the strobe lights have liquid glycerin inside the lens to help cool the unit. Newer models may not have the glycerin.

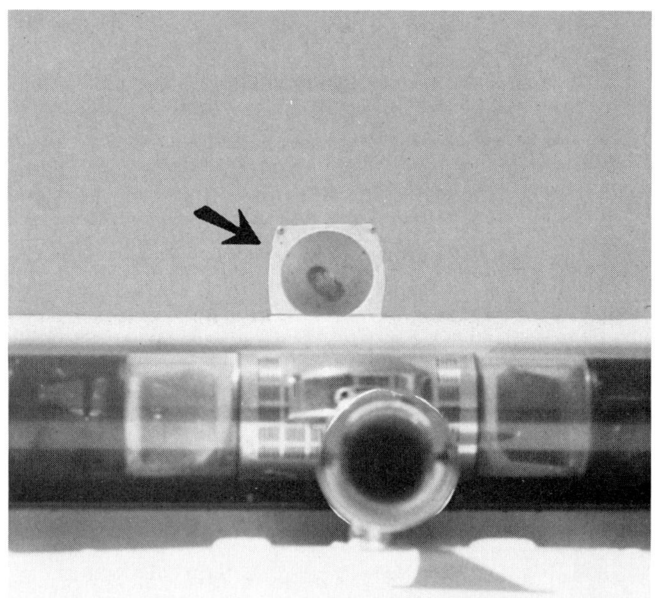

Fig. 9.2a Electronically controlled traffic light systems allow lights to be changed by using strobe lights mounted atop emergency vehicles.

As the emergency vehicle, with its Opticom strobe activated, approaches an intersection where an Opticom sensor system is in place, the sensors, usually at several locations along the route, "see" the high-frequency strobe and begin to cycle the traffic light. [Highway engineers will determine the best places for these sensors. Frequently they will be mounted on the arms that suspend the traffic signals themselves. In addition, a sensor may also be mounted well ahead of the signal, so it can see the approaching vehicle early on.] Once the sensor identifies the emergency vehicle, it will cycle all of the signals at the intersection to allow the vehicle to pass. An example of a "tripped" light would give the oncoming emergency vehicle a green light in both the through lanes and the left turn lane. All other lights at the intersection, including the oncoming traffic lanes, would see red lights. Since a given amount of time (determined by traffic engineers) is required to cycle all of these lights (green-to-yellow-to-red), the emergency vehicle must not approach at speeds in excess of the time required to change the lights. Additionally, some time should be allowed for tardy traffic to clear the intersection. Typically a traffic signal used in a 30-35 mph zone would require 7 seconds to cycle. The approaching speed of the EV would be about 28 mph. This speed is less than the designated speed limit but insures the light will have changed, thus providing safe passage through the intersection. One word of caution, even with a functional Opticom system and your emergency warning devices in operation, there is no guarantee that a motorist won't blow the light.

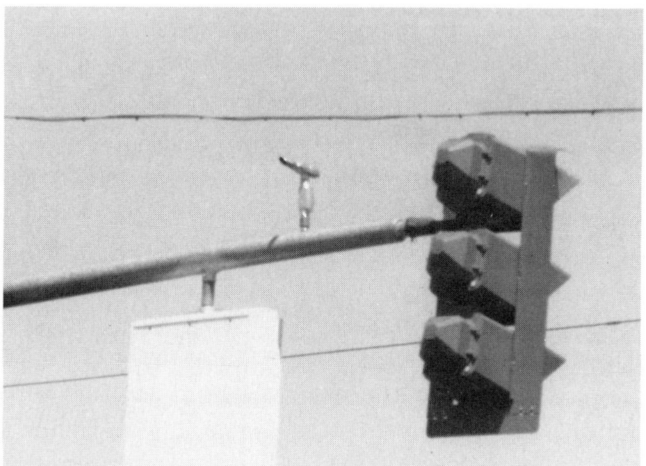

Fig. 9.2b Sensor mounted next to traffic signal receives strobe pulses and changes accordingly.

When properly installed and used, Opticom systems can make your travel on major prearranged response routes much safer and more efficient. If such a system exists in your community, travel routes may need to be adjusted to utilize the system even if it requires occasional backtracking. The time saved and reduced chance of an intersection collision make the additional time spent a worthy investment.

Maps. Every ambulance should carry as a standard tool adequate maps with street indexes of their potential coverage area. No matter how well the crew knows their area, the map still seems to get used. Additionally, the crew should study the maps from time to time. There is nothing like a map to put things in perspective. Some extensively traveled roads may be found to curve out of the way more than realized, or perhaps may be found to be more direct than previously thought.

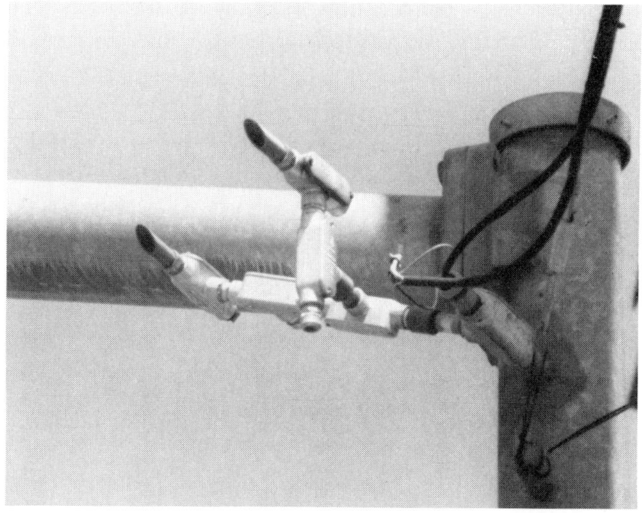

Fig. 9.2c Some Opticom systems use two sensors with one acting as a pre-sensor.

All maps should contain an indexing system which will assist the navigator to quickly find every street. Added to the index should be any local names used by the people in the community that might not otherwise appear on the map. Many roads have had name changes but are still referred to by the locals by their old names. Others have slang names given to them such as "Gasoline Alley," "The Boulevard," or are referred to by the name of the family who first lived on the road. As many as possible of these local names must be available to the crew.

When the map is used while responding to a call, the EMT who is not driving becomes the navigator. It is never advisable for this person to try and show the driver the route on the map. Instead, the navigator must become adept at interpreting the map and then telling the driver precisely where each turn will be and in which direction. It is extremely helpful to the driver for the navigator to give the names of the two streets prior to each turn. The driver can then identify the first street name given without having to slow the ambulance. The second street acts as a backup and as a countdown to the target street. When this system of street identification is used, the driver can maintain speed without having to slow for each street sign.

Once the map is opened, it should be left open for quick reference in case the route of travel has an unforeseen obstruction. Besides, there is nothing as distracting to a driver as someone who has trouble folding a damn map. A map-book which illustrates small segments of the community on each page is preferred to large fold-out maps.

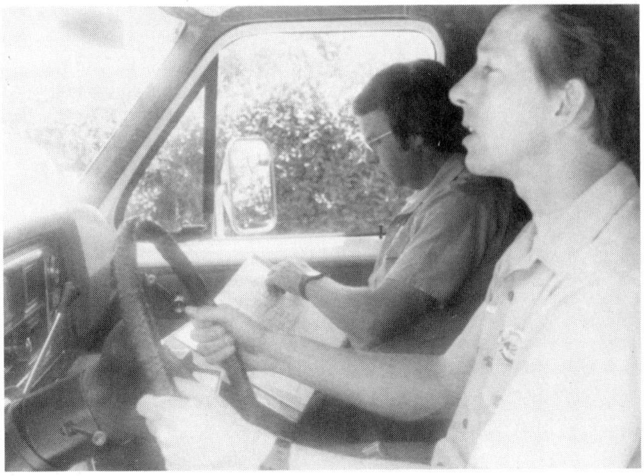

Fig. 9.3 The EMT who is not driving should read the map and become navigator, verbally directing the driver to the scene.

In order to perform his mission properly, the ambulance must take into consideration both speed and safety and then be able to quickly determine the most expedient route. The driver must also be able to quickly alter the route should conditions necessitate a change. By knowing these rules, quick route planning will be made much easier.

Use of Helicopters

In areas where helicopters may be called for assistance, ambulance crews must become familiar with how to read legal descriptions on a map. Obviously, helicopters cannot swoop out of the sky to check the name of a road on the sign. Helicopter pilots navigate by plotting square miles. These show up on a map as RANGE, TOWNSHIP, and SECTIONS. Range and township identifications are easy to find since they are printed along the border of a map. Section numbers often are not printed on the map, so the user must count them himself. To count section numbers, the user must begin in the upper right-hand corner of each township (townships are usually delineated by bolder lines). He then counts from that corner across the township to the other side, right to left. Upon reaching the other side of the township, he drops down one row and counts back in the other direction (left to right), again dropping down and counting back when reaching the end. Each township contains 36 section squares, each representing a square mile. To make navigation even easier in rugged terrain, the informant might indicate that the helicopter is needed in the "northwest corner of the southwest corner" of the specific section. This information indicates the location is toward the center of the section but slightly to the southeast.

In order to better understand how this mapping system works, an example follows. A logger has been injured on an unnumbered road off Black Rock Creek. The ambulance crew has a leader who meets them at the junction of Union Creek Road and Road 242. Upon arriving at the scene, the crew determines a helicopter is needed to evacuate the logger. His injuries won't tolerate the ride out on the logging road. Looking at the map, the crew can determine they are within RANGE 1, EAST, and TOWNSHIP 27, SOUTH. They then count sections to find their location which is in SECTION 21. To make the location even easier to find within the rugged terrain, they can indicate that the patient is in the southwest corner of the northwest corner of SECTION 21.

Blazing a Trail

In calls such as the logging accident mentioned above, it is not unusual for more than one emergency vehicle to respond. A first-response unit, mountain rescue team, or sheriff might also respond with the ambulance. Often wilderness roads are not adequately marked. The first arriving crew will take any available leader with them to the scene, leaving those following to fend for themselves. The later arriving emergency personnel's task of finding the scene can be made easier if the first crew in will leave a flare behind at any intersection where they turn. The flare should be placed just a few feet down the desired road so the crews will know in which direction to turn. Keep in mind the potential fire hazards associated with the use of flares. Even dry dirt in some areas will burn.

Facilities Crucial to Route Planning

Along with knowing their way around the streets of a community, it is important for the ambulance crew to know the location of major facilities. These facilities often stand by themselves as landmarks. Such landmarks are often easier to use to identify locations than a simple

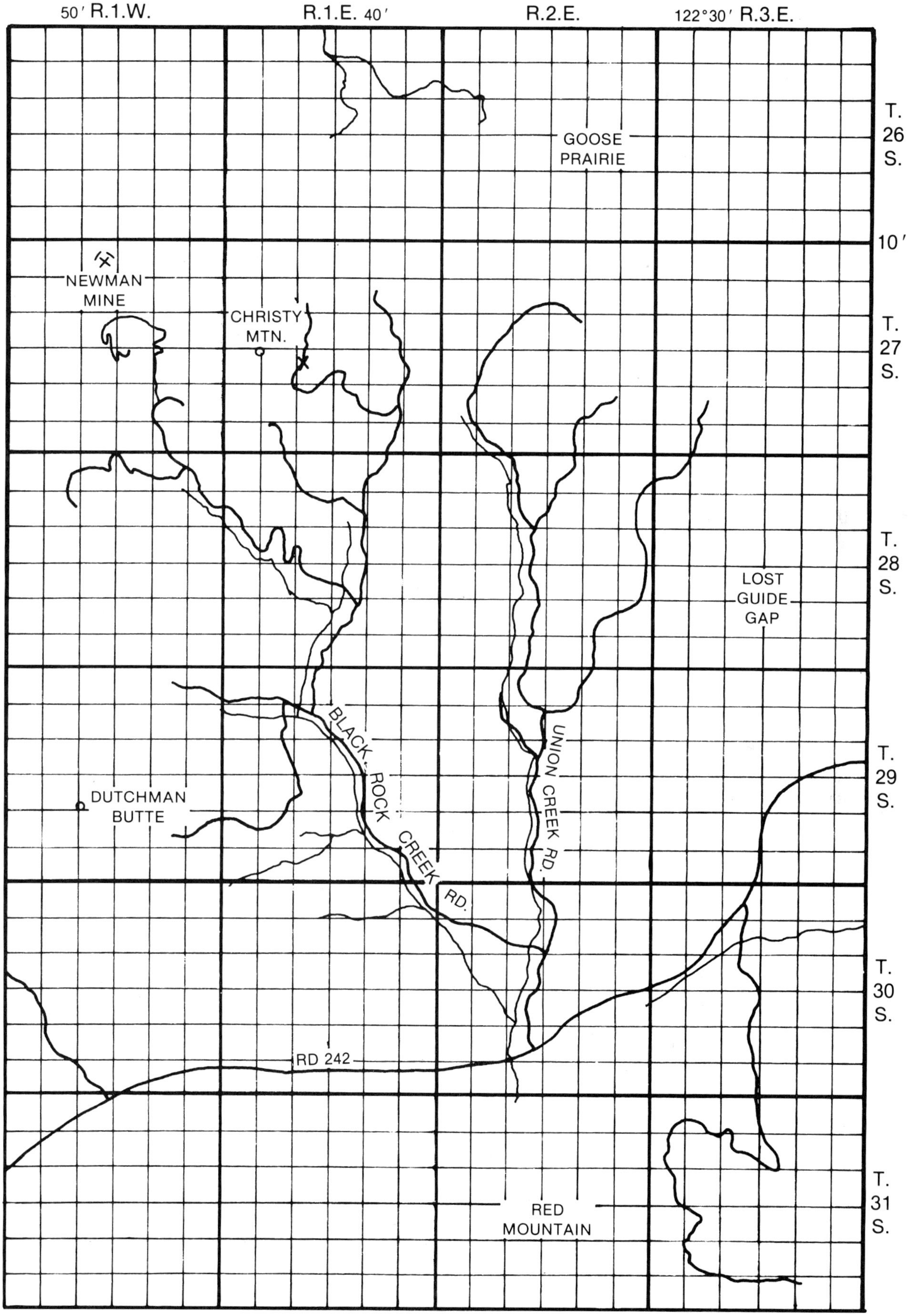
50′ R.1.W.
R.1.E. 40′
R.2.E.
122°30′ R.3.E.
T. 26 S.
GOOSE PRAIRIE
10′
NEWMAN MINE
CHRISTY MTN.
T. 27 S.
T. 28 S.
LOST GUIDE GAP
BLACK ROCK CREEK RD.
UNION CREEK RD.
T. 29 S.
DUTCHMAN BUTTE
T. 30 S.
RD 242
T. 31 S.
RED MOUNTAIN

street name. Landmarks may also be areas of periodic high density population, which will increase the likelihood for an emergency response to them. These facilities may also be more hazardous, again increasing the likelihood for a response.

One common denominator can be expected to exist when major facilities or landmarks are found within your coverage area. People calling for assistance will expect you and the dispatcher to know where they are without giving a street address or nearest cross street name. A caller might easily report a traffic accident by saying that it is in front of the "Middlesex School" and not give the dispatcher the opportunity to obtain any further information. It is then incumbent on the dispatcher and the crew to know where the Middlesex School is located. Such might also be the case with a church where a member is having a heart attack, a community center, auditorium,-concert hall, or stadium. Landmark names should be listed in the map index system with either the address or nearest cross streets referenced.

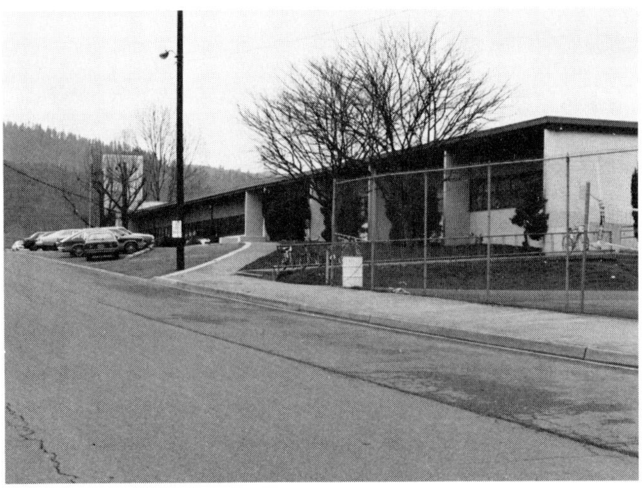

Fig. 9.4a Those calling for aid will expect the dispatcher and ambulance driver to know where they are simply by using landmarks. Ex.: "It's in front of the Middlesex School."

Many of these landmark-type facilities will also require the crew to know something about their layout in order to respond most efficiently. As an example, it would not at all be unusual for a caller to give apartment #85 of the Northridge Apartments and then expect the responsible public safety agency to not only know where the Northridge Apartments are located but also how the numbering system is laid out. Mobile home parks are especially confusing since space numbers are located in a different location for each park. Some numbers might be posted on the front of the home or on a lamp post in the front

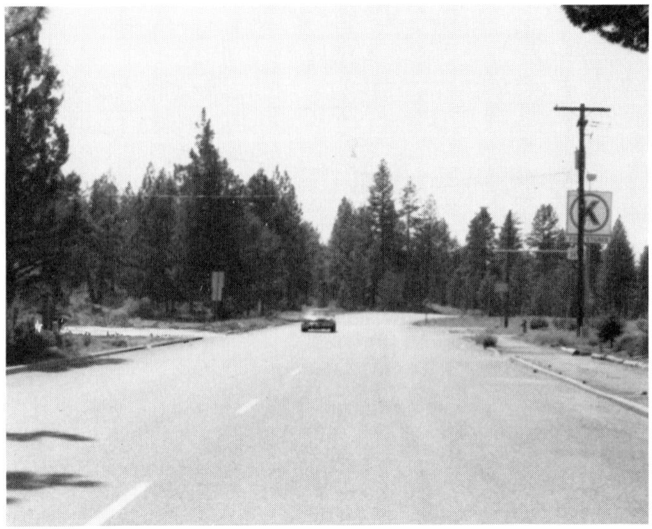

Fig. 9.4b Typical directions might consist of "It's at the driveway across from the Circle K."

yard, or they might be painted on the curb. You may even find the space number painted atop a carport. To assist the crew in knowing such information, the mapping system can have supplements which could include apartment and mobile home complex layouts. Large factories and mills should also have general areas of activity mapped out so if a call is received to, let's say, the loading dock, your response can be more direct. Shopping malls, often with several floors of small shops, should also be mapped out so you may park at the most appropriate entrance.

Maps alone are not enough to insure rapid response to these facilities. Ambulance crews, much like fire suppression crews, should have a general idea of the building or facility layout. This familiarity is obtained by touring each facility. Such a first-hand tour may expose little problems like an alley drawn on a map which is actually too narrow for an ambulance to pass through safely and other access problems that might not be apparent on a map. Whether the crew gets a chance to tour a facility or not, they must know how to get to a landmark facility with nothing more to go on than the facility's name.

Vehicle Height

Often an ambulance crew is asked to drive into a parking structure or under low overhangs to reach a patient. In each case, the driver must be able to determine rapidly whether the vehicle can safely pass. Such structures are frequently posted with a sign designating vehicle clearance limitations. If the ambulance has its height conspicuously printed on the dash, the driver can

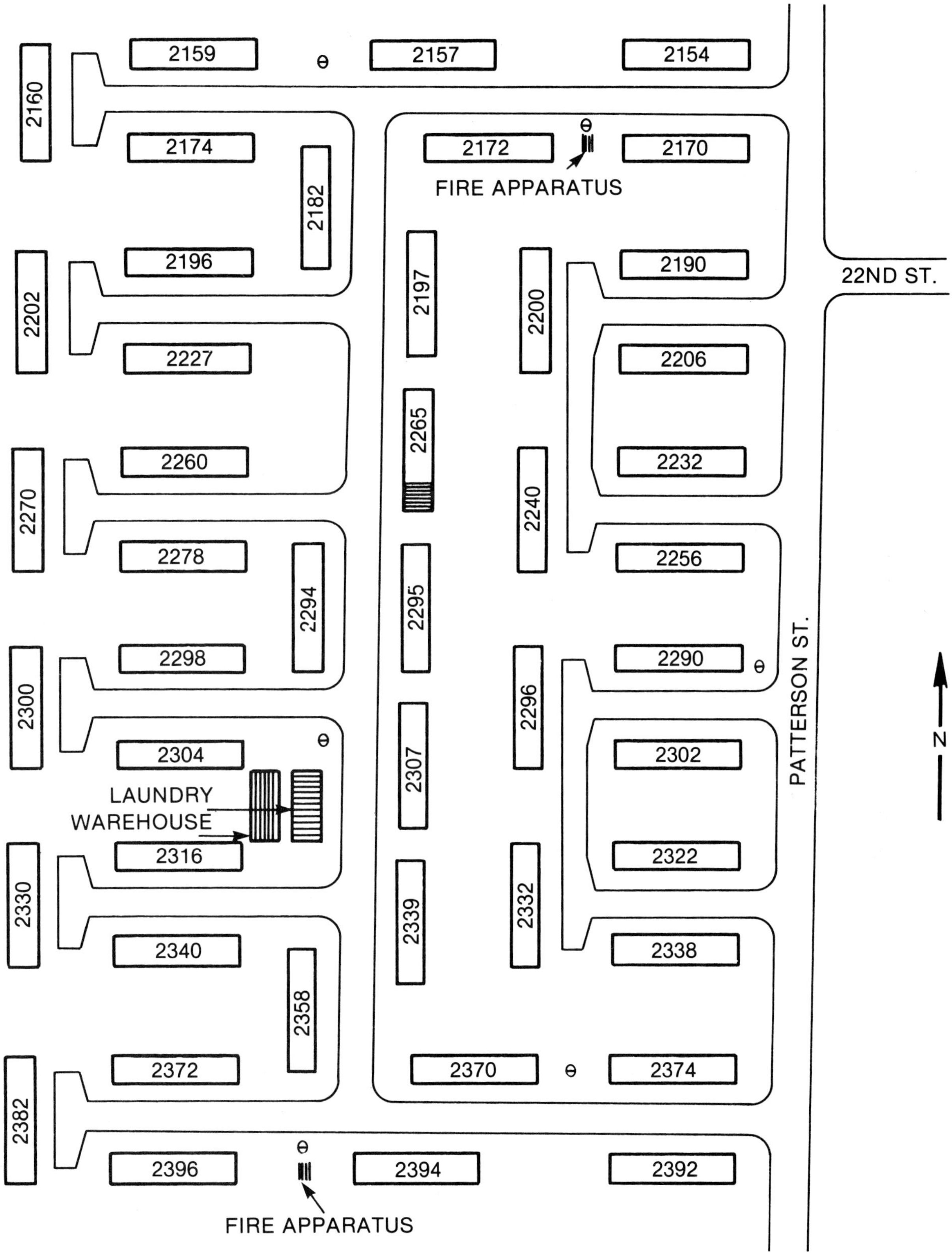

BURTON APARTMENTS

248 UNITS
SPEED LIMIT 12 MPH
θ = FIRE HYDRANT

Fig. 9.5a Some large facilities require the crew to know something about their layout so that the crew can respond efficiently. Apartment maps can be invaluable.

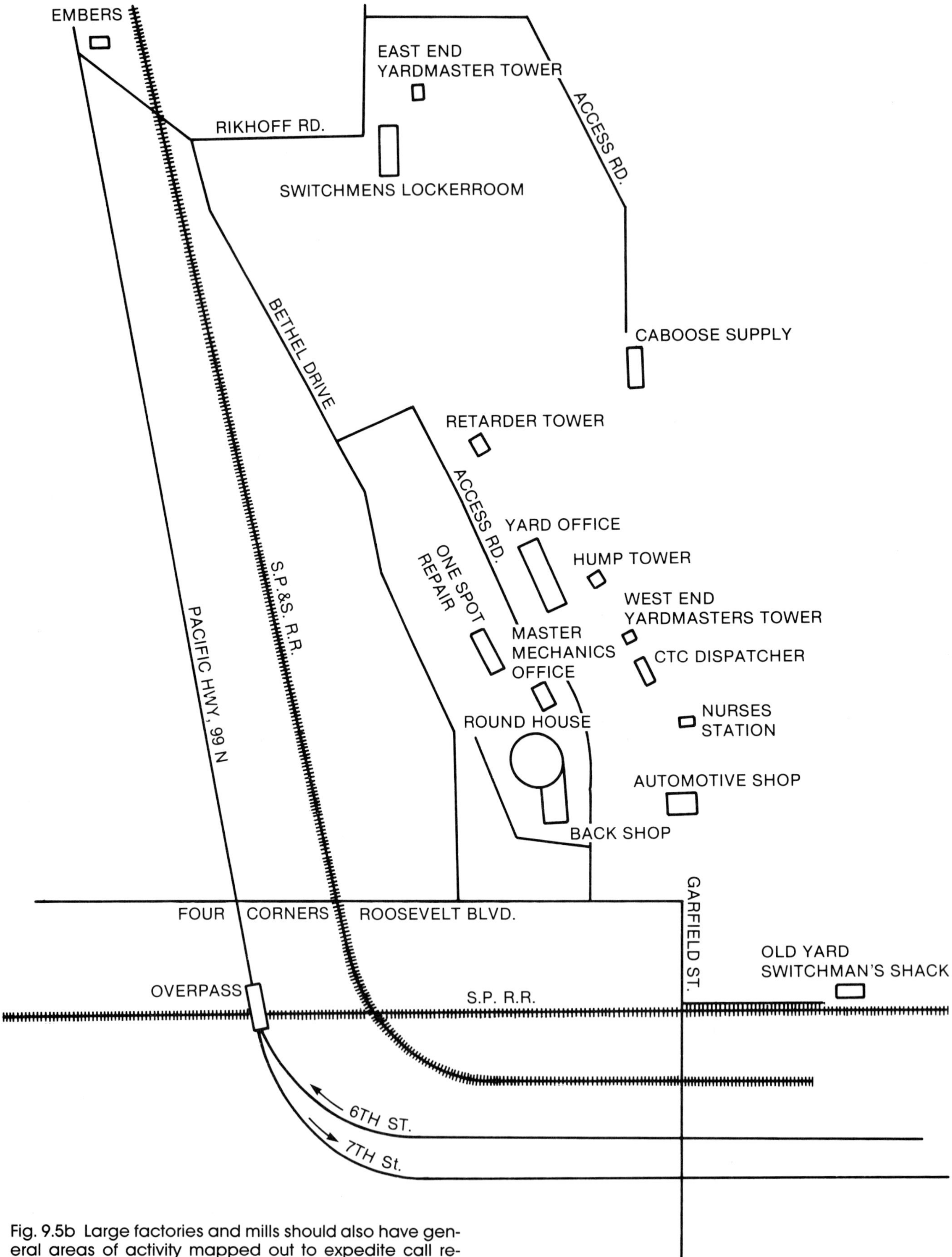

Fig. 9.5b Large factories and mills should also have general areas of activity mapped out to expedite call response.

easily determine if he has adequate clearance or must choose another route or park and walk to the scene.

Friends in The Sky

It seems as though nearly every city now has at least one "in the air" traffic reporter who broadcasts on a local radio station during the rush hours. Obviously, these reports can help motorists avoid the scene to which you are responding. More importantly, the ambulance crews on duty can monitor these radio stations during the rush hours and thus, keep abreast of unusual traffic conditions, before having to encounter them during an emergency response.

Know the New Stuff

It seems as though most communities have new developments that are constantly being undertaken. It is this development that identifies a healthy community. The development of new industry often calls for more housing and shopping centers. It is the duty of the ambulance crews to tour such projects, learning firsthand the location of all major structures, and then to map the area for future reference and reinforcement.

A good time to start learning new developments is while they are under construction. The nature of the construction itself is often dangerous, and so it is likely that the crew may have to respond during this period. Also, it is often easier to find out information about a complex that might be important later while it is under construction. An example of such information might be a shopping complex where alternative hallways exist. They are much easier to locate before they are closed off to the public.

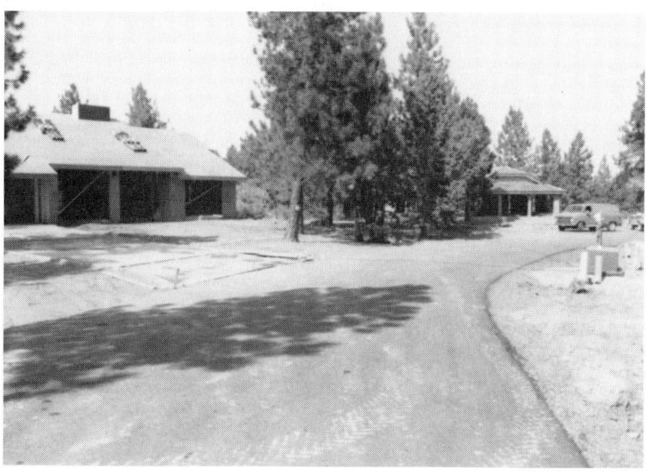

Fig. 9.6 Learn new street names and addressing systems before new homes are occupied.

Subdivisions often have streets that meander about and have many new names to be learned. It is a great help for the crew to have adequate time to begin learning the streets, their names, and their relationship to each other before a call is received. This extra time can be gained by beginning to familiarize yourself with the neighborhood before homes are occupied.

Familiarization tours should not be restricted to just one visit. Each duty crew needs to go back as often as necessary to fully learn the complex. It is especially important for the crew to visit a complex after it is completed. It is at this time that the landmarks, which will be referred to by future callers, will become apparent. Example: Playground on the Common. Only when the colors and trappings of completion and use are in place can a person get a proper mental image that will be useful when an emergency call is received.

Temporary Changes

Events are always occurring that can change the route to the scene of an emergency. In order for the driver to do anything about these changes, he must first be aware of them. Even when the ambulance driver has familiarized himself with his response area, he can't sit back secure in that knowledge. The area will change from day to day and even hour to hour. In order to really be able to know his area, the driver will have to understand those changes, what causes them, and where they will most likely be found. A well-prepared driver will then have alternatives in mind to deal with any change encountered. Example: The major route of travel to the hospital might be partially blocked by construction. The driver must first be aware of the situation and then analyze its effects. Are there alternative routes available? What are they like? If the alternatives entail rough roads, residential neighborhoods, or lengthy backtracking, the driver must be able to weigh these factors against the congestion, and uneven terrain of the construction zone in order to select the best route.

Major events, such as football games and shopping center grand openings, will almost always call for the modification of routes of travel. The EMS agency that takes these events into consideration ahead of time is way ahead of the game when a call is received during those heavy traffic periods. Some situations might even require a temporary change in the basing of the ambulance. Traffic congestion and crowds go hand in hand to increase the potential for illness or injury. During such an event, emergency medical access to someone attending it may be difficult and lengthy. By stationing crews closer to event sites ahead of time but not in the expected mainstream of traffic, access to an attendee may then be quickened.

Weather factors can cause a driver to alter the normal route of travel. The ambulance driver must know the whereabouts of the steep hills and if alternative routes exist so they can be avoided during icy conditions. In addition, the driver should also be familiar with where high winds are the most prevalent. These areas, along with bridges and overpasses, will be the first to freeze. Some streets may become more slick from rain than others; these should be avoided. Any street with low spots that may fill with water or roads across low lying lands should also be avoided during wet weather.

Adverse weather conditions can slow traffic into certain areas, again making temporary redeployment of ambulances an alternative worthy of consideration.

It is imperative that good communications be maintained between the ambulance dispatch center, or 9-1-1, and the street and highway maintenance departments, police agencies, and the weather bureau so that relevant information can be given to the crew as soon as problems are detected. This line of communication will help the crew to select alternative routes, even before an emergency response is required.

Local Characteristics

While this text can discuss in general terms what is needed to efficiently navigate and predetermine routes of travel, each crew member must have specific knowledge of his own coverage area. For instance, many areas are laid out in one-way grids. Each street in the core area has traffic flowing in only one direction. Such patterns usually alternate, with one street heading north and the next one south, or one heading east and the next west. Such engineering seems to work well for moving large volumes of traffic, but can create problems for the emergency vehicle driver.

When operating within such a grid system, the driver must know the addressing system of the area to avoid lengthy backtracking. Example: The crew is responding to an address in the 600 block of a one-way southbound street. The address numbers become higher as the street continues south. By approaching this street from the south, the crew will have to find a through northbound street and travel to a point beyond the 600 block, then double back. This may be easy, or it may make for considerable backtracking as you will learn later in this chapter.

Additionally, knowledge of addressing systems becomes important to the crew when determining such locations as the particular portion of a segmented street. The crew also needs to understand on which side of the street to find the odd and even numbers to make the finding of a specific address quicker. Where appropriate, using mnemonics such as ONE for odd north and east may be helpful. This particular mnemonic means that the odd numbers are on the north and east sides of the street. To help you find an address quickly, the public should be encouraged to post numbers conspicuously on contrasting backgrounds where they may be easily seen.

Many areas have expressways available for traveling between different parts of the community. While expressways are great for use by most motorists, they should be avoided by the ambulance when not responding to a call. Here's an example that will illustrate why. A crew working from a substation is asked to move to a location that will cover both their own response area and that of the main station. All the main station ambulances are committed. The crew decides to use the freeway as the fastest route to that standby point. After driving for a couple of miles they receive a call to a traffic accident not far from their substation. It is now another three miles to the next interchange, which means the crew will have to travel six miles out of their way, three going to the interchange and three more while doubling back. For this reason it is then usually better to avoid driving on the freeway when in service but not responding to a call. Additionally, any time spent on the surface streets will help the crew to REFRESH themselves with the streets and addresses in the less familiar area.

Freeways can present problems for the crew when the call is on them too. When a collision occurs on the freeway, traffic usually backs up severely. Entering the freeway too soon may put the ambulance into more traffic congestion than they can negotiate. For this reason the crew must be familiar with where all the entrances and exits are located in order to be able to get close to the accident without encountering excess traffic. On some rare occasions, the ambulance may have to enter the expressway from an off ramp and travel the wrong way to get to the scene. Such occurrences should only take place when the collision totally blocks all oncoming traffic.

It is very helpful for the crew to know in which lanes the collision has occurred. This information may make a difference in how they will access the expressway and from which direction. If the ambulance approaches from the opposite direction, one crewperson can jump out and go to the scene while the driver continues to the next exit to access the proper lanes. This cannot happen if the collision occurs on a multidecked bridge. On a multideck bridge, the traffic flows in one direction on one level and in the opposite direction on the other level. When such bridges are found in the coverage area, it is imperative for the crew to be familiar with all access points, including any stairs between levels.

In some larger metropolitan areas, certain portions of expressways are used strictly for one-way through traffic either to the core area or completely bypassing the core. These express lanes travel in one direction during the morning rush hours and in the opposite direction in the evening. Since these roadways change direction and often have VERY limited access, it is essential that the dispatchers and ambulance crews be completely familiar with these characteristics. Should an accident occur on the express lanes during limited-access periods, it may be necessary to dispatch a unit many miles "upstream" rather than one a few blocks away, since the closer vehicle will be unable to efficiently reach the scene.

The time of day can present the ambulance driver with specific traffic problems which he should take into account before choosing a route. Most everyone is aware of the typical rush hour traffic experienced on major roadways between 7-9 a.m. and 4-6 p.m. There are other rush-hour conditions that can create smaller areas of traffic congestion. The times that schools open and close can create a temporary jam, especially around high schools. A large factory or mill may employ three shifts, creating three rush hour periods each working day. If your preplanned route takes you past such an area, it would be advisable to have alternate routes chosen for these congested periods.

Every area has its short cuts, and the ambulance driver should know where they are. The use of short cuts won't always work for every driver. Most motorists tend to feel more at ease in the flow of the traffic within a sort of comfort zone. Short cuts only work for drivers with a certain amount of aggressiveness. An ambulance driver must have this quality, being careful to stay within the bounds of courtesy. For example, a short cut might allow the ambulance to slip into an opening that might present itself rather than to line up in the long line of cars trying to access a bridge. The hazard comes when some nonaggressive motorist tries to use the route and ends up blocking it for a long period while waiting for an extra long gap in traffic.

Keep in mind that if you use short cuts, you run the risk of creating ill feelings with the public you serve. Shortcutting should only be done during an emergency response and must be performed with great caution.

Routing Problems

Using the map and the following text, we can demonstrate a few examples of route problems that may be encountered. Once you have become familiar with the map and the response area, the text will develop some examples of preplanned routes.

This is a map which includes a segment of the city within the coverage area of your station. For the purposes of this exercise, your station is at 922 F Street, a two-way street. F Street becomes a one-way street one block north of your station. The hospital is in a residential neighborhood at 511 Jackson. Jackson is a through street for the area. The area between 1st and 8th and A and K Streets is primarily commercial with one-way streets. Highway 12, which becomes 1st and 2nd, is a major east/west arterial. Although Highway 12 is easily traveled, it usually becomes congested with traffic when the city basketball team is playing at home in the Tyler Pavilion. Additionally, Highway 12 is heavily congested during rush hours. Another west-to-east one-way arterial is 8th Street. It too becomes clogged during rush hour. Twelfth Street is a major two-way east/west arterial. Because 12th is out of the commercial core area, it does not become as congested as the other east/west arteries.

The major north/south arterials are Milford Road (two-way) and E and F Streets, each one-way until they meet south of 8th. A major residential area exists in the Hill Drive area. Direct access from your station to the Hill Drive subdivisions is across the railroad tracks. It's a high-call-volume area.

Grove is the link to the neighboring town and is bordered by several industrial complexes.

Now that you have learned some of the characteristics of this response area and its traffic patterns, let's develop some preplanned response routes.

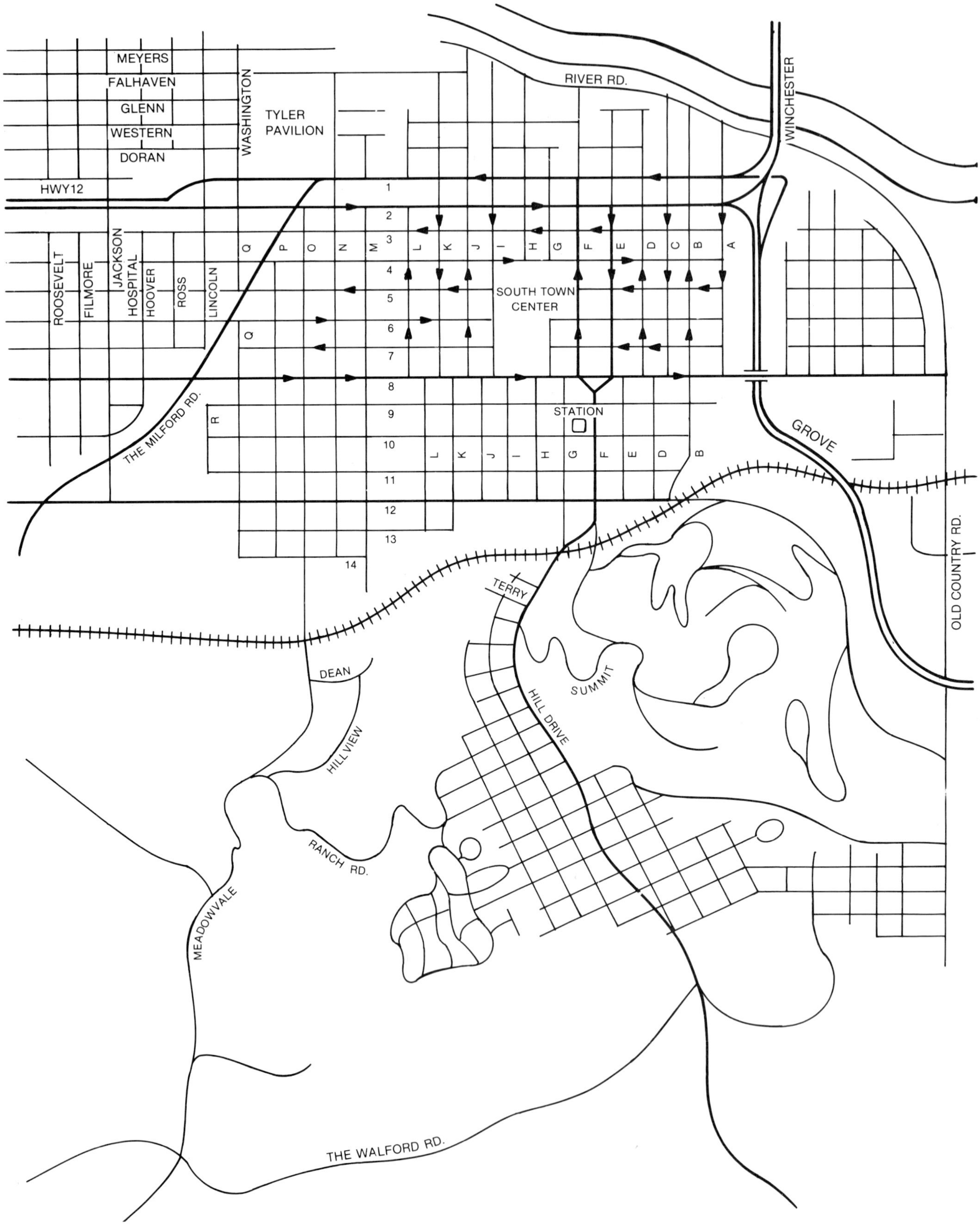
MEYERS
FALHAVEN
GLENN
WESTERN
DORAN
WASHINGTON
TYLER PAVILION
RIVER RD.
WINCHESTER
HWY12
ROOSEVELT
FILMORE
JACKSON HOSPITAL
HOOVER
ROSS
LINCOLN
SOUTH TOWN CENTER
STATION
THE MILFORD RD.
GROVE
OLD COUNTRY RD.
TERRY
DEAN
HILLVIEW
SUMMIT
HILL DRIVE
RANCH RD.
MEADOWVALE
THE WALFORD RD.

Route Planning Examples

Here are some examples of route planning. Refer to the map and keep in mind the conditions noted in the previous section.

Example 1. While traveling on Grove Avenue near the Old County Road, you receive a non-emergency call that will take you north out of the city on Winchester Road. It is 5:30 p.m. and you know from experience that the ramp that will place you onto Winchester from Grove backs up several blocks with traffic trying to get north out of the city. An alternative route might very well be to take Grove north around to 1st Street and then turn left onto A, then left onto 2nd Street which will take you over the Winchester Bridge. Such a diverse route will often work best because most motorists will not want to try to access arterial traffic from a side street. If the driver knows how to gauge traffic intervals well, accessing an arterial can be done with little problem.

Example 2. From the hospital on Jackson Street at 5th Street, you receive a call to 445 D Street. First, you need to realize that D Street is a one-way street running north and so the best way to access it with a minimum of doubling back is from 8th. By taking 2nd to E Street, you would have to go south past the intended address by two blocks to 6th Street and then turn back north on D Street. As an alternative you could take 2nd Street to C Street and then take 5th to D Street. Still you would be traveling three blocks north to 2nd, one block beyond the designated street to the east, one half-block beyond the address to 6th, and then the half block on D to the address. All of this turning of corners, even if the emergency equipment is used, takes time in urban traffic.

Example 3. Segmented streets can also present problems in forming a route of travel. On the map, 7th Street has three different segments. The only way then to formulate a route of travel is to know which addresses are contained in each segment. It is very helpful if the dispatcher can obtain a cross street as a reference.

Example 4. Returning to your station, eastbound on 12th at L Street, you receive a call to 419 H Street. The first inclination would be to continue on 12th to H and take H north. But, as you can see on the map, this would force a considerable detour around the shopping center. In order to get to the scene quickly you must take L or K to 8th and then take J Street to 4th.

Example 5. It is a Thursday evening, about a half hour before the basketball game is to start at the Tyler Pavilion. You receive a call to Glenn and Roosevelt. Under normal traffic conditions, it would probably be best to take F north to 1st Street, then west to Jackson and north to Glenn, leading into Roosevelt. Since there is game traffic, 1st Street will be heavily congested with slow traffic trying to get to Tyler Pavilion. In this case, it would probably be better to go south to 12th Street and then west to Jackson even though this route would cause you to double back four blocks.

Example 6. The railroad yards lie between Meadowvale and Hill Drive and can be accessed from M, Dean, and Terry Streets.Which route would you travel to get to the switchman's shack? Without knowledge of the shack's location, you would be lost unless the dispatcher had obtained that information. A separate map drawn by the ambulance crew or, better yet, one provided by the rail yard would be of benefit.

Example 7. Where streets do not line up properly and a one-way grid is in place, additional problems may be encountered. Returning to the station eastbound on 12th at L, you receive a call to 340 J. Your first inclination might be to take J straight through from 12th to the address. Through careful evaluation of your map, you can see that J Street doesn't align properly and that this route will actually force you to travel a considerable distance out of your way. You will also have to contend with the mall traffic due to the additional restrictions imposed by the one-way grid on 8th and J Streets.

From the examples above, it should be apparent how knowledge of the coverage area and route planning go hand in hand. When these two components are properly united, the speed and efficiency of the emergency response is greatly increased. So, too, is the safety of the mission when high-density traffic areas and uncontrolled intersections are avoided.

10 EMERGENCY DRIVING

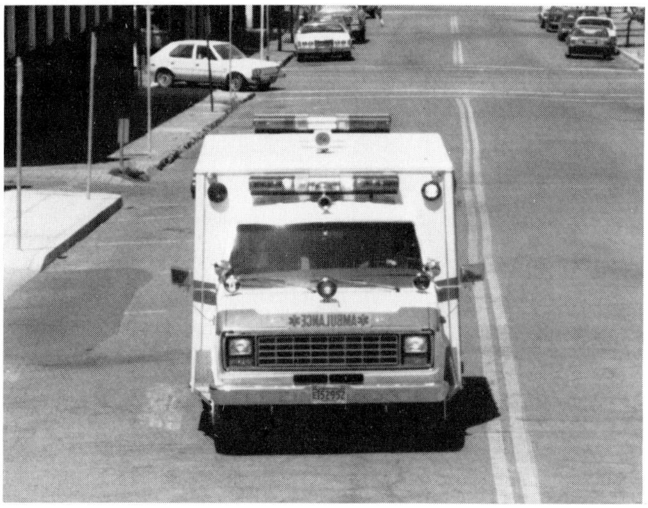

The term ambulance driver, used frequently in this text since it is a text on driving the ambulance, is nevertheless looked upon with disdain by many EMTs. It refers to the day when ambulance attendants had no training in emergency medicine and were often hired merely for their ability to drive. Since the attendants couldn't provide proper patient care, the only activity for them to perform was to rapidly transport the patient to the hospital. Those pre-EMTs can be forgiven for that attitude, and their ignorance of what such an ambulance ride was doing to the patient. But today, EMTs can provide prehospital care for the patient, and do far more than just drive the ambulance. The role of driving the ambulance obviously exists even though many look upon it as a secondary task, or try to avoid it altogether. Since ambulance driving not only exists but has grown as a profession since the 1960s, EMS professionals need to reevaluate ambulance driving skills. The many advancements in patient care have overshadowed one of the EMT basics—transportation of the sick and injured.

Emergency ambulance driving and high-speed driving are two distinctly different activities. High-speed driving may seem heroic, a desperate attempt to save a life at all cost, but it is in fact dangerous for the patient, the crew, and everyone else on the road. The jeopardy placed upon all of these parties is far greater than the potential loss of the patient's life. Even when responding to the scene of a medical emergency, there is NO justification to drive at excessively high speeds and endanger yourself and others on the road.

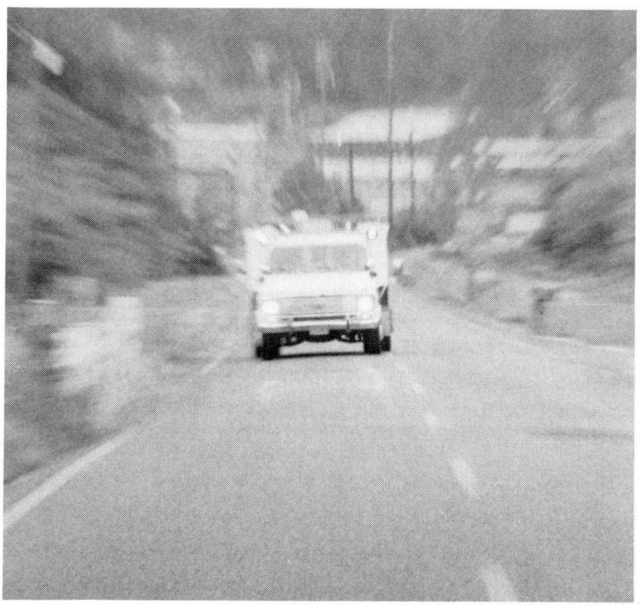

Fig. 10.1 Ambulance drivers should become aware of the difference between emergency and high speed driving.

The use of the emergency lights and siren can in no way guarantee safe, unobstructed passage. No matter what any law states, the emergency signaling devices only serve to notify the public of your presence and to request the right of way. If the public does not yield to the ambulance, you must continue to drive in a safe, courteous manner. Usually, the public will yield to an emergency vehicle if given sufficient time to (1) realize that it is there, (2) make a decision as to what to do, and (3) carry out that decision. The public must have sufficient time provided to them which is not available if the vehicle is traveling at high speed. Even during an emergency response, there is time for courtesy, and in fact, if you take the time to let a motorist make a rational decision as to how to best help you, your response time to your destination will most likely be quicker. Understand, it takes a panicked driver longer to overcome his panic and react properly than it would if he wasn't frightened by a blaring siren while an ambulance tried to drive up his tailpipe. No one in his right mind would attempt to pass such a motorist while he is still in a state of panic. In short, time is lost while this driver gets his act back together.

The use of emergency signaling systems actually increases the danger of collision. Other motorists and pedestrians may not react in the manner you expect; reasonable speed gives them time to react and, if needed, time for you to counteract any inappropriate response by the public.

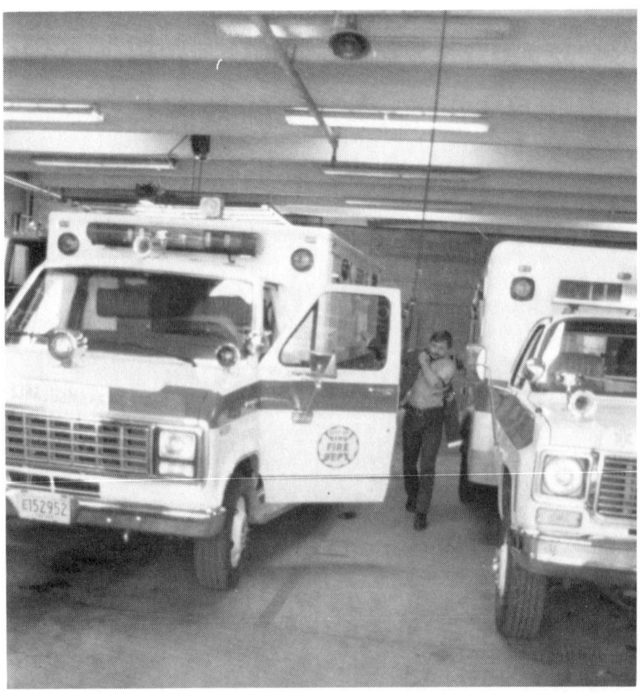

Fig. 10.2a Running to the ambulance saves little time in the long run and may produce an "adrenalin rush" that's hard to control.

Speed limits are designated with normal traffic conditions and the quality of the road in mind. To think that one can take an ambulance which is larger than the average vehicle and drive it significantly faster while the road quality and traffic remain the same is dangerous. Instead, emergency ambulance driving provides a method of getting through clogged traffic, not by weaving around through it, but by methodically moving it from your path, while maintaining a wide margin for error between you and others. You must always give consideration to road and traffic conditions, since basically you cannot change them. This is not to say that you can't drive expeditiously; you can, but always within the confines of what the road and traffic conditions will safely allow. When the lights and siren are used judiciously, and with courtesy, the general public will feel good about their EMS system and be more willing to lend it support, and you will find that your job becomes much easier.

Response Time

Public safety agencies frequently go to elaborate lengths to shave a few seconds off response times, often to the detriment of the employees and those around them. While there is a need to economize time as much as possible, when carried to extremes, such methods can have harmful effects. Examples of activities to save time include leaving the ambulance door open to save that second it takes to open it, or running to the vehicle instead of walking. Obviously, running will get the old sympathetic nervous system working and increase the adrenalin flow. This "fight or flight" reaction becomes hard to overcome and soon you will find yourself driving faster than you really intended. Finding yourself in that predica-

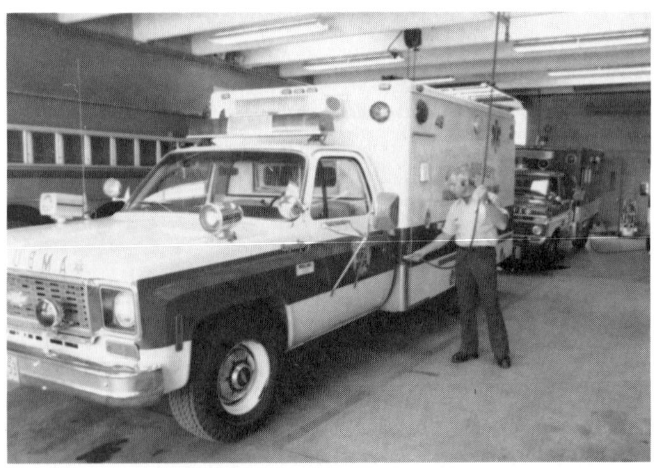

Fig. 10.2b Approaching the ambulance smartly and relaxed will make for a more organized and careful response.

ment, hopefully you will attempt to slow down. But, as stated before, once a certain speed is attained it is much harder to slow and keep the speed down for an appreciable amount of time. Such an attempt will result in a feeling of going too slow and the driver will again subconsciously start increasing speed. As the speed increases, events begin to occur faster than you can deal with them, increasing driver tension. You will begin to grip the wheel, stare, and lose your proper visual habits. Such occurrences become a vicious circle, as poor visual habits fail to identify occurring events, and tension increases dramatically.

Imagine arriving at the scene in such a tense state. You run to the patient's side, out of breath and with frayed nerves. It may become difficult to concentrate on the matters at hand, and you appear confused to the people relying on you for help. You may also find it easy to take information for granted. Your patient interview and exam will suffer. If the call came in as a heart attack, you may try to fit the patient's signs and symptoms to your preconceived notions rather than trying to determine the problem through his signs and symptoms.

What is really gained by such time economizing? Seconds, and at the most a couple of minutes. Ask yourself, "Will the patient really exsanguinate in that brief time saved?" "Will that savings really help the patient with severe abdominal pains?" In the vast majority of cases, the slight time savings will probably not matter. Even in the very rare cases where a minute or two quicker response to the patient's side will make a difference, the time saved by a high-speed response cannot justify the jeopardy to which the general public is exposed.

The Emergency System

The emergency lights and siren are often thought of as a warning system and are so described. Rather, it is an audio/visual system which alerts others to the presence of an emergency vehicle. As an alerting system, each component has specific manners in which it can be used to obtain the greatest efficiency. Each component also has several limitations. The two components of the alerting system, the emergency lights and siren, will be discussed individually.

Emergency Lights

Turn on the emergency lights at the base station and they will appear very bright to you. That is because you have a specific interest in the action of emergency vehicles. Even when you are off duty, emergency lights quickly gain your attention. In reality, the emergency lights used have severe limitations which hinder their ability to be seen by the public. Although they appear bright and easily discernable, this just is not the case.

Location. The first concern with emergency lights should be their placement on the vehicle. Lights placed only on the top of the vehicle can go unseen. This is especially true when the ambulance approaches small cars from behind. Instead of gaining the driver's attention in his rear view mirror, the light beams pass overhead.

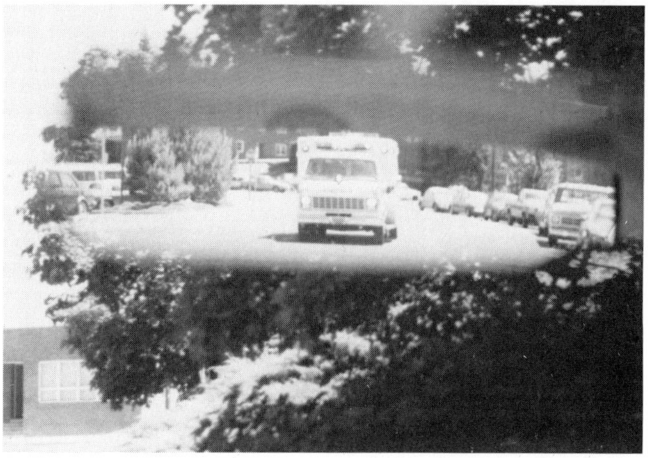

Fig. 10.3a Lights placed high on a vehicle are visible above traffic and may be seen by those you are trying to alert.

A more desirable placement of lights would be to have the main lights high on the vehicle with additional lights mounted low, either on the hood or in the grill. Low-mounted lights can then be seen better by small car drivers.

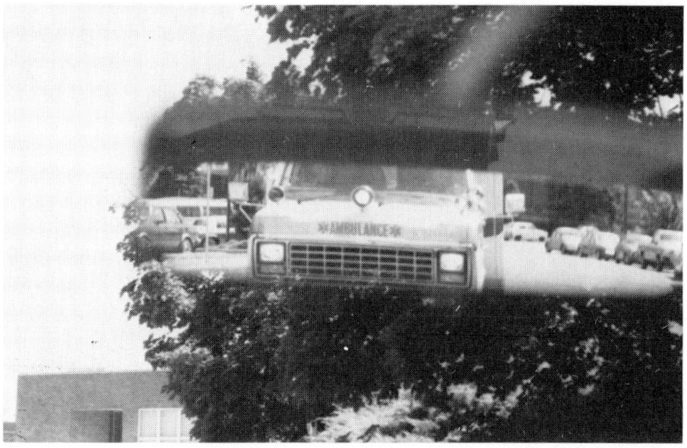

Fig. 10.3b Extra lights should be placed on the cowl or in the grill to be seen in a rearview mirror at close range.

Too Many Lights. Some ambulance operators apparently think the more lights used the better. Most ambulances are equipped with many more emergency lights than other emergency vehicles, such as police cars and fire apparatus. The number of lights in use may actually be causing problems.

When observed at a distance, an ambulance with several emergency lights flashing at different frequencies can present a very confusing picture. Although other motorists may recognize that there is a problem ahead, they may become confused about how to deal with it.

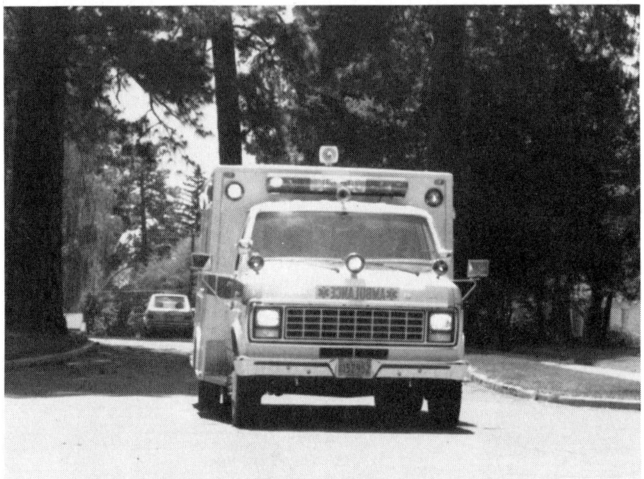

Fig. 10.4 Too many lights on a vehicle can create confusion at a distance and panic at close range.

Viewed at close range, the emergency lights will present another problem. The number of lights will overwhelm the driver's visual senses and thus, he will be much more likely to panic.

The reason for these problems is that the light flashes are not coordinated. The overheads may or may not have a coordinated flash frequency, and certainly they will not be synchronized with the other lights, such as those mounted on the cowling or the side flashers. Additionally, the lights are often of more than one color, again lending to confusion.

While the need for the low-mounted as well as the high lights has been stated, having them the same color and the flashes coordinated will help reduce others' confusion. A vehicle equipped with only a few emergency lights may actually be better able to move traffic from its path. Fewer lights will also reduce the power demands on the vehicle while parked at emergency scenes.

Glare

Obviously the emergency lights are not going to be as easily observed in daylight as they are at night. During periods when the sun is low on the horizon, it can overpower or "wash out" emergency lights. A driver looking into the sun will be unable to detect the lights. Unfortunately, such periods often correspond with rush hour traffic.

While it is easy to understand the visual problems experienced by a driver looking into the sun, you may not realize that a motorist traveling at an angle to the sun or even away from it might also be blinded. Sunlight reflecting off the polished metals, windows, and the mirrors of other vehicles, storefronts, or light-colored walls can be every bit as bright as the sun itself. Even if glare does not partially blind the driver, it may keep him from being able to use his rearview mirror.

Use of Lights. Of the many lights mounted on the ambulance, which should be used and how? Certainly the headlights should be used, even in the daytime. Even though there is a risk of adding to others' confusion, the white light of the headlights will often be seen before the red lights of the emergency system. This is because the frequency of white light allows for greater broadcast at a lower candle power than red or blue. While the headlights do not serve notice to others of an emergency, they may draw just enough attention to your vehicle for other drivers to then be able to see your emergency lights. The results of one extensive study showed that driving with headlights on low beam during daylight reduced head-on collisions by 50%.

When the headlights are used, they should only be used on low beam, since high beam tends to mask the emergency lights both in daylight and darkness.

Some ambulances are equipped with headlight flashers which, when utilized, flash the headlights alternately. Again, while there is a risk of confusion, such a system may be helpful during an emergency response in daylight for the same reason that headlights are used. The benefit is that the flashing lights are more likely to draw attention than steady lights. When the vehicle is equipped with flashers, they should be connected to a separate switch isolated from the other emergency lights. The headlight flashers should not be used at night as their use may actually contribute to driver vertigo, since they will limit and confuse your night vision. Of course at night, the high beams should be used as much as possible. Remember, even during an emergency response, you must dim the brights when approaching other vehicles. Keep in mind that although you are requesting the right-of-way when operating emergency signaling devices, you do not own the road.

The four-way hazard flashers are often used by some ambulance personnel, perhaps theorizing that more is better. However, these lights do not have sufficient power to lend help to the emergency lights and only serve to add to the confusion. When the four-way flashers are activated, the turn signals will not work. The emergency lights will be of little value if other motorists do not have any idea of your intentions. Thus, the turn signals should always be used.

The ambulance should also be equipped with spotlights. Such tools are invaluable when searching for addresses on dark streets and rural roads. Judicious use of the spotlight can also help to move traffic. However, great care must taken when using a spotlight since its powerful beam can easily blind other drivers. The light should be turned away from all traffic before it is turned on. It is then swept rapidly across the rearview mirror of the driver ahead. Take care not to allow the light beam to linger on his mirror. The intent is to flash the light across the mirror, thus getting the driver's attention. The light should not be visible by the time the driver can lift his eyes to his mirror. At this point, he will be able to see your flashing emergency lights. Any lingering light on the mirror will almost certainly temporarily blind the driver or mask your emergency lights, defeating your intentions.

The spotlight on the left side of the ambulance should be used. This is because it provides the best angle to hit the leading vehicle's sideview and rearview mirrors. By quickly flashing the light across the rearview mirror in a direction toward the right side of the road, you will keep the light from being directed into the eyes of oncoming drivers. This act is much more difficult if the left outside mirror is used as a target.

The danger of blinding oncoming drivers with the beam is another reason to use the spotlight located on the driver's side. Certainly such spotlight techniques should not be performed routinely. The spotlight should only be used as a last resort in gaining the lead vehicle driver's attention.

Light Preference. The ideal emergency light system will include a light bar, utilizing only one color of lenses, mounted on or near the top of the vehicle. The bar should have both sides flashing in a synchronous pattern so the vehicle can be recognized at a distance. A light bar is preferable to individual rotator lights because of the synchronous flashing. In addition, emergency lights should be mounted lower on the vehicle so as to be seen at relatively close distance by drivers of small vehicles. Two lights mounted on the hood or in front of the grill work well. These lights should also be synchronized with one another. The only other recommended emergency lights would be flashers on each corner of the sides of the patient compartment. These are mounted below the roof line. The same type of flashers should also be mounted on the back of the patient compartment. All of the lights should be the same color, which will reduce confusion. The only exception might be the use of amber-colored lights for the patient compartment flashers facing towards the rear.

Today, strobe lights are also commonly used on ambulances. Because strobes flash with such high intensity, many operators believe that they can catch someone's attention easily. While strobes may look great in the garage, they are not any more effective on the road than the regular emergency light systems. Strobes flash so rapidly that their light is gone before other motorists can determine from where the flash is coming. Additionally, there is a problem with strobe lights triggering seizures in some people, even if they are without prior history of seizures. Strobe lights are of little or no benefit when used on moving vehicles and may actually be more dangerous than valuable.

The Siren

The siren seems to be the least understood component of the emergency signaling equipment. Why? Perhaps because you can see the lights and where they project their beams. The same is not true of the siren. Therefore, many emergency vehicle operators expect it to be heard by other motorists under conditions where they cannot possibly hear it. Additionally, many ambulance operators expect others to immediately recognize the siren for what it is and take immediate and proper action. For some people's subconscious, the siren builds an invisible force field around their ambulance, shielding it from other vehicles on the road. Obviously, the siren is not this omnipotent, and in fact the opposite is true. Instead of eliminating all potential for trouble, the siren invites trouble.

While the crew often views the use of the siren as indispensble while trying to get through traffic, EMTs must realize that it has only negative effects on everyone concerned. It doesn't matter how experienced the driver may be, the sound of the siren will have a tendency to cause him to drive a little faster than he otherwise should. The siren's rhythm constantly reminds him of the urgency at hand and excites the sympathetic nervous system. This outflow of adrenalin may in turn cause the driver to take risks he ordinarily wouldn't take. The siren can also cause a kind of hypnosis. This hypnosis can cause the driver to become less attentive to the task at hand. Thus, he will not recognize potentially hazardous situations until it's too late.

The sound produced by the siren occupies the same audio frequencies as human speech. Thus, siren use can make verbal communication within the vehicle difficult. During its use, the driver may have difficulty differentiating similar sounds, not even realizing it. He may think the dispatcher is telling him seven thirty-four for an address, while in reality it may be eleven thirty-four, an error of four blocks. The same type of hearing problems can occur during conversation between crew members. At times, only portions of conversation will be heard distinctly. The faster the siren cycles, the more apparent such problems become.

If the siren can have deleterious effects on the crew, even when conditioned to it, what kind of effect will it have on the general public? Talking with motorists forced to the side of the road by the siren revealed statements like: "You almost caused me to have a wreck, comin' up behind me and blowing that siren like you did." The siren can create tremendous anxiety in other drivers. They may then perform irrational acts such as impulsively pulling into a congested intersection or changing lanes without looking. It is not at all uncommon for a frightened motorist to stop dead in his path, his senses overwhelmed. These inappropriate actions occur when others hear the siren. Conversely, other motorists may respond with statements like: "How was I to know you were behind me? Your siren certainly wasn't loud enough to hear." Such diverse conditions create a dilemma for the ambulance crew. While the siren is easily heard by the crew, sitting right underneath the speakers, it may not be easily heard by the motorist you're trying to alert to your presence.

Modern technology would easily allow louder sirens to be manufactured for the ambulance. Unfortunately, louder sirens could permanently injure the hearing of those frequently in its close proximity (e.g., the crew). Most electronic sirens in use today are as loud as safety will allow (approximately 95 decibels (db) of sound at 100 feet). Of that 95 db, as much as 30 db of intensity can be lost as the sound passes through the window glass and insulation of another motorist's vehicle. If people are talking in the car at 60 db (normal speech), you can easily understand why there is little chance for the siren to be heard by others, and this is only the beginning of the problem. Vehicles traveling in the same direction as the ambulance are actually pulling away from the sound produced by the siren. The 95 db figure given earlier is registered at 100 feet. If your ambulance is traveling at 60 mph and following at a safe distance from the car in front, the siren's sound travels much further than 100 feet to reach the vehicle ahead.

During experiments conducted by the authors, a "target vehicle" traveled at a constant 60 mph to determine siren recognition. Routinely, the ambulance had to be within four to five feet of the "target vehicle's" bumper before its occupants heard the siren. Additionally, it didn't seem to affect results whether the driver's window was open or closed. Apparently, the wind noise created by the open window offset the sound insulation value of the closed window. For these

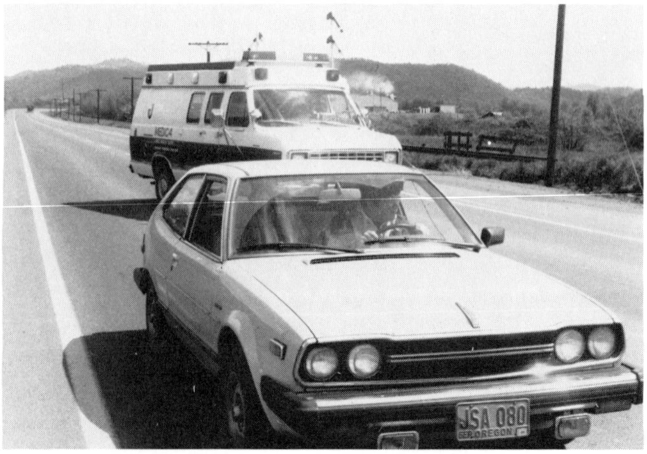

Fig. 10.5 At 55 mph, motorists you intend to pass may not hear your siren until you actually pass them.

reasons, it is obvious that the emergency vehicle driver must do everything possible to insure efficient use of the siren.

Sound is most easily detected when it changes frequency. Just as a blinking light draws attention faster than one constantly on, sounds changing pitch will draw attention similarly. Therefore, the ideal siren sound will be one that changes pitch. Many tales are told about the efficiency of the old mechanical siren (growlers) and how well it moved traffic. In reality, mechanical sirens do not produce as efficient a sound as the modern electronic devices. Additionally, mechanical sirens require a tremendous amount of power to operate which is not always available.

The sound emitted from the mechanical siren is created by a spinning impeller. Pitch is changed by spinning the impeller faster or slower. The higher frequencies are produced by faster revolutions. Impeller speed changes cause a change in the decibels delivered. While the mechanical siren can match the electronic devices for decibels at the higher frequencies, the db's rapidly diminish as the siren winds down. The wind-down produces the "growl" sound which many believed gained the most attention. In actuality, it is the higher frequency sounds which we hear better. The sound produced by the mechanical siren is also impure. It is made up of many different frequencies which can become lost in the presence of surrounding noise, lessening the siren's overall effects. In contrast, the electronic siren's frequencies are more pure. Electronic sirens deliver the full decibel rating to each frequency emitted at any given moment.

Sound waves travel in a straight line, but are readily deflected or "turned" by bouncing off objects. This deflection distorts the sound, creating confusion for the listener as to the exact source of the sound. In urban areas where there is an abundance of buildings and traffic, siren sounds ricochet off the multitude of surfaces, making it impossible for the listener to determine its source.

The effects of siren sound deflection can be reduced somewhat by careful placement of the speakers. Mounting the speakers as high on the vehicle as possible will allow them to project their sound "over" other traffic, reducing deflection off other vehicles. Care should also be taken not to mount other objects (e.g., Opticoms®, MARS lights, etc.) in front of the speakers.

Siren Use. The purpose of the siren is to gain attention to the emergency vehicle. The siren has absolutely no value once this attention is gained. It will create anxiety in drivers, and therefore frequently cause undesirable reactions by other motorists.

To gain attention, the typical electronic siren has several different sound modes. Since we recognize sound easiest by changes in pitch, the more frequently that change occurs the more readily the sound will be heard. Unfortunately, the more frequent the change, the more negative effect it will have on the crew and others. Therefore, the crew should select the siren mode that will do the best job of gaining others' attention while being the least detrimental on themselves. Additionally, by varying the mode, the crew can avoid the hypnosis that is often associated with the siren's use.

Wail. When using the siren, the "wail" mode should be used the majority of the time. It changes frequency often enough to gain others' attention but does not create the anxiety that a faster (yelp) mode might. Therefore, it is considered the standard operating mode. Changes to other modes can be made when the wail does not adequately gain attention.

Yelp. The "yelp" mode changes pitch about three times per second, the most efficient rate at which to gain attention. Of course, the yelp mode will also cause the most stress, its rhythm driving hard at people. Its fast cycle will also create the most interference with voice communications since its sound crosses speech frequencies three times per second. The yelp is best used when the ambulance is moving quickly, or is some distance from the traffic in front. Special emphasis on pitch changes may be needed when the traffic in front does not readily move from your path while using the wail at intersections, road construction, or when a change in traffic patterns occurs. The yelp also works well when approaching pedestrian areas. Remember, the yelp should only be used for short periods of time. The siren gains attention by the change in sound, thus changing from wail to yelp will help gain attention.

Manual. With the other modes to choose from, the manual position is often overlooked. Some emergency drivers may feel that it doesn't seem to be able to do anything the other modes can't and requires more effort. Actually, the manual mode is very effective. When traffic is moving slowly, and the ambulance is close, the siren can be readily heard. By turning the siren to manual, and just depressing the siren button occasionally, the traffic ahead can be made aware of your presence or reminded occasionally without creating the anxiety associated with the other modes. This approach will allow other motorists to deal more rationally with the situation. A wailing or yelping siren simply assaults others when they may not have a safe or appropriate place to drive as they attempt to yield to your request for passage. On the open road where there isn't any other traffic to make aware of your presence, the siren serves no function. Under such conditions, it may be turned to the manual mode so it is readily available if needed.

High/Low. The high/low mode is probably the least effective of the siren modes. Because it produces only two frequencies, it is less likely to be heard than other modes. Additionally, it is easy to lose one-half of the siren's two frequencies to background noise or to a driver's hearing deficiency. Occasionally, an unattentive driver may "tune out" the other modes, yet may respond to the high/low's less familiar sound. This mode is less stressful than the other modes mentioned and may be a good selection to use when there is no traffic to alert, but the traffic laws require that your siren be activated.

Public Address (P/A). The Public Address position of the siren is also often overlooked. It can be quite effective when used to direct confused or panicked motorists from the ambulance path. The crew can simply switch the siren to P/A and courteously request: "Will the driver of the green car please pull to your right."

When Not to Use the Emergency Equipment

The use of the emergency signaling equipment is a privilege, not a right. If EMS personnel abuse the privilege, it will be taken away. Over the years, such revocation of emergency status has taken place in several states. The privilege can also be taken away by society in a more subtle manner by simply not yielding to the emergency signals produced by the ambulance. For these reasons, the privilege must not be abused and the ambulance must always be operated with due regard for others.

The siren should not be used when it will be ineffective, unless required by law. For example: Open-road driving has been discussed. The siren can actually become an outright liability when activated on multilane expressways. Since it is difficult to hear the siren at higher speeds, motorists won't hear it until the ambulance is nearly upon or actually passing them. Suddenly startled by the siren, a motorist may respond with a violent turn of his head to see what's going on and will turn his steering wheel in the process—right into your vehicle. On the expressway, almost every driver is used to being passed, and your silent passing should not affect others. Therefore, the only times the siren should be activated while traveling on an expressway (unless required by law) is when you have a motorist in the left lane who simply will not move over for you or when you approach a scene and traffic is stopped. This is because many drivers will instinctively stop their car, throw their door open, and jump out to see what is the cause of the traffic blockage. An ambulance, traveling upon a shoulder or safety lane, can suddenly be faced with a possible accident since it will not have an escape route available.

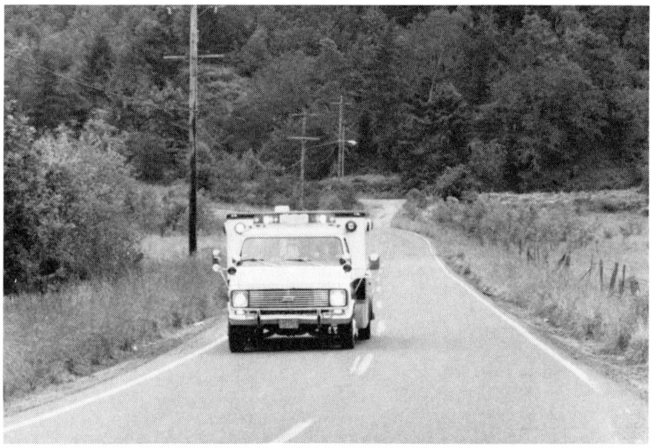

Fig. 10.6 Unless required by law, using the siren when there's no traffic to alert serves no purpose.

Although the siren may not be activated, it must always be turned on when the ambulance is driven with its emergency lights activated. The idea of running a complete emergency response with no intention of using the siren is dangerous. An ambulance operator should intend to use (activate) the siren anytime he overtakes another vehicle (except for those conditions previously noted) and certainly at every intersection at which you would not normally have the right-of-way. If you are transporting a patient whose condition warrants the use of emergency lights, that patient's condition also warrants use of the siren.

When TO and when NOT to activate emergency signaling equipment requires judgment on the driver's part. Certainly, motorists will tend to become confused if the emergency lights are frequently switched on and off. Such acts also increase the probability of the traffic ignoring the ambulance. But the siren may be activated and then its use discontinued. Again, care must be exercised since such acts tend to confuse others as they momentarily hear the siren and try to locate its source, only to immediately lose it again.

The emergency signaling equipment should not be used when the ambulance is traveling slower than the other traffic. Such a condition occurs when your patient's condition requires a slow ride, as it almost always does. It may also occur on a steep grade when the ambulance is unable to keep pace with lighter, faster passenger cars. Use of the emergency equipment insinuates that the ambulance is traveling faster than others on the road. When the ambulance is not traveling faster, the use of the emergency signaling equipment will confuse following drivers who are unsure if they can or should pass. Drivers in vehicles ahead of the ambulance will also become confused, not knowing if they should yield or accelerate. Such confusion can certainly cause accidents.

If the ambulance speed is so slow that the driver feels that he needs to, in some way, warn other motorists, the hazard lights should be activated since they are better recognized by the motoring public for this purpose.

Adverse weather, too, can indicate the discontinuance of the emergency equipment and therefore the emergency run. In fog, the emergency lights do not project far enough to adequately alert others of your presence and can create a dangerous vertigo which the crew may experience. For this very reason, aircraft are forbidden to use navigation lights in fog. Use of the siren in fog will also create additional confusion since the other drivers will not be able to identify its source. Additionally, thick fog should force the prudent driver to slow his speed as he picks his way along. At this point, the vehicle is then traveling nonemergency.

And then there is ice. It's already established that the use of emergency equipment can cause the motoring public to react improperly. When this occurs on ice and a motorist suddenly jams on his brakes or whips the steering wheel, he is likely to go into a skid. Most drivers have enough with which to cope without this additional burden. The ambulance, also traveling on the same icy surface, doesn't need to be doing much passing, or other maneuvering either. While the use of the emergency signaling equipment may need to continue under such circumstances, it must be used judiciously.

On the Road

The goal of emergency ambulance driving is to move slow traffic out of the way and pass through intersections as safely and easily as possible. In essence, you are trying to open up the road. This can best be done by positioning your ambulance where it can be easily seen by as many motorists as possible as early as possible. Proper positioning of the vehicle will telegraph your intentions to others, thereby making their decision on how to yield easier. Since the traffic you will have the most trouble with and therefore the most concern for is that which you are attempting to overtake, we will examine how to gain its attention first.

In order to safely overtake or pass a vehicle, the ambulance must first be seen by the leading driver. The device most of these people have for seeing the ambulance is their interior rearview mirror. For that reason, you must make an attempt to be easily seen in it. Unfortunately, there are some problems associated with this mirror. Many vehicles, such as vans and trucks, do not have a rearview mirror since its view would be blocked. Even a vehicle with a rearview mirror may have its view obstructed by cargo or passengers seated on the back seat. Additionally, the rearview mirror also becomes misadjusted quite readily. Misadjustment may occur when the driver wants to see those in the back seat or when a passenger in the front seat wants to adjust makeup or comb hair.

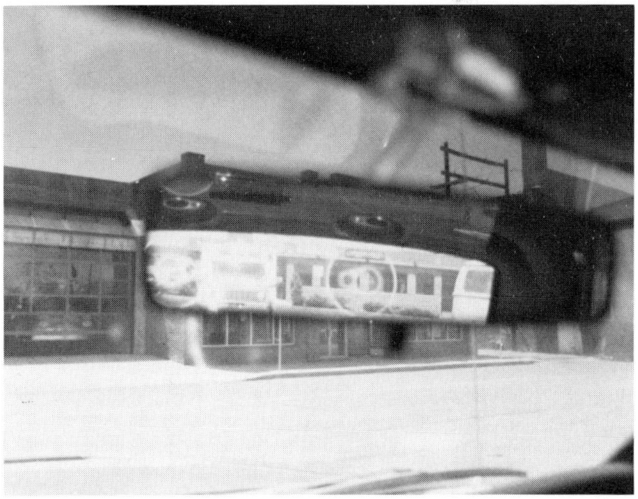

Fig. 10.7 Although you want to be seen in a driver's interior rearview mirror, the mirror has severe limitations (such as reflections in the rear window).

While trucks and vans have mirrors on the right side of the vehicle, most passenger vehicles do not. Therefore, the mirror the ambulance driver should strive to align with is the left outside mirror which is required on all vehicles. Such positioning of the ambulance also allows you to be seen by those ahead of the car immediately in front of the ambulance, as well as those coming toward you. This positioning has the additional benefit of telegraphing to others your intention of passing.

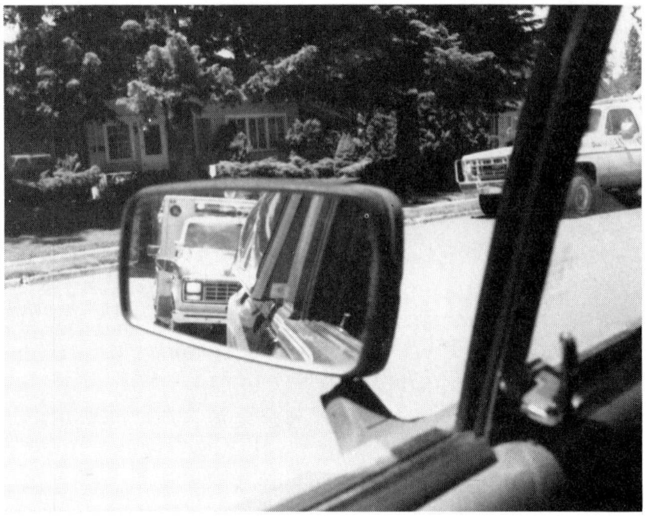

Fig. 10.8 Maneuver the ambulance so that it can be seen easily in the left hand rearview mirror of the driver ahead.

A cardinal rule of emergency driving is to pass on the left. This is for the reasons just stated, as well as the fact that many states' motor vehicle laws direct drivers who encounter an emergency vehicle traveling in an emergency mode to pull to the right hand curb or shoulder and stop. This is a natural reaction for most drivers. Therefore, if the driver of an ambulance attempts to pass on the right, he is exposing himself to an extreme probability of being struck by the vehicle he is passing since the ambulance will be in the lead vehicle blind spot.

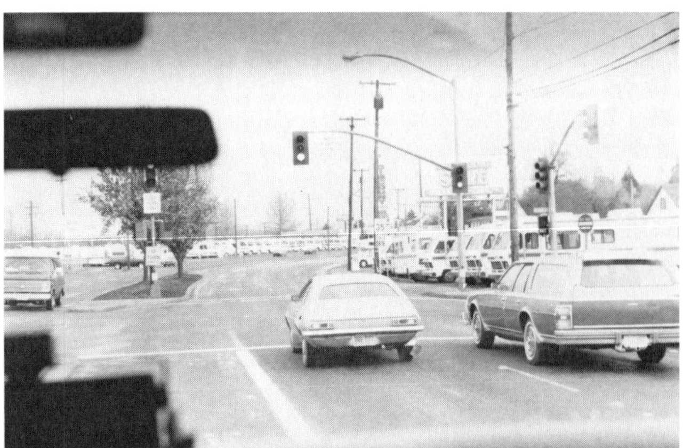

Fig. 10.9 A cardinal rule of emergency driving is to pass on the left.

There are rare occasions when it will be impossible for the ambulance to pass on the left. At such times, the ambulance driver may decide to pass on the right. But to do so, he must use extreme caution. It may actually be safer to temporarily turn off the siren and wait for the other driver to make a move than to pass on the right. Such a decision can only be made after each situation is evaluated by the ambulance driver. More importantly, the ambulance driver should allow as much room as possible between his vehicle and the one he is overtaking, while traveling at a reduced speed. The combination of the reduced speed and escape route will allow you to react if the leading driver should decide to pull right.

While passing is routinely performed by most vehicles on the open road, ambulances cannot do so as easily while in the emergency mode. Here are several reasons why this statement is true. While passing, the emergency lights may be observed by a more attentive driver in the vehicle in front of the car you are passing. This observation may cause the more forward vehicle to pull to the side of the road. The driver you are passing, who does not realize why the other driver pulled over, might then attempt to pass him, pulling into the ambulance. There is also the problem of the siren not being heard well. The lead driver, unaware that he is being passed, may not hear the siren until the ambulance is actually alongside. The result can easily be a violent turn of the driver's head followed by his hands on the steering wheel moving in the same direction.

For the ambulance driver to safely pass others, he must obtain two things from the driver in front.

First: The ambulance driver must have **eye contact** with the driver he is passing to be sure that the driver is aware of the ambulance's presence. Ideally, eye contact is obtained by watching the other driver's eyes in the rearview mirror. In reality, it may only be obtained by watching the lead driver's head move as he looks in the mirror and recognizes the ambulance. (Characteristically, the driver will hold his eyes on the mirror longer than usual when he recognizes the ambulance.) Without eye contact, a move on the part of the other driver can be misinterpreted by the ambulance driver. The lead driver's head action or steering may simply be an attempt to avoid an obstacle in the road, or worse, be pulling to the right in order to have more room to turn left.

Second: The ambulance driver must have **a commitment to act** from the other driver. Of course, this occurs when the lead driver makes a deliberate attempt to clear a path for the ambulance. If the ambulance driver attempts to pass a vehicle without this commitment to action, he is relinquishing valuable room on the road he may later need to use. Also, the ambulance driver has no idea of what action, if any, the other driver will take. Since such action is often delayed and not always favorable, the ambulance driver is exposing himself and others to a much higher probability of an accident.

Fortunately, most drivers will take some action to get out of the way once they see an ambulance. If the ambulance driver does not observe eye contact and commitment to act, he then must realize the inherent danger of passing. His only recourse is to slow down, and allow as much room between vehicles as possible.

Sometimes it is not easy to wait for the proper time to overtake another vehicle. The urgency of the emergency response and the rhythm of the siren all pressure the driver to pass. Such impulse must be resisted. The safe emergency vehicle driver can and must wait until all factors are in his favor. There is absolutely no rule that says he must pass others or drive unsafely.

For some reason, most drivers tend to pull over to the right but keep driving when an emergency vehicle is trying to pass. This act makes passing even more difficult for the ambulance driver. Even though the car has pulled to the right, passing will often force the ambulance to cross the center line if proper distance is maintained between the vehicles. By not stopping, the car in front makes the time spent in the oncoming traffic lane much longer. Therefore, if there is oncoming traffic, hills, curves, or intersections which may hide danger, the ambulance cannot pass. Even with the emergency lights and siren activated, driving three-abreast on a two-lane road is not comfortable. Again, the ambulance driver should hold back and wait; a condition which is frustrating for the driver who is to be passed as well as for the EMTs.

Emergency driving does not allow you to drive any closer to the vehicle in front than you would normally. In fact, use of the emergency signaling equipment dictates that you allow an extra second following distance. The closer you are to the vehicle in front when its driver first sees or hears the ambulance, the more likely he will be to panic. Typically, the first reaction by a driver to such a situation is for him to hit the brake (not good if you're sitting on his bumper). By staying back, you also make it easier for others approaching you to see your lights. This extra margin gives him a head start in yielding the right of way. Consequently, an ambulance traveling in an emergency mode should avoid following the vehicle in front by any less than a three-second margin.

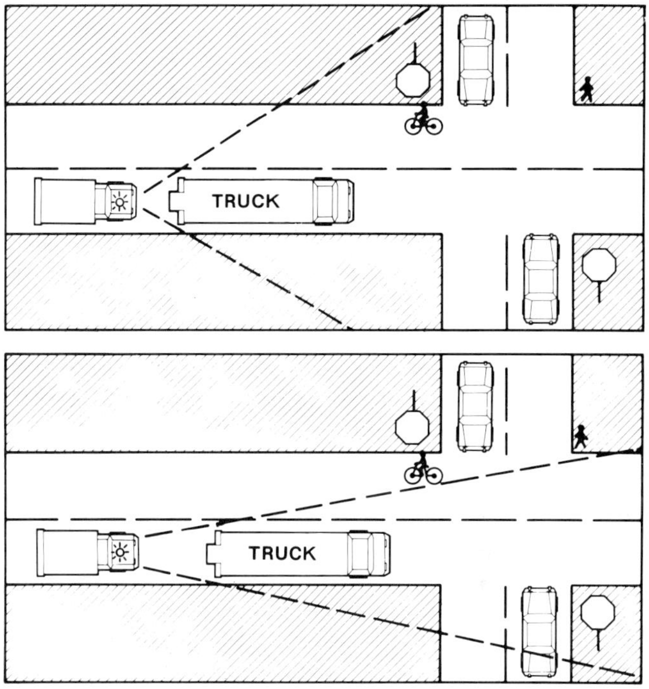

Fig. 10.10 The closer an ambulance trails behind another vehicle, the less visible emergency lights become.

The term expedite seems to be used frequently in public safety. It's usually used when a problem overwhelms the first units on the scene. Being asked to expedite should not affect the ambulance driver's speed or clearances. The word expedite should only serve to confirm that indeed the patient's condition is serious. Just because the emergency is confirmed or the problem overwhelming does not change the conditions that the ambulance must be driven safely and with due regard for others.

Occasionally, while the crew is loading a critical patient, a police officer will suddenly say, "Follow me, I'll escort you to the hospital." While the officer's intentions are well-meaning, the crew should try to avoid such "help." Most motorists observing an emergency vehicle (especially law enforcement) will pull to the side of the road and yield. But once they realize the officer is not pulling them over, they will quickly whip back onto the road and attempt to see where the officer is going. Often this act will occur without the motorist looking in his mirrors, since he expects all other traffic to pull over as well. If the ambulance is following closely behind the police vehicle, these curious motorists may pull out in front of it. The results are obvious.

Such caution is also extended to fire department ambulances and fire suppression apparatus as well. Many fire apparatus are equipped with a warning sign on the back of the vehicle which cautions others to stay back 500 feet. This same rule should also be followed by the next piece of equipment responding to the same call.

When you must drive behind other emergency equipment, it is wise for each vehicle to use a different siren mode. This will help others (public and other emergency vehicle operators) on the road to distinguish that there is more than one vehicle present.

Railroad crossings and emergency response deserve special attention. It is very difficult to hear a train over the blare of the siren. Controlled railroad crossings, equipped with mechanical warning devices, are not 100 percent safe, and must not be relied upon for clear passage. Anything mechanical is subject to malfunction. Ever consider a power failure at the crossing? To safely negotiate a railroad crossing, the ambulance driver must also slow down and look in both directions carefully. If conditions permit, the siren should also be turned off to enable you to hear an approaching train, especially if visibility down the tracks is impaired.

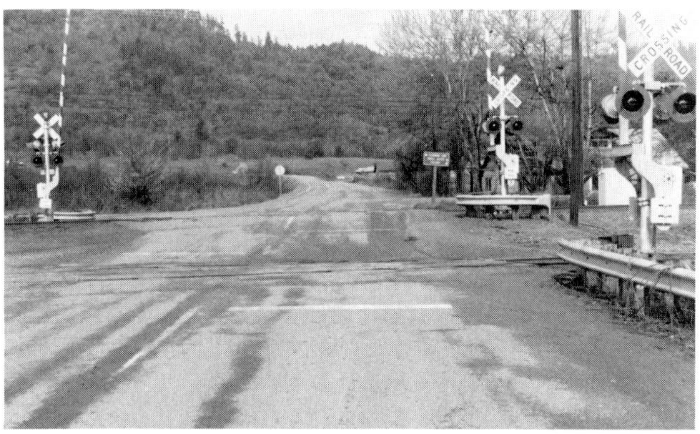

Fig. 10.11 Pay special attention at railroad crossings—deactivate siren momentarily and *look both ways.*

Most states require emergency vehicles to stop for a school bus displaying its flashing red lights, regardless of whether or not the E.V. is on an emergency response. This policy should be followed even if your state's laws do not clearly require such action. The school bus driver should observe your vehicle approaching, account for the children's safety, close the bus doors, turn off his red lights and wave you past. While waiting for the bus driver's actions, deactivate the siren since it will only add useless noise to the situation and excite the children.

Intersections

A certain law of physics can be paraphrased to say something to the effect that two vehicles cannot occupy the same intersection at the same time. When you consider the number of motor vehicle accidents to which you respond at intersections, obviously the intersection is an unsafe environment. Statistically, 37% of all traffic accidents occur at intersections. Nearly 50% of all ambulance accidents involving two or more vehicles occur at intersections. The higher rate is probably due to ambulance drivers attempting to force their way against the control devices (stop signs, red traffic lights, etc.). Another factor which contributes to accidents at intersections is that although the ambulance driver may signal his intent to turn, it seems other drivers expect the ambulance to go straight through an intersection. These intersection accident risks can be minimized when the ambulance is driven in a proper and courteous maneuver.

Negotiating the intersection, even more than the open road, requires the ambulance driver to think ahead. Some cardinal rules of driving intersections: Whenever possible, you must approach the intersection in order that you can overtake on the left. If you are planning to turn at the intersection, you should signal well in advance. If you are to go against a red light or stop sign, you should come to a complete stop at the intersection before passing through it.

Before an intersection can be safely negotiated, the ambulance driver MUST have eye contact and a commitment from ALL of the other drivers. Since an intersection has more traffic traveling in several directions, gaining eye contact and commitment will take longer than on the open road. Keep in mind, too, that a driver can very easily look right at the ambulance and not have it register in his mind. He may be thinking of the tasks ahead at the office or activities coming up at home and not see your lights. Thus, the commitment to let you pass becomes extremely important when negotiating intersections. Obviously, this contact with each driver requires time. It cannot be done while blazing through the intersection at 30 mph.

Although it is normally not acceptable for a vehicle to stop in the crosswalk, this is the best place for the ambulance to stop at intersections while on an emergency run. Actually, it is best to stop just before the crosswalk, insure that it is empty, and then roll into it and stop again. By doing so, the ambulance driver can accomplish three things: First, he makes his ambulance easily

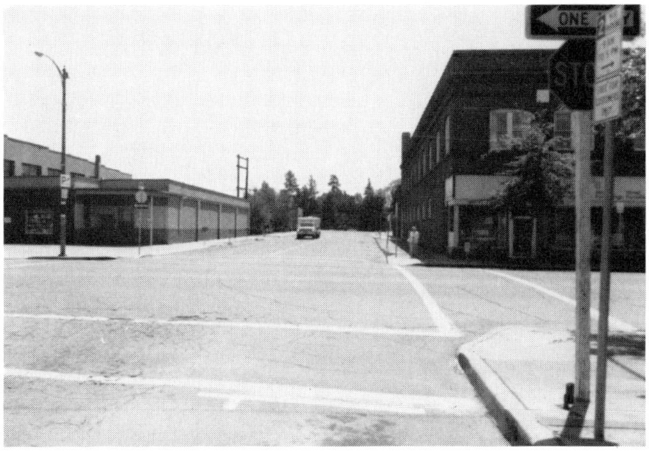

Fig. 10.12a Blind intersections are especially hazardous.

visible to others approaching the intersection. Second, he keeps pedestrians on the curb, and third, he also lets the other traffic know the urgency of the situation and of his intention of occupying the intersection.

As the intersection is cleared and the ambulance driver looks briefly at each of the other drivers, he must also realize that a vehicle might be hidden from his view by a larger vehicle. (If you can't see them, they can't see you!)

The intersection where the traffic light is about to complete its cycle is especially dangerous. It is very common for motorists who have been timing the lights for several blocks to enter an intersection early, before the light has actually changed in their favor. And, of course, drivers attempting to get through an intersection on a yellow light often end up going through on the red. The only way to avoid collisions with these drivers, as well as those who just aren't paying attention, is to slow down at all intersections, and gain eye contact and commitment before proceeding.

Ambulances need to pass through intersections quickly, yet they are notorious for poor visibility to the right. Responding to a call can be made easier if the crew has a system whereby the second crew member observes the right side of the intersection. As the intersection is approached, the second crew member scans the right side to make sure HE has eye contact and a commitment from each driver. If he has contact, he states loudly, "Clear right!" If traffic is slow to respond or he is unsure, he states loudly, "Traffic!" Such assistance only serves to make clearing the intersection a little quicker. The DRIVER of the ambulance is still responsible for his vehicle's operation and must quickly double check his path.

When the crew is planning on turning right at an intersection, they must still overtake traffic on the left. This will best allow everyone else on the road to see the ambulance. To make this turn safely, the driver must pull well into the intersection before making the right turn. Once again, a cushion of time and space must be provided between the ambulance and the other vehicles. The second crew member can further assist by sticking his hand out the window on his side, indicating to the traffic at his right to hold their position until the ambulance has safely passed.

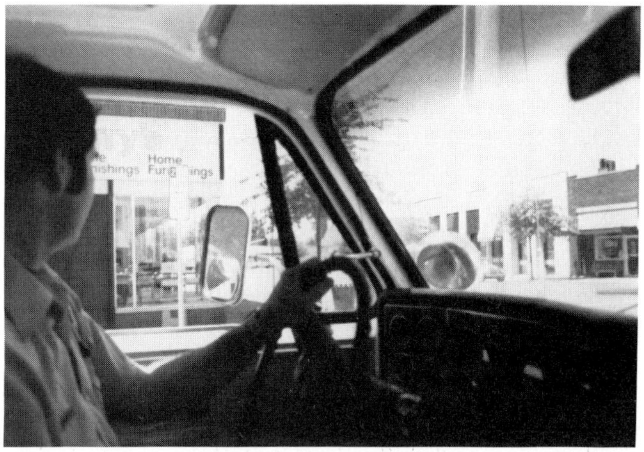

Fig. 10.12b As a driver approaches, he cannot see to the sides until almost into an intersection.

Probably the most dangerous situation in emergency driving occurs when an E.V. attempts to pass a vehicle that is signaling to turn left. Coming up behind this motorist, the ambulance driver simply CANNOT KNOW what the other driver will do. By passing this vehicle on the left, the ambulance driver is inviting a collision. It is very common for the lead driver to decide to complete his left turn to get out of the way of the ambulance. Such a reaction is even more likely if

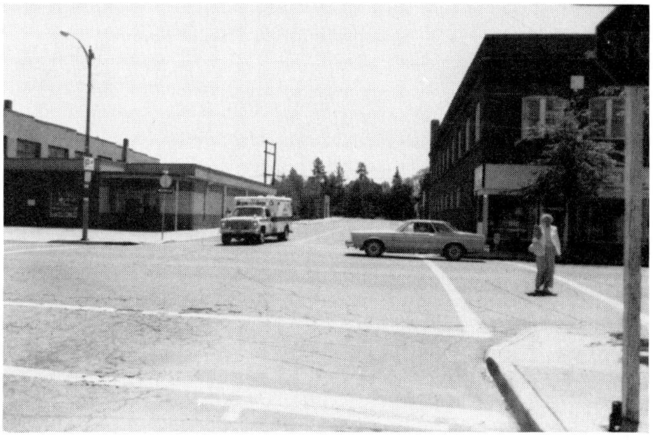

Fig. 10.12c If an ambulance driver doesn't slow and stop, it may be too late when cross traffic is observed.

oncoming traffic slows or pulls over for the ambulance. The lead vehicle driver might then misinterpret their action as courtesy towards him and complete his left turn. You can't pass this vehicle on the right side either. This driver could also pull to the right when he sees the ambulance. The only safe alternative is to STOP and WAIT this driver out! Make him turn left or pull right before you proceed.

Almost every emergency ambulance response will have more than one piece of emergency equipment responding with it. If it's a motor vehicle accident, police and fire units will probably respond. Typically, an aid unit or fire apparatus will also respond to medical calls. These vehicle operators will approach intersections with the same attitude as the ambulance driver, each expecting traffic to clear for their passage. Other sirens will be drowned out by their own. Remember, two emergency vehicles cannot occupy the same intersection simultaneously either. Always be watchful for OTHER emergency vehicles at the intersection.

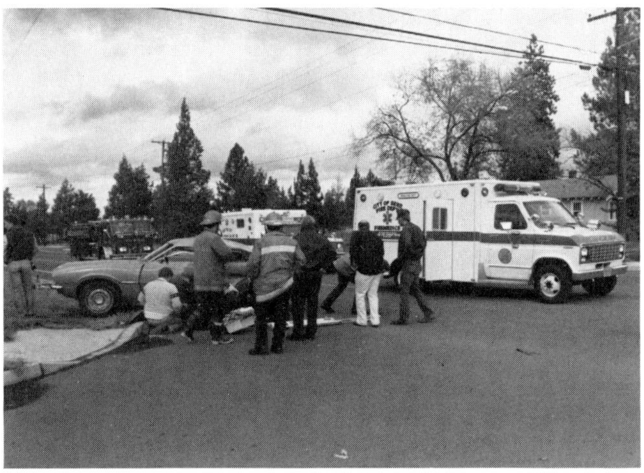

Fig. 10.13a Multiple response by emergency vehicles from several directions (note engine company to the rear acting as barrier vehicle to protect rescue workers).

The only way to drive an emergency response is with caution. Caution does not mean you can't be as expeditious as possible; it only means that you can't accept any additional risk. There is no law that states that you can't slow down and even stop during an emergency. Take the time to acquire eye contact and a commitment from each driver on the road. The time required to gain this can be kept short by placing the ambulance where it can be seen, and by telegraphing your intentions so the other driver can make a sound decision as to what to do to yield to you.

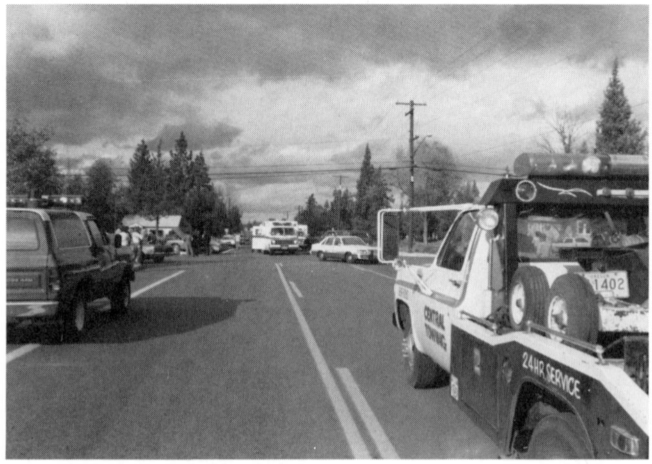

Fig. 10.13b Nearly every emergency ambulance response has several pieces of equipment responding, so, be watchful for other vehicles at intersections. Note Police Unit Serving as barrier vehicle.

Several illustrations of specific conditions follow to help you better understand emergency ambulance driving techniques.

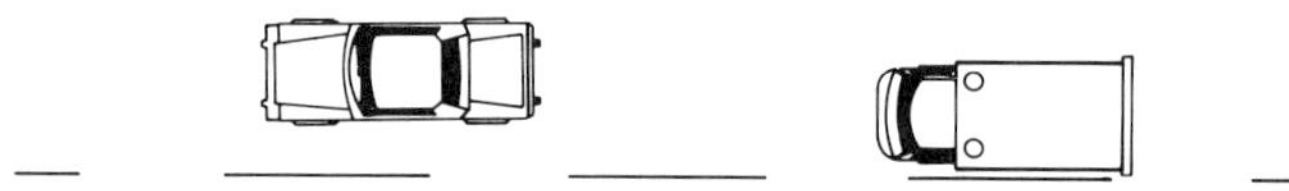

Figure A

Crowding the center line when driving on a two-way street. This position accomplishes three things at once: First, it places the ambulance in the optimum position to be seen in the left side-view mirror by the driver ahead. Second, it tells him your intention to pass, and third, it places the ambulance in a position to be most easily seen by the drivers ahead of the vehicle in front of you and those approaching from the other direction.

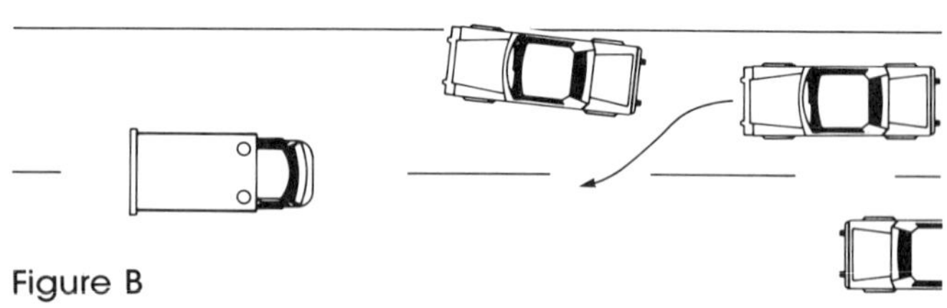

Figure B

Many emergency vehicle drivers actually straddle the center line, using it as a third lane. This position forces oncoming vehicles and those you are overtaking to pull to their respective shoulders. While this position works quite well for moving traffic from your path, it does create added dangers. One: If an oncoming vehicle yields to you, the vehicle behind him may not see you (poor visual habits) and attempt to pass—pulling into your head-on path. Two: You want to avoid having to pass between two vehicles at the same time, a situation that is more probable with this technique.

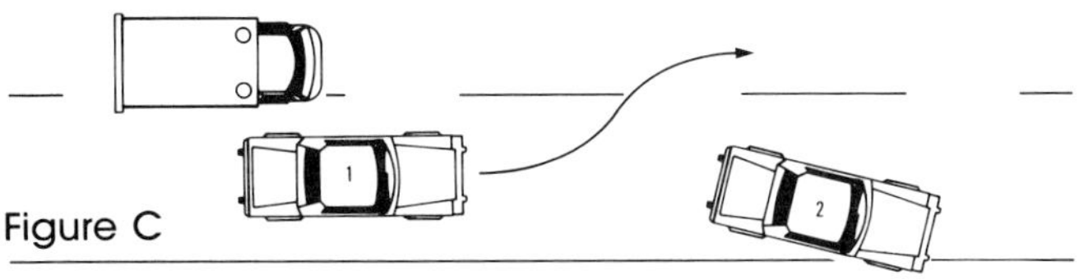

Figure C

By pulling around driver #1 ahead, the emergency signaling equipment system may alert a more observant driver, #2, to pull over. If driver #1 is not aware of your presence, he may attempt to pull around vehicle #2 and into your path. Additionally, many drivers will not hear the siren until it is almost right beside them. When this occurs, they may turn the wheel as they whip their head around to determine the source of the siren. You must have eye contact and commitment before you execute a pass.

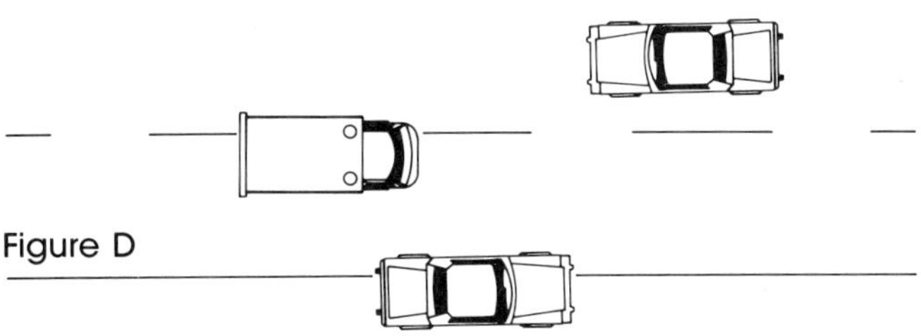

Figure D

Passing three-abreast does not leave you an out. If one of the drivers should do the unexpected or experience a mechanical malfunction, a collision is likely. Avoid this situation whenever possible.

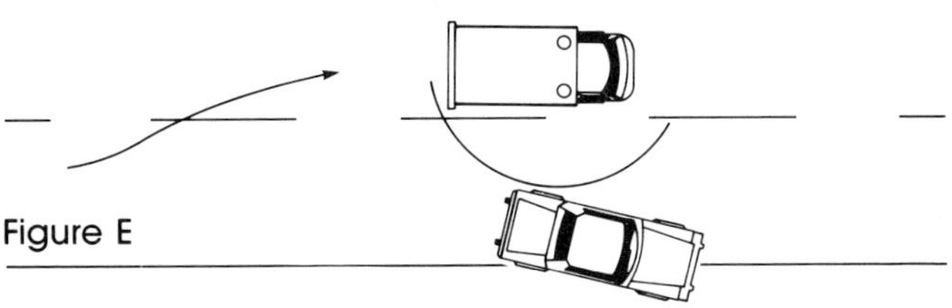

Figure E

When overtaking another vehicle, the ambulance driver should slow down and allow as much room as possible between the ambulance and the vehicle being overtaken. This margin or escape route will allow you time and space to react if the other driver should suddenly do the unexpected.

Whenever possible, avoid overtaking vehicles as you approach intersections. Other drivers

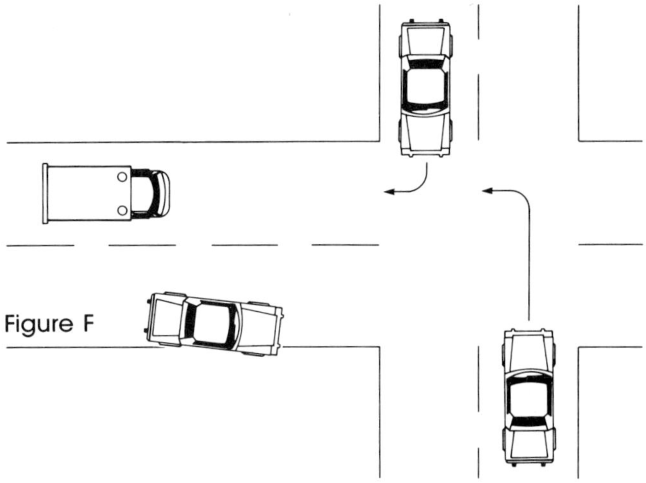

Figure F

typically turn from cross streets into this lane of traffic without looking for oncoming traffic.

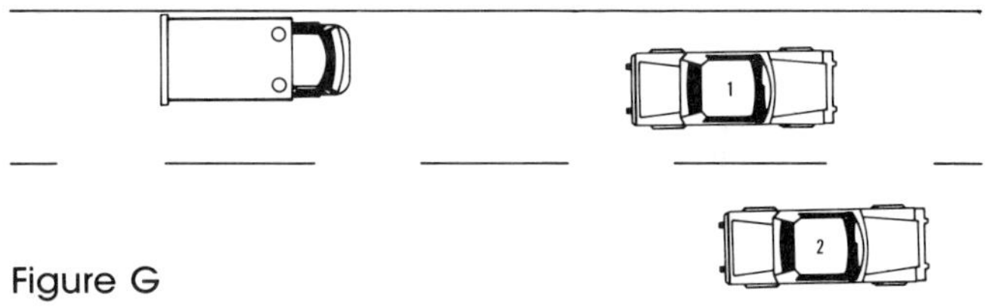

Figure G

When traveling on a one-way street, drive as close to the left shoulder as is safely possible. This action should force driver #1 to pull to the right. Care should be taken to remain a good distance behind the other traffic (#2), so your lights can remain visible. This extra distance will also prevent driver #1 from having to move over hastily and perhaps sideswiping another vehicle. While your intentions should be to overtake all vehicles on the left, some drivers may pull to the closest curb, especially if the right lane is blocked by traffic. If this occurs, you are forced to pass on the right. You can never be guaranteed that driver #1 will remain stopped and since you will be overtaking on his blind side, leave as much room as absolutely possible between the ambulance and his stopped vehicle.

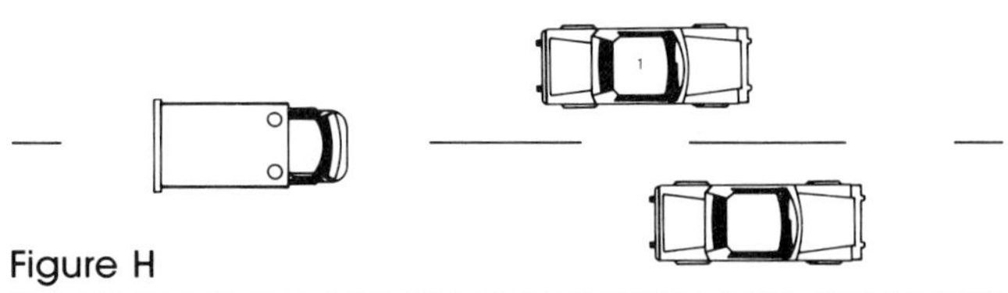

Figure H

Many ambulance drivers attempt to straddle the center line while traveling on a one-way street in an attempt to force the traffic to both shoulders and open up a lane down the center. While still far back from the traffic, this position has some advantages since it will allow traffic in both lanes to better see you. As the ambulance gets closer, you will be driving in the left vehicle's (#1) blind spot, reducing your chances of being seen. This forces you to pass on his right side without eye contact or a commitment.

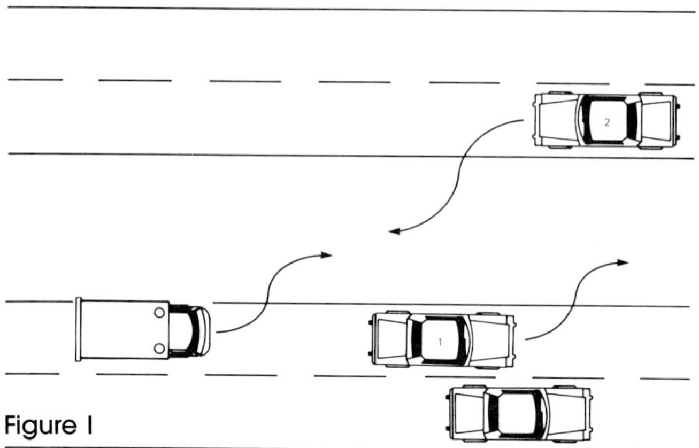

Figure I

Many streets have a center median that is used as a left turn lane. Upon first examination, this lane may seem like an ideal place to drive the ambulance, since there is little or no traffic present. Closer examination reveals that the center lane may not offer the opportunity first seen. This area quickly fills with debris from the road such as gravel, sand, glass, and anything else that may find its way onto the road—not a safe surface on which to drive. More importantly, the motorist (#1) you are overtaking may suddenly attempt to use the lane for a left turn. This maneuver is frequently performed by drivers without considering that someone could be trying to pass. Additionally, oncoming traffic (#2) may also use the lane without looking far ahead (poor visual habits).

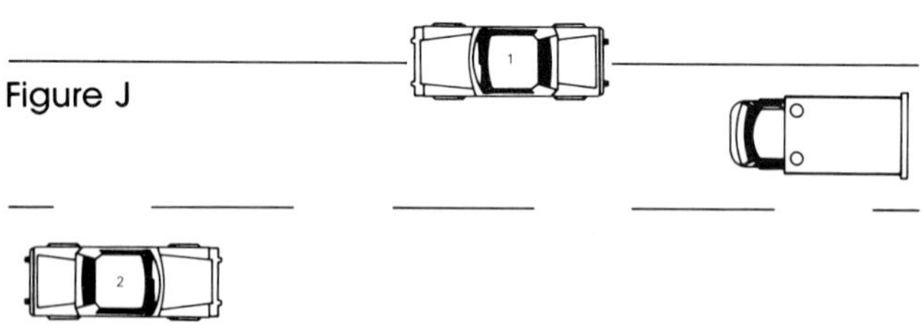

Figure J

Even though the driver (#1) in front of the ambulance has pulled over, you can't safely pass when faced with oncoming traffic (#2), intersections, hills, or curves that might hide traffic.

The ambulance driver must approach each intersection in such a manner as to allow his vehicle to be seen and telegraph his intentions. He must also gain eye contact and a commitment from every driver at the intersection before pro-

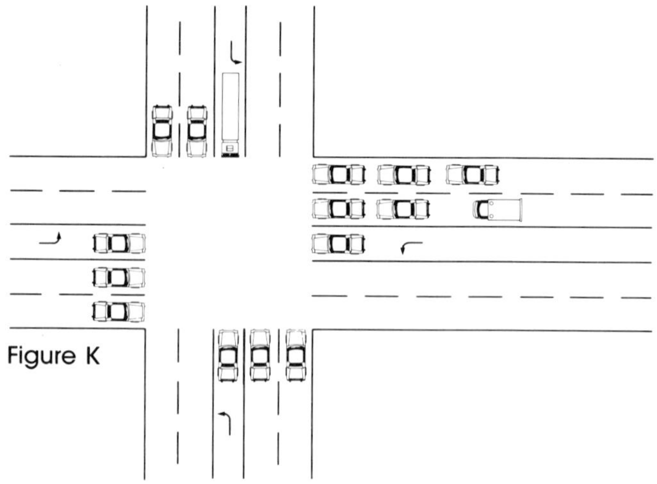

Figure K

ceeding (something that can't be done while blazing through at 30 mph). Note the two cars in the blind spot created by the tractor/trailer.

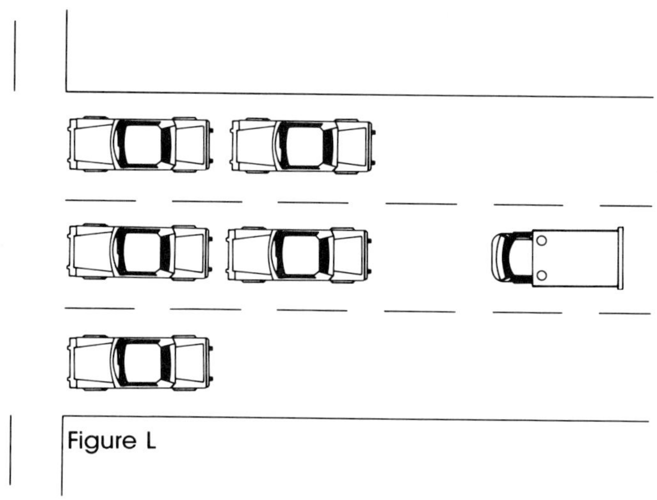

Figure L

When access to an intersection is blocked by traffic on a one-way street, it is best if the ambulance driver stays well back to take advantage of any openings the traffic might offer. Continued use of the siren in this situation may panic drivers

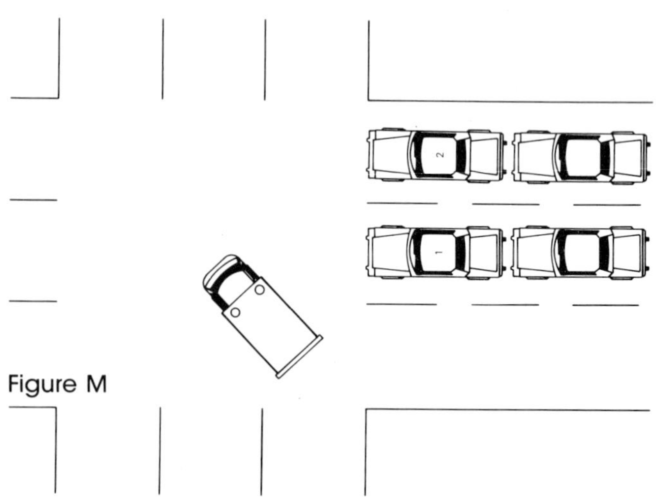

Figure M

and cause them to impulsively pull into a busy intersection. Instead, the siren can be used on manual and "rolled over" or "bumped" occasionally to remind others of your presence.

When you are required to turn right in front of stopped traffic, you should drive very slowly and leave as much room as possible between your vehicle and others. In addition, you can have your partner signal to the stopped vehicles (#1 and #2) to hold their position. Your partner can accomplish this by rolling down his right side window and using a hand and arm signal.

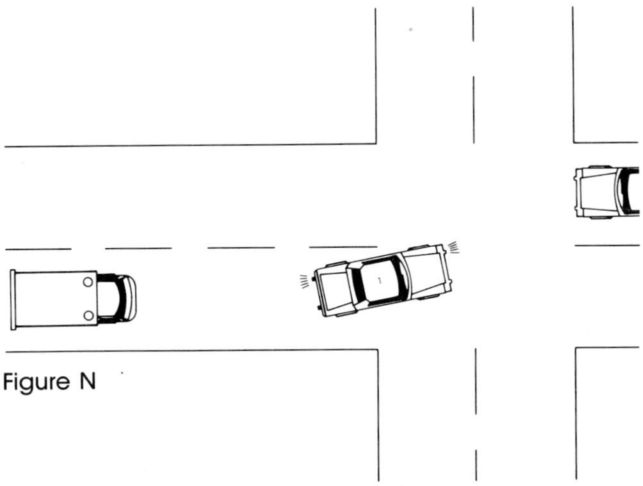

Figure N

The most dangerous situation an ambulance driver can face is trying to pass a vehicle while it is attempting to turn left. Passing on the left may very well result in a collision if the driver (#1) decides to complete his turn. Conversely, by passing this vehicle on the right, the driver (#1) may decide to pull to the right as required by law. The safest way to handle this situation is to hold back and force the driver to move one way or the other before you proceed.

Parking at The Scene of An Accident

Perhaps the most challenging of parking situations an ambulance operator will encounter will be that of parking at the emergency scene. As the driver approaches the scene he will be faced with several immediate concerns.

Among these immediate concerns will be any hazardous conditions present such as fire, chemical or radiation spills, the immediate needs of the patients and of course, a safe efficient place to park the ambulance.

In order to more quickly meet the patient's needs, many ambulance drivers simply abandon the ambulance at the first opportunity. However such action may actually cause more delay as care of the patient progresses and access to the ambulance becomes lengthy or dangerous.

The emergency scene can become extremely confusing at times. There is no need to make it more confusing by parking the ambulance inappropriately. By asking himself four questions, the driver can quickly pick the most appropriate location to park the ambulance.

1. Is the Vehicle and Access Around it Safe? At most accident scenes, traffic flow will deviate from its normal path. As emergency vehicles arrive, the traffic will often be forced to deviate even more from its normal path. When an accident occurs, everyone wants to take a look as they drive past; people are naturally curious. These two conditions, travel different than the normal path of traffic and curiosity, combine to make the scene extremely hazardous. The risk of additional collisions occurring within the vicinity of the accident scene is greatly increased. With this in mind, it is important for the ambulance operator to attempt to locate the ambulance in as protected an area as possible. While looking for such an area, the driver must keep in mind that access to the ambulance will probably have to be made during the course of the activities at the scene. Obtaining additional medical equipment, loading the patient, and helping passengers to board the ambulance are activities which require access to the ambulance. These activities must be carried out in an area as free of traffic as possible. An ambulance parked on one side of the street while the scene is on the other inhibits safe access. With all that is occurring at the scene it is easy for an EMT, or another individual intent on helping, to head for the ambulance to retrieve equipment without looking for cross traffic.

2. Does the Ambulance Placement Block Traffic? The dangers of the vehicular traffic present at the scene have been established. Even with normal traffic patterns intact, motorists attempting to see what is happening become less attentive to their driving. Add to these conditions the problems encountered when the emergency vehicles at the scene further impede traffic flow and the dangers of collision increase dramatically. At the same time a parked emergency vehicle cannot impede traffic flow without placing at least one side of the vehicle body in close proximity to traffic. This proximity to passing traffic makes access to that side hazardous.

3. Can an Easy Departure be Made From the Scene in the Direction of the Nearest or Most Appropriate Hospital? This is the parking consideration that most often gets overlooked. The crew, anticipating the immediate needs of the patient, often fails to consider the likelihood that the patient will eventually be transported. By assuring that the ambulance is placed so departure can be made quickly and easily, the patient may actually arrive at the hospital more rapidly.

4. Is the Ambulance Close to the Patient? The EMS mission is patient care and transportation. It stands to reason that the ambulance will provide that transportation. Additionally, efficiency dictates that the patient care equipment must be placed as close to the patient as is reasonable. Most patient care equipment and the patient's loading will be accessed through the back of the ambulance. Therefore, it is the location of the back doors of the ambulance that should be considered when parking the ambulance. Unfortunately, the idea of placing the ambulance close to the patient can often override the other three considerations of parking at the scene. One word of caution: Avoid backing the ambulance when it is in close proximity to patients as the risk of an accident is greatly increased.

Many people advocate parking a vehicle between the scene and the moving traffic in order to protect the scene, its patients, and rescue workers. This vehicle is placed as a sacrificial barrier in the event a passing motorist isn't paying attention and runs into the scene. It is the ambulance that is going to transport the patient to the hospital. Because of this role the ambulance should not be placed as a barrier in this situation. If the ambulance becomes involved in a collision, patient transportation, perhaps even patient care, will be compromised. It is also possible that a collision could occur while the patient is being loaded. In the event of such a collision, the patient's condition could be made worse and the crew would quite likely also be incapacitated.

Police vehicles are the best sacrificial barriers. Little activity takes place around a police vehicle once it has delivered its officers to the scene. In the event that the police have not yet arrived, a fire truck would be the next best barrier vehicle. Although the engine will have activity going on around it, it will not be required to transport patients. A fire engine makes a formidable barrier.

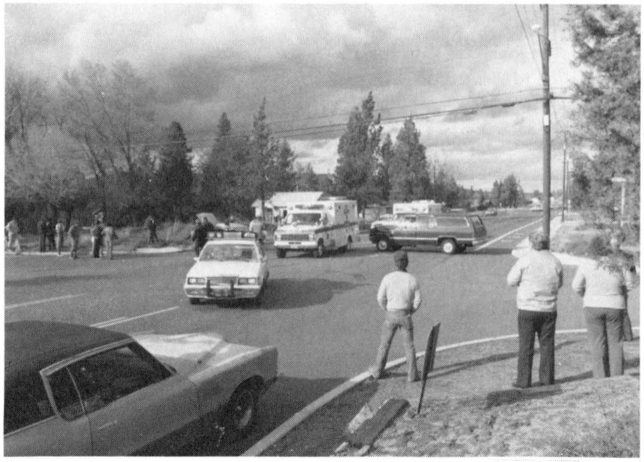

Fig. 10.14a Police vehicle at this scene is well placed to act as a sacrificial barrier.

Any barrier vehicle should be placed to provide a safe corridor between it and the scene in front of it. The barrier vehicle should also be parked in an offset manner to allow another corridor alongside of the barrier vehicle.

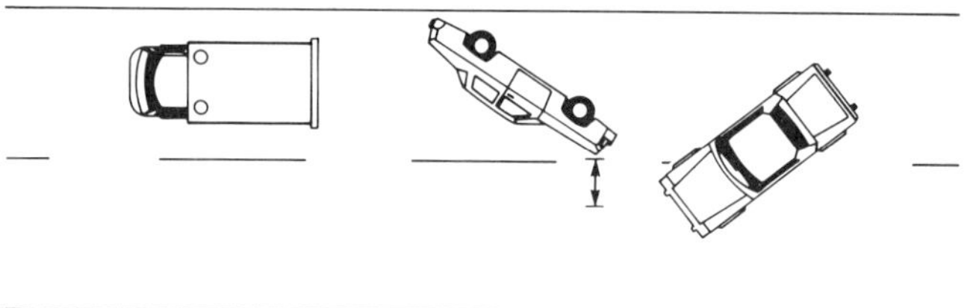

Fig. 10.14b Barrier vehicle should be placed to provide a safe corridor between it and the scene in front.

Generally, there are four areas in which to park the vehicle at the scene: the area immediately preceding the scene, the area to either side of the scene, and the area just beyond the scene. Each should be evaluated with regard to the four previously mentioned considerations for parking.

Prior to The Scene. This parking location may or may not have access around all sides, but it is likely. If the accident is predominantly on the right side of the road, the vehicle can easily become a barrier vehicle. It is important to note that the area that would be exposed to the oncoming traffic would be the patient loading area. Parking the ambulance prior to the scene puts it more or less in line with the accident and generally won't additionally restrict traffic. While the front of the vehicle is close to the patient the rear can be quite a distance away when considering the perils of having to go around the vehicle on the traffic side. Such positioning may at times be appropriate. When the hospital is in the direction from where the ambulance approached, this location may be the easiest for leaving the scene. Occasionally, the scene will completely block the road, making this the only parking alternative. If the accident scene is on the left side of the road, this location may be the most protected area in which to park.

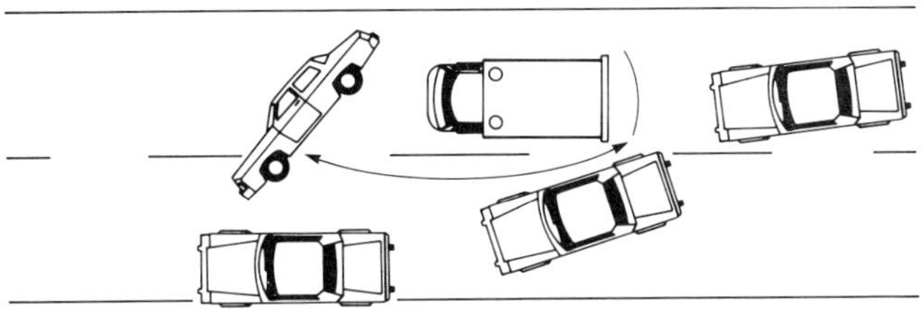

Fig. 10.15 Parking in this location makes the ambulance a barrier vehicle and puts the patient loading area in jeopardy.

To the Traffic Side of The Scene. At most accident scenes, traffic is diverted to one side or another. Only rarely will traffic be diverted around both sides of the scene. The traffic side is rarely a good place to park the ambulance except in those situations where the scene is located completely off the road and the ambulance is parked on the road shoulder. Otherwise, the ambulance on the traffic side will severely restrict traffic, and make one side of the ambulance almost inaccessible because of the close proximity of the vehicles passing by on what little road is available for travel.

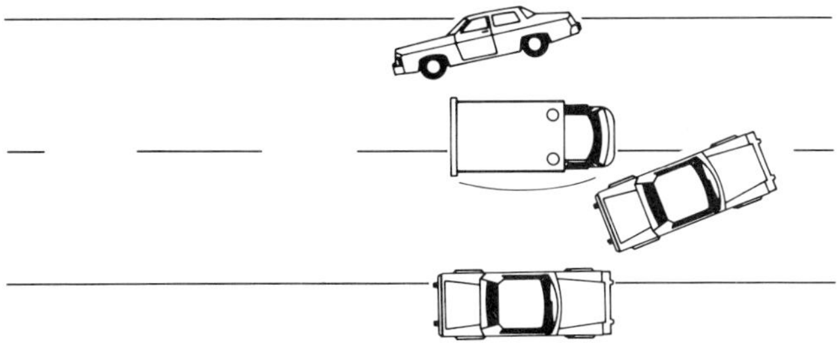

Fig. 10.16 Parking on the traffic side will almost always further restrict traffic and limit access to other side of the ambulance.

The Off-Traffic Side. A shoulder that isn't being used for traffic diversion is one of the better places to park the ambulance. Unfortunately, there is rarely room for parking in such a position without encroaching on the scene or restricting access to the ambulance because of guard rails, shrubbery, or other hazards along the side of the road.

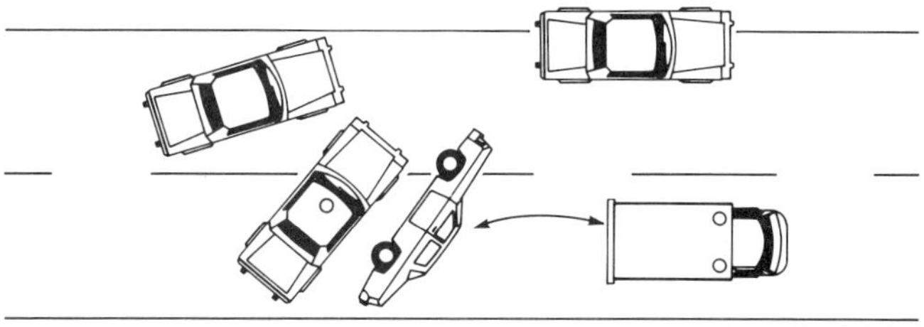

Fig. 10.17 The best place to park is beyond the scene—it protects ambulance from traffic and puts the patient loading area nearer to the patient.

Beyond the Scene. As a rule, beyond the scene is the best place to park an ambulance. The ambulance will be in line with the scene and so access around it should be fairly easy. Because it is in line with the scene, the ambulance usually won't further restrict traffic flow. More importantly, the back of the vehicle is close to the patient and a safe loading area is provided. If the scene occupies the left side of the road, the ambulance may again become the barrier vehicle if parked beyond the scene.

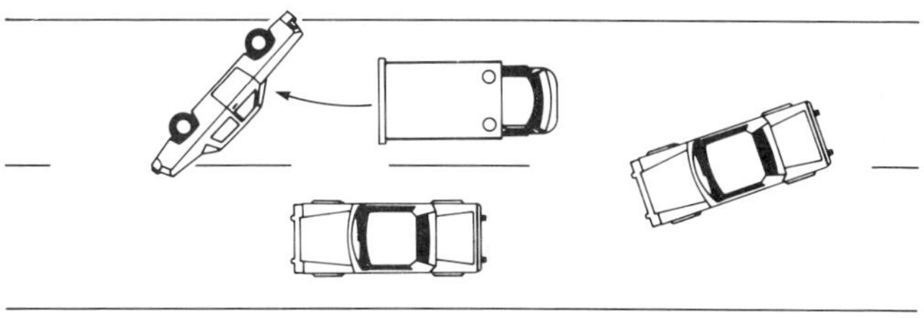

Fig. 10.18 If the scene occupies the left side of the road, the ambulance may, again, become a barrier vehicle, if parked beyond the scene.

Traffic restriction at the scene of an accident is an extreme concern. The ambulance driver must do everything he can to avoid further restricting traffic flow. On divided highways, the ambulance driver should avoid parking on one side of the highway and walking across to the other side to the scene. The police have enough problems with the traffic flow on the one side without having to be concerned with traffic flow from the other direction.

Parking at A Home or Business. Many ambulance responses will be to a home or business. Normally when someone goes home they simply drive in the driveway and park. An ambulance with its greater size and different needs introduces several elements which must be considered. If the house is reasonably close to the road, as in most suburban neighborhoods, or if the driveway is steep, it is better to park the ambulance on the street, perhaps at the foot of the driveway. The patient can easily be brought to the ambulance parked on the street. Keep in mind, a residential neighborhood is one of the more risky places to back an ambulance.

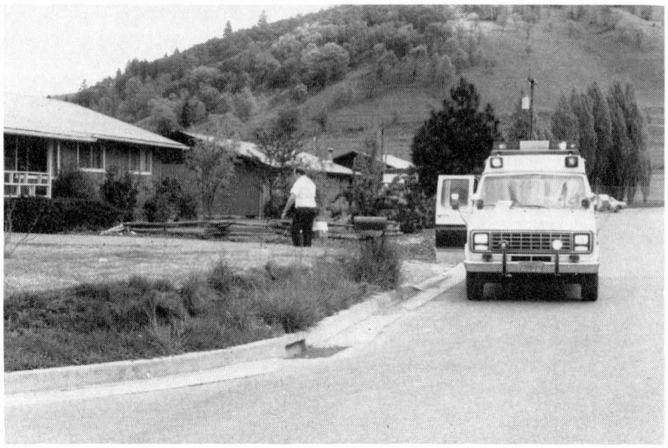

Fig. 10.19 If a house is reasonably close to the road, it's better to park on the street rather than back into or out of the driveway.

Should the ambulance driver decide to park in a driveway, it is usually better to back the vehicle into the driveway, using his partner as a spotter. This maneuver avoids the situation of having to back into the street without a spotter (now providing patient care), and the associated problems of seeing the traffic through mirrors.

Backing into a driveway can present some hazards. In a residential area, children are likely to be present and nothing attracts children like an ambulance or fire engine. Frequently, the driveways encountered are narrow and shrubbery or grass is often backed over while attempting to get into these driveways. Such an occurrence tends to upset the homeowner even if an emergency exists.

Emergency parking in a business district may require the ambulance driver to double park or otherwise inconvenience other motorists. Although such situations often can't be avoided, every effort should be taken to minimize obstructing traffic. Unfortunately, the public is often more concerned by a traffic inconvenience they might experience than the mission of emergency personnel.

When the ambulance first arrives at the scene, the driver is often confronted by someone trying to direct the ambulance to a parking spot that he thinks is appropriate. Should these directions be given by law enforcement officers or fire personnel, it is usually best to follow their directions since they have already evaluated the scene. When directions are given by a bystander, the ambulance driver should quickly make an analysis of the scene and choose a parking location, even if it's against the bystander's wishes. Time and safety for all are the concerns of the driver. His training will allow him to choose the best parking location at the emergency scene.

Frequently, the driver will park and leave the ambulance and then allow someone else to relocate it later. This situation should not be allowed to occur. Typically the throttle is set up to increase engine speed while the ambulance is at the scene. Another person attempting to move the ambulance may not be familiar with the higher engine speed and could get into trouble. When the parking brake is released, the ambulance will tend to move much more rapidly than a passenger car. The ambulance is an expensive and complex piece of equipment. A lay person or one unfamiliar with ambulances should not be allowed to drive it, especially around a congested emergency scene.

Once the ambulance has arrived at the scene, the first order of business is for the other crew members to assess the scene and get to the patient's side. The driver can then park the ambulance in a safe and efficient location, even though it may keep the driver from providing patient care for a few extra moments.

Once the vehicle is properly positioned the driver must then insure that the parking brake is firmly engaged and that the transmission is in park. The driver must then shut down any electrical systems that won't be immediately needed.

The driver should determine if all of the emergency warning lights are needed and turn off any that are not while parked at the scene. He should also shut off the heater or air conditioners and any other auxiliary electrical systems which are not needed. The driver should then engage the throttle to increase the engine speed. This will allow the alternator to better handle the electrical load currently being used. If the ambulance is parked facing oncoming traffic at night, the headlights should also be turned off to reduce some of the visual confusion for other motorists. Wheel chocks can then be placed against the tires for added safety.

While it is common for the doors of the ambulance to be left open at the scene, it is better to close them. The doors are usually left open because of the EMT's concern for rapidly getting the equipment to the patient. However, it only takes a second to close the doors. By doing so, you can better protect the equipment left behind from tempting sightseers present at the scene. In addition, you can better control the interior temperature, and limit the amount of dust, rain, or other debris from entering the unit. With the doors left open, traffic flow is also further interrupted, since it is presented with an additional obstacle. Even when the ambulance is parked well away from vehicular traffic, pedestrian traffic by rescuers and others may be hampered by the open door. When closing a door, be sure that it isn't just shoved and then abandoned, since this will cause extreme wear on the hinges and especially the latching mechanism. It only takes a second to grasp the handle and firmly shut the door in the proper way.

The act of finding the appropriate place to park does not take more than a brief moment. The alternatives should be weighed in comparison to the four parking considerations and then the location selected. This simple act can save loss of property and possible injury to the many public safety personnel working around the ambulance.

Warning Devices

The scene of an accident on a roadway is often dangerous and must be protected by warning motorists of its presence so they will know what is expected of them to avoid additional accidents. Ideally, warning devices will be placed to define the accident scene and mark temporary traffic lanes.

Typically, placement of warning devices and securing the scene from further accidents is performed by law enforcement or fire suppression personnel.

Seldom will EMTs be involved in the placement of elaborate warning device patterns. Occasionally, the ambulance crew will find themselves as the first public safety personnel at the scene and, typically, bystanders will already be directing traffic. When faced with such a scenario, one ambulance crew member should quickly assess the scene to determine if any hazards are present while the driver parks the ambulance. Once the scene is determined to be free of hazards, a crew member can distribute warning devices to one or more of the bystanders, giving them some brief instructions on the use and placement of the devices. This will usually be the limit of the crew's involvement in controlling traffic. Their primary responsibility is patient care and they simply have little time for further concern with traffic flow. The flow of traffic is not to be confused with securing a safe scene. Law enforcement personnel are charged with the responsibility of getting traffic rolling again.

Generally, there are two types of temporary traffic warning devices in use today, flares and warning triangles. Each will be discussed with emphasis on proper usage and placement with regard to identifying an accident scene.

Flares. The procedure for starting flares may seem confusing to some, but the process is actually quite simple.

It is important that the procedure for starting flares be learned before it comes time to use them at a scene. The flare has two sections, the flare itself and a plastic cap at the top of the flare. The cap contains a striker that is used to ignite the flare. This striker is protected under a small lid on top of the cap. To start a flare, hold the flare in one hand and pop the lid off the cap to expose the striker. Next, remove the cap by giving it a sharp twist and pull it off the flare body. Reverse the cap and strike the black knob that is now exposed at the top of the flare with the cap.

Extreme care should be taken when igniting a flare; strike it away from the body. Once lit, the flare should be held away from your body. The materials used in the flare burn at extreme temperatures and freely drip from the flare. If the flare is struck in a direction toward the body, this burning material can come in contact with skin or clothing, causing severe burns.

Flares are manufactured in several sizes —lasting from 5 to 40 minutes. If the scene will require flare protection for a longer period than the duration of the flare, additional unlit flares can be placed for extended use. Simply lay the burning flare on the ground and place the second flare, with its cap removed, on top of the base of the ignited flare. In this way, the first flare will ignite the second flare just before it burns out. As many flares as necessary can be placed in such fashion.

Extreme care must be taken when flares are used. Because of the flame and heat produced by the flare, anything in proximity to it that is combustible may ignite. Certainly, flares should be kept well away from the

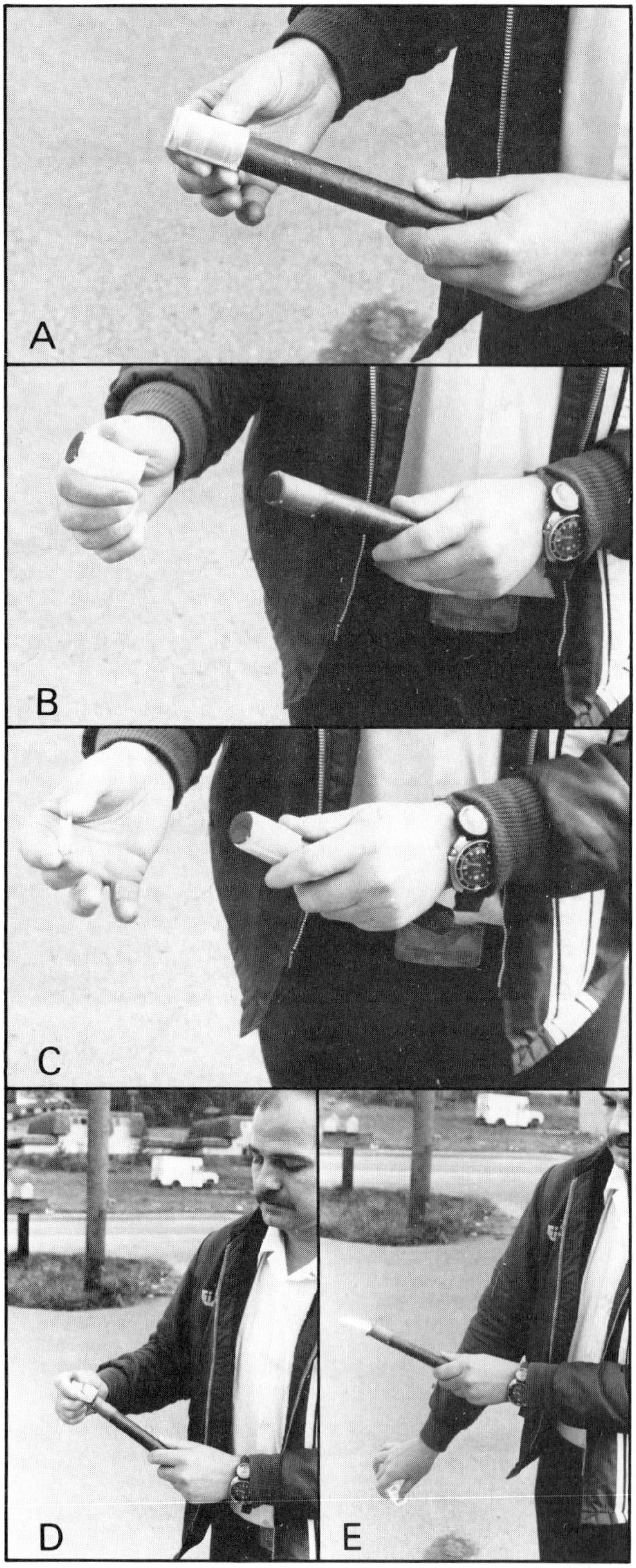

Fig. 10.20a To start a flare, hold it in one hand and use the other to remove the cover.

Fig. 10.20b Pop the lid off to expose the striker.

Fig. 10.20c Remove cap by twisting it sharply and pulling it off the flare body.

Fig. 10.20d Strike the black knob (exposed at the top of the flare) with the cap.

Fig. 10.20e Take care to strike *away* from the body to avoid splattering hot materials on you.

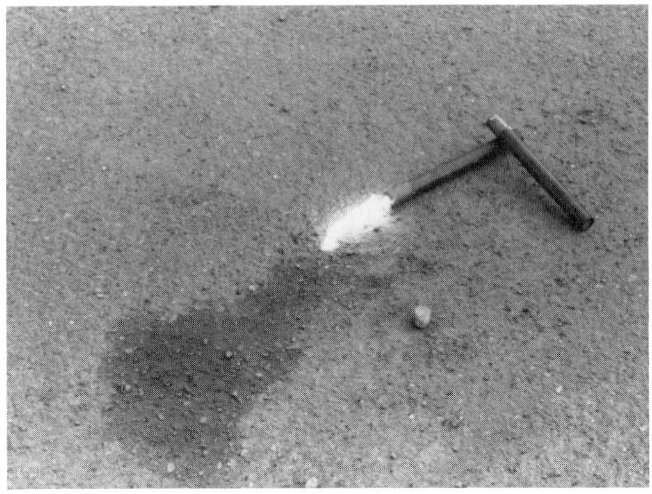

Fig. 10.21 To extend flare protection for a longer duration, simply place an unlit flare with its cap removed on top of the base of the lit flare.

scene when fuel, oil, or any other highly combustible liquids or *vapors* are present. Keep in mind that gasoline VAPORS are heavier than air and may be present downhill/downwind from a wreck.

Care must also be exercised when placing flares to insure that they are not placed where washdown hoses will extinguish them or cause them to roll, still iginited, into something combustible.

Warning Triangles. The large, reflective orange-red triangles often used by truck drivers to mark their parked vehicles are especially effective warning devices. These devices are also safe to use when there is an odor of gasoline or any possibility of fire present at the scene.

Placement of Warning Devices. The placement of flares and reflective triangles is essentially the same for most situations. When warning devices are used to mark a disabled vehicle or an accident scene limited to one side of the roadway, the devices should be placed in the following order. One device should be placed alongside the scene or vehicle. A second device is placed approximately 150-200 feet towards approaching traffic. A third device should be placed about 300 feet from the scene. This distance can be estimated by counting your steps as you walk quickly. Typi-

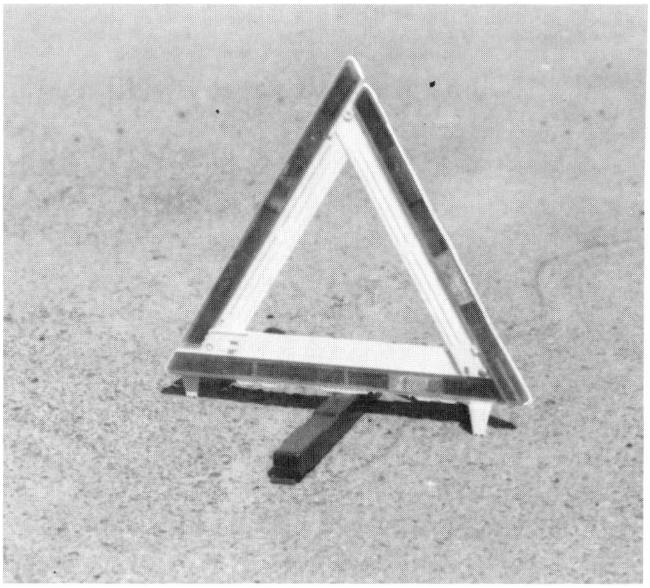

Fig. 10.22 Warning triangles are another means of alerting drivers to a scene.

cally, the average pace is slightly more than two feet. Placement will also depend on whether or not the roadway is obstructed. If a vehicle is off to the side of the road, it may suffice to place warning devices at the edge of the roadway. If a traffic lane is blocked, the warning device should be placed in the center of the affected lanes. These placement guidelines are offered for straight, flat roads. The presence of hills, curves, or other obstructions to the vision of approaching traffic will require more creative placement of the warning devices. The speed of approaching traffic will also be a factor in determining adequate distances for placing flares or warning triangles.

Summary

Regardless of the reason for the emergency response by the ambulance crew, several concerns must be addressed. A true emergency must be perceived; the vehicle should always be driven cautiously and courteously. The ambulance driver must always exercise due regard for public safety when he drives in an emergency mode. The vehicle must be positioned on the road so that it can be seen by others. The emergency signaling equipment only requests the right-of-way. You must have eye contact and commitment by all other drivers before overtaking or passing through intersections.

Keep in mind that you are responding to someone else's emergency, not your own. Such an attitude will allow you to slow down and drive with everyone's safety in mind.

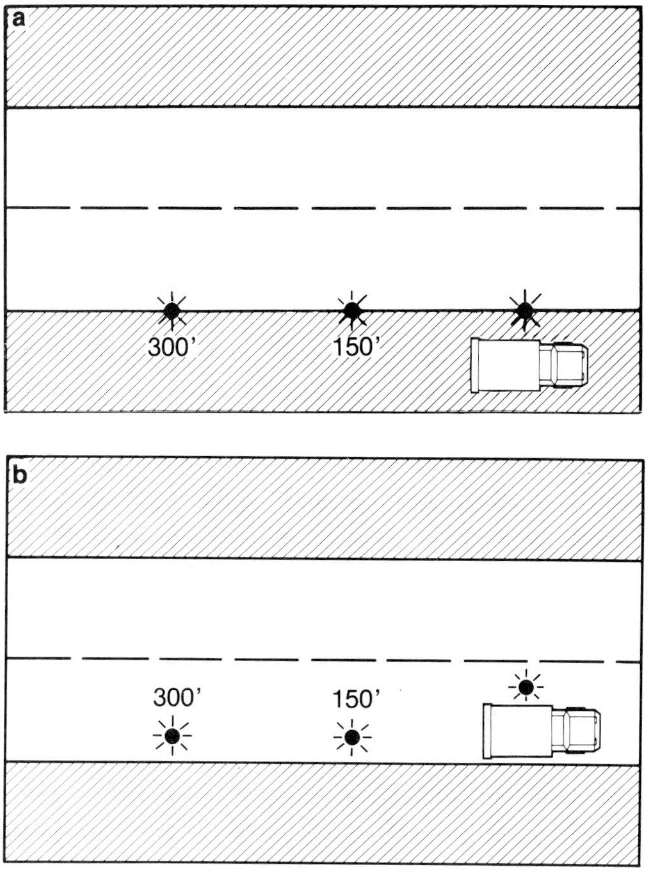

Fig. 10.23 Place warning devices as follows: one along side the scene, a second 150 to 200 feet toward approaching traffic, a third at about 300 ft. and possibly a fourth 150 to 200 ft. in the other direction.

11 ADVERSE CONDITIONS

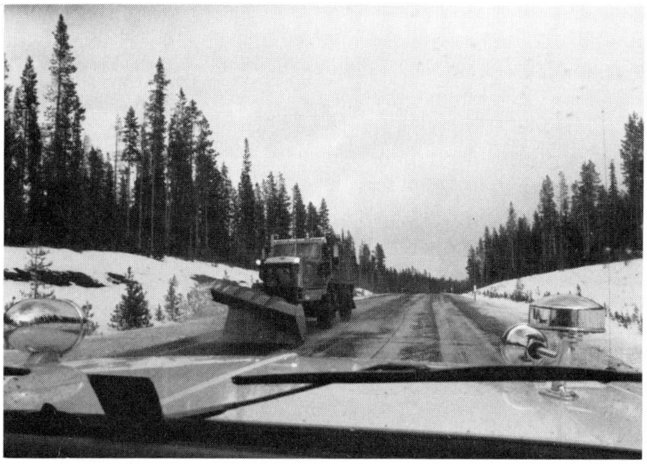

Anyone who drives for very long will soon find himself driving in adverse conditions. Adverse conditions can range from simply driving at dusk to driving in a freezing rain which is making the streets all but impassable. Many motorists shy away from such adverse conditions and refuse to drive in them. Of course that is a luxury the ambulance crew cannot afford. While driving under such conditions can be extremely frightening and dangerous, both of these elements can be reduced by learning a bit about how to handle each condition. With experience, the driver can look upon adverse conditions as a challenge. When he encounters something different from that which he sees everyday, his mind will be livened, his reflexes quickened, and generally he'll be more aware of what is happening around him. These intensified feelings can be very good. The runner is said to experience such feelings. So too does the mountain climber and others who are involved in risky sports. This is not to say that the driver goes in search of such conditions, and then drives with reckless abandon. Rather, this is a time to exercise all caution. The challenge comes in taking on such a dangerous situation and driving safely within it. The same philosophy holds true for the mountain climber. Although some people might believe that the urge to climb is some sort of death wish, in reality, the climber rarely has such a feeling. Instead, he looks at the challenge of making a dangerous situation as safe as possible. The reward for succeeding is a sense of self-awareness and accomplishment; confidence that one can meet the challenge. By viewing driving in adverse conditions in this same manner, the driver will realize that he must learn as much as possible about each condition, and then practice driving them in a safe manner.

Once the driver accomplishes these tasks, he'll be less frightened when faced with adverse conditions. At the same time, his knowledge will also reduce some of the danger associated with driving under such conditions.

Types of Adverse Conditions

Adverse conditions come in a variety of forms including such things as ice, snow, fog, and darkness. Adverse conditions can be separated into two categories: those that affect vision and those that affect traction. Those conditions which affect traction are certainly the more dramatic, the ones that everyone thinks of first, but adverse visual conditions are more prevalent. Although they may go unnoticed, they certainly cause significant driving problems.

Before any type of adverse condition can be driven safely, everything must be in good working order.

The Vehicle

As discussed earlier in the text, the vehicle's condition is always important. Additional discussion on a few important aspects of the vehicle follows.

The Windshield. It is imperative that the windshield be kept as clean as possible in anticipation of driving in adverse conditions. Any vision problems encountered during adverse conditions will be magnified by a dirty windshield. Keep the windshield clean by using a commercial windshield cleaner. Commercial cleaners make the windshield more slippery so moisture runs off easier. The cleaner reservoir should also be kept filled with the same cleaner, diluted according to the manufacturer's recommendations in water, so it is readily available for use while driving.

In addition to commercial windshield cleaners, products are available that coat the windshield to make it more slippery. Such products enable dirt to more readily come off and also allow water to run off to the point that wipers need not be used as frequently, thus reducing wiper blade wear.

The inside surface of the windshield must also receive frequent attention. A thin film will be created on the inside of the windshield if smoking occurs in the vehicle or if the vehicle is parked in direct sunlight for long periods. Many of the interior components of the vehicle such as the dashboard and seat upholstery will give off a gas which will coat the inside of the vehicle's glass and create a film similar to that which is found in a smoker's vehicle. While not appreciably affecting day vision, that film will reduce night visibility. Additionally, lights of the oncoming traffic hit this film and are refracted into a multitude of sparkles which will cause the pupils to dilate and constrict rapidly or fibrillate.

Under some conditions, the windshield may not defog as well as it should. This condition can go unnoticed at night or especially in fog since vision is already diffused. In humid weather, the air conditioner may actually work better to keep the windshield clear than the defogger since the air conditioner moves a greater volume of air. In chilly weather, the air conditioner can be used without passenger discomfort by moving the temperature selector to the warmer settings.

Windshield Wipers. The windshield wipers should always be in good repair. As mentioned earlier, they should be replaced each fall. They should also be inspected, and if necessary, changed after any frost, ice, or unusual heat. Ice and frost tend to tear the edges of the blade as it moves across the windshield, thus reducing the right angle of the edge which is so important for the squeegy effect on glass. Heat will actually allow a small portion of the rubber edge to melt and adhere to the windshield. Since the windshield reflects sunlight and the black wiper blade absorbs it, little heat is required to cause blade deterioration.

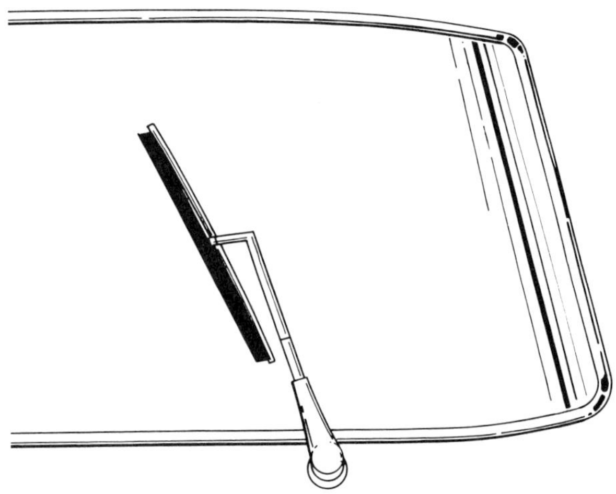

Fig. 11.1 Ice, frost and heat deteriorate the wiper blade's edges, thus reducing the right angle of the edge. Efficiency is lost.

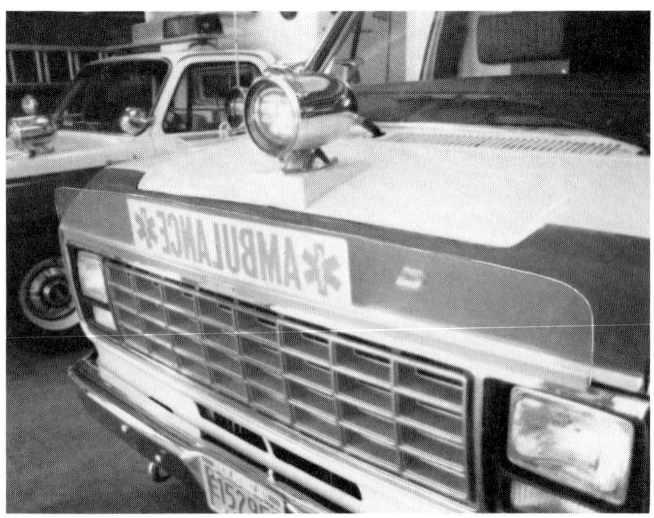

Fig. 11.2 Insect screens or wind deflectors redirect air currents passing over the hood and reduce the accumulation of bugs on the windshield.

Bug Screens. Bug screens or wind deflectors are found on the front of many vehicles which are intended to reduce the accumulation of bugs on the windshield. These plastic guards sharply deflect the air current coming over the hood of the vehicle, causing bugs and even rain and snow to be directed upward, missing the majority of the windshield surface.

Headlights. Driving in traffic will invariably cause the lights to become dirty, as debris from other vehicles is thrown up in your vehicle's path.

Of course this condition becomes worse when the roads are wet. The resulting film of dirt significantly diminishes the projection of the lights. Snow can build up very rapidly, also causing lighting problems. Therefore, the headlights should be monitored closely and cleaned as needed.

Be Prepared

The vehicle is not the only thing that must be ready for the adverse conditions—so must the driver. A driver who is ill or fatigued will not have reactions as sharp as one who is healthy and well-rested. In addition, illness will tend to adversely affect a driver's night visibility.

A driver must also stay relaxed! This one condition is the key to driving in adverse conditions. Most drivers get into trouble because they "psych" themselves out so much that they cannot possibly relax before they actually start to drive. Driving in such conditions will often require the driver to consciously get relaxed before pulling out onto the street. If such effort is required, then that is what simply must be done before driving. Once relaxed, the driver must constantly monitor himself to make sure he stays relaxed. It is interesting to watch a nervous driver in fog. As he drives, he will slowly move his head closer and closer to the windshield, until he reaches a point where his chin is over the top of the steering wheel and his arms are very flexed. Presumably, this position helps him to see further down the road. This, of course, is not true. However, this posture does diminish the driver's ability to control the vehicle and fatigues him very quickly.

By relaxing, the driver can steer the vehicle, accelerate, and brake much more smoothly—critical tasks when driving on ice or snow, since a driver tends to drive faster the more tense he becomes. Relaxing also makes driving slow much easier.

A light grip of the wheel should be maintained. In order to keep the tension from developing, the driver may actually hold the wheel only with the fingertips. Steering with your fingertips will allow the wheel to be turned rather than whipped, a desirable trait.

Of course, an extremely important part of preparing for driving under adverse conditions is the development of proper visual habits. Proper habits will allow the driver to see in the most difficult conditions, and will also help him to relax.

Driving at Night

Although night driving may seem routine to many drivers, to others it is something they dread. Under any conditions, night driving is more dangerous. While only 30% of all automobile accidents happen at night, 47% of the fatal accidents occur at night. There are a number of reasons for these statistics. People driving at night are generally more fatigued, and the percentage of those drivers who are under the influence is also much higher. Additionally, the eye cannot see as well at night, which contributes to accidents.

How the Eye Works. Understanding how the eye works will allow you to get the most out of it and improve your night vision. The eye has two receptors, cones and rods. Cones, named for their shape, are used primarily during daylight or times of high ambient light. Normal daytime vision is called photopic. Cones are color-sensitive, they allow us to see color. Located near the center of the retina, cones allow us to see with the full eye.

Rods, again named because of their shape, are used primarily for night vision (scotopic vision). Rods see shades of gray, without color, and are generally located around the periphery of the retina. During the day, eye strain can decrease the scotopic vision.

The change of use from the cones to the rods has a peculiar effect called the Purkinje Shift. This is the phenomenon whereby dark colors are more readily seen during the day. As darkness comes on and vision changes to the use of the rods, dark colors drop from sight. This is significant since dark colors are not readily seen in daylight because they can often be camouflaged by background colors. At night these same dark colors blending with the background often become nearly impossible to see.

Let's examine why light affects our night vision to such a great degree. The rods are made up of molecules of Vitamin A, attached to protein. Bright light causes the two to separate causing a momentary loss of function until they can be reunited. Such a condition might therefore indicate to some that drivers need to take more Vitamin A to increase their night vision. However, nutritionists indicate that most Americans already consume enough Vitamin A and that additional amounts will not perceptively change night vision. There is a subtle warning contained here. Keep in mind that you are sharing the road with some drivers under the influence of alcohol. Alcohol and Vitamin A are metabolized in the liver; however, the liver likes the alcohol more and will metabolize it while avoiding the Vitamin A. This metabolization action will, of course, reduce the scotopic (night) vision of a person under the influence of alcohol.

How to Drive at Night. Driving for long distances at night can cause a driver to develop a false sense of security as the night envelops him like a cocoon. It is at night that one often becomes more introspective without the visual distraction of things that are seen during daylight. Since visual factors are reduced, drivers often discontinue the use of their proper seeing habits and instead begin to stare straight ahead.

Equipped with the knowledge of how the eye works, you can understand that at night, more than ever, you need to keep the eye moving.

Since you see more with your peripheral vision (where the rods are located) at night, concentrate on shapes rather than colors. You can see the shapes of different shades of gray. Therefore, you should look for changes in the shade of gray against the darker background.

While most drivers only look in the field of vision illuminated by their headlights, a good driver will look beyond his lights for the shapes not yet illuminated. He will also use the lights of other vehicles on the road to aid vision. The lights of an oncoming vehicle will show shapes that may not be apparent beyond your lights. The taillights of the vehicle in front of you can also create shadows of objects in the road that are between the two vehicles. The headlights of the vehicle in front of you will also illuminate a portion of the road that your lights cannot reach. By looking as far ahead as the leading vehicle's lights broadcast, you may be able to see hazards much earlier, which will help you to prepare for them.

All drivers should realize that light does not bend. For this reason, it is harder at night to see around a curve. Therefore, you should slow additionally when negotiating curves at night. Often, you can get an idea about the amount of curve to be encountered by watching the reflector posts along the side of most roads. These will, when properly placed, appear closer together on sharper curves. Learn how to read these clues. In lieu of reflector posts, power poles and lines can be used as clues on long, sweeping curves.

Depth perception is also greatly distorted at night. A truck pulling out in the distance will appear much further away at night. Some of this distortion can be attributed to the fact that, in the daytime, the entire truck can be seen in its relationship to the environment. At night, only the truck's lights can be seen without reference to the environment. Additionally, scotopic vision does not lend itself to good depth perception. Therefore, when driving in darkness, you should allow extra room for passing or pulling out at intersections.

How to Maintain Night Vision. Since bright light causes the Vitamin A to separate from the protein, it is obvious that you want to avoid looking at bright lights whenever driving. The first step in reducing light is to turn the dashboard instrument lights down as low as practical (not so low that you have to strain to see them). Next, limit the use of any light in the interior. Quite often maps will be used to aid the ambulance crew in finding the scene. When maps are read at night, a small light should be used by the second crew person, aimed well away from the driver. Certainly care should be taken that the light never shines right at the driver. It is curious that red light does not separate the Vitamin A from the rods like other light does. Therefore, a red lightbulb should be used by the map reader when possible.

Obviously, you should avoid looking at the headlights of the oncoming traffic. By looking at them, the eye will be flooded with light, and the scotopic vision will be disturbed. Instead, you should look at the white line painted along the side of most roads, often called the fog line. This will reduce the amount of light entering the center of the eye. Then, using your peripheral vision, you can watch the oncoming vehicle and its relationship to the center line.

Certainly you don't want to blind an oncoming driver with your bright lights; you still must get them to dim their lights when you approach. You can do this by quickly flashing your high beams and dimming back to low beams. This should alert the oncoming driver of the need to dim his lights. The idea of "that driver isn't going to dim his lights so I'll blind him with my lights" is immature and extremely dangerous! Blinding the oncoming driver only increases the risk of collision. The quick flash is dangerous enough, and should only be done as a last resort, and not repeatedly.

It is easy to assume that when you are traveling in an emergency mode other drivers will be pulled over to the side, so you need not dim your headlights. Such an assumption can eventually cause a collision since oncoming drivers will be blinded and may cross the centerline. As mentioned before, even when traveling in an emergency status, you should be courteous to others. This is one situation where courtesy is a must. Additionally, use of your bright lights will actually mask sight of your emergency lights. Lights should be used on bright as long as possible to facilitate night vision, but they must be dimmed at least 500 feet ahead of an approaching vehicle and 300 feet behind a vehicle you are following. In addition, the headlights should be dimmed before entering any right-hand curve since they will instantly blind anyone coming around the curve. You should become accustomed to watching for the projected light beams of oncoming vehicles on curves and hills in order that you may dim your lights before the vehicle is actually seen.

Twilight

Driving in twilight is actually more dangerous than night driving. Almost one-third of all motor vehicle accidents occur during the brief period of time between 4 p.m. and 8 p.m. More than one-quarter of all fatalities and one-third of all pedestrian accidents occur during twilight. Children, because of their size and the driver's inability to see them under such circumstances, are twice as likely to be hit at twilight as they are during daylight hours.

Twilight is that condition which occurs twice a day, starting when the sky begins to first lighten in the morning and continuing until the sun rises. In the evening, it begins at the time the sun sets and ends with nightfall. Twilight conditions vary from 24 minutes in duration in the southern United States to all night in the winters of Alaska. The 48 contiguous states generally experience 24 to 30 minutes of twilight each evening and morning.

It is during the evening twilight that it is most dangerous to drive, since the light is continuously diminishing. The morning twilight evolves as a constantly increasing light which allows a driver's vision to constantly improve. During the evening twilight, the eye, having just been bombarded by the brilliance of the sun setting on the horizon, suddenly experiences a condition where the ambient light fades faster than the eye can adjust. Additionally, the sky will continue to stay bright for some time as the light from the sun is refracted into the atmosphere. The eye receiving this light from the sky cannot simultaneously adjust to the fading ground light, so seeing problems are encountered.

Under such diverse conditions, resolution decreases rapidly as the colors fade. The eyes, which require five minutes for scotopic (night) vision to surpass photopic vision, cannot keep up with the light changes experienced during evening twilight. The resulting lack of contrast and reduced depth perception can disorient the driver.

Often there are additional hazards present when you consider that twilight occurs about the time the roads become flooded with drivers traveling home from work. Many of these evening drivers will be suffering from a phenomenon known as "twilight narcosis." These people have put in a long day at work, are tired, and are anxious to get home. They often become impatient with the mass of traffic surrounding them and become prone to rash movement. The presence of these drivers, combined with the worst lighting conditions possible, make the evening twilight period the most dangerous time of day to drive.

How to Drive in Twilight. Use of the sun visor in such light conditions can be a great aid to the eyes. Use should start while the sun is still above the horizon, shielding the driver's eyes from its brilliance. By continuing the sun visor's use after the sun sets, the bright blue of the sky will be hidden from the eyes so that they may more easily adjust to the changing shadows of twilight.

Although this practice may seem foreign at first, it really does help to improve your vision during twilight. A properly adjusted sun visor should be just low enough to block out the direct view of the sun or at a level even with the horizon during twilight. When adjusting the visor, swing it past its lowest point so it is swung toward the windshield, not the driver's head. In the event of a collision, the driver's safety belts should restrain him so his head will not contact the visor if it is placed in such a forward position.

Sunglasses, if worn during the sunset, are often forgotten; they must be removed. Although by law the headlights don't have to be used until one-half hour after sunset, it is wise to start using them once the sun starts to set. Although the headlights will not help you to see, they will allow others on the road to see your vehicle against the brilliance of the sun. When the headlights are to be used, the low beam lights must be used, not the parking lights. Parking lights are too easily missed by other drivers as their eyes do battle with the sky. Additionally, if parking lights are used, it is easy to forget to turn on the headlights when they are needed, since your dash lights are already on. High beam lights should not be used during twilight since they will not help you to see the road any better, and instead will only serve to further blind other drivers. Since the effects of high beams cannot be readily seen in twilight, it is also easier to forget to dim them. Always look for the high beam dash light indicator when headlights are first turned on.

Since visibility is so reduced during twilight, the driver must slow down and allow extra time for recognition and then reaction. Certainly, you must exercise proper visual habits and be especially watchful for pedestrians during the twilight periods.

Fog

Fog is an interesting phenomenon that greatly reduces visibility. It occurs when moist air hangs over ground that is colder than the air temperature. The effects of fog can be startling, not the least of which is having the car in front of you suddenly disappear, leaving you with only a vague idea of where it is and its speed. Questions suddenly pop into your mind, like: "Did they jam on the brakes?" or "Did they change lanes?"

One of the most frightening effects of fog is the distortion it causes in depth perception. Most observers estimate objects to be much further away than they are in reality. Tests have shown that an object at 15 yards will appear in fog to be 30 yards away. This effect increases as the distance increases, which is interesting when you consider that the size of a familiar object is one of the determining factors of distance perception. Due to the many water droplets suspended in the air, fog magnifies objects so they actually appear larger than life.

The overpowering factors involved in the estimation of distance are the brightness of an object and its contrast to its background. Of course, both of these factors are significantly reduced in fog so an object will appear further away. In fact, when the contrast between the object and its background is reduced enough, the object will disappear even when lit.

When the eyes have nothing at which to look, they tend to focus at a very short distance in front (usually about ten feet). When an object gains enough contrast to be seen, the eye still may not see it because it is focused very closely and the contrast is not enough to bring attention to the object. This phenomenon occurs because the brain shuts down when it has nothing to do. When the eye has little to see, the brain only functions at minimum capacity for that sight. As a result, when an image appears, the brain may not wake up in time to react for its presence.

For the reasons just noted, it is easy to see that visual habits take a beating in fog. At the same time, good visual habits become all the more important to combat the effects of the fog.

How to Drive in Fog. Just as in any other adverse driving condition, you must slow down. However, you must also be careful that the slowing process does not occur too rapidly so you aren't rear-ended. Don't stop on the road in fog. If you must stop, pull well off the road and activate the hazard flashers. If your vehicle will be parked for an extended period, properly place warning triangles or other safety markers.

Certainly the headlights should be used, but only on low beam. This knowledge seems common enough, but many drivers still continue to use their bright lights in fog. Presumably, the reason for their use is that the high beams tremendously increase the light, almost to the point that it may seem like daylight. This brilliance is the result of the light being reflected off the water droplets in the air. This brilliance creates a glare that increases light but actually reduces depth of field. Sometime at night try pulling up to an object in the fog with the low beams on. Stop just as the object first comes into view. Then change to the high beam. The object will usually drop from sight or at the least blend more into the background.

Fog lights are a great help. They should be mounted low on the vehicle in an attempt to cast their light under the fog. In addition, fog lights should be amber colored. Such a color has a frequency that does not reflect as easily as white light, and therefore will penetrate further into the fog.

In fog, tiny water droplets will build up on the windshield similar to those found on the inside of the vehicle when it fogs up. This buildup of moisture can easily go unnoticed because of the poor quality of contrast present in fog. This buildup can make the fog appear thicker than it is in reality. To avoid this subtle problem, the windshield wipers, along with the defroster on the inside, should be used.

The road itself can be very difficult to see in fog. It is here that the often-used fog line really becomes a great helper. By keeping the fog line in sight, you can keep yourself lined up with the road. It will help you to maintain your lane and reduce your fear of crossing the center line.

The emergency equipment should not be used in heavy fog. Since you cannot see adequately, their use will not allow you to get to the scene any quicker. The emergency lights will create vertigo for the driver, as the many beams twirl about and may cause severe disorientation.

The siren will be refracted by the fog, causing confusion for everyone else on the road. Refraction occurs whenever sound waves slow down. Sound produced by the siren in clear air will suddenly be refracted when it meets fog. This also occurs as sound encounters different densities or layers of fog. The result of this refraction is that other drivers will become extremely confused by the siren and will be unable to determine the direction of its origin. The confusion is amplified by the fact that the other drivers are unable to gain a visual "fix" on the siren's location, since vision is so greatly impaired by the fog.

Impaired Traction Conditions

Rain

Rain is probably the most common condition a driver faces that impairs traction. Because rain is so common, many motorists don't give it the respect they should. It is interesting to note that six times as many people are killed while driving on rain-slicked streets as are killed on snow and ice-covered streets combined. The fact of the matter is that it takes twice as long to stop on a wet street as it does to stop on a dry one. Of course, if stopping traction is reduced, so will be cornering traction. Therefore, not only does a driver have to drive slower in rain, he also has to take corners slower.

A driver needs to be extremely careful right after a rain starts, especially if there has been a long, dry spell prior to the rain. The reason for this extreme care is that as vehicles travel over the streets and roads they deposit small amounts of oil and other debris. Debris can be in the form of oil-soaked dirt that may fall from underneath the vehicle. Gasoline may vent out and spill, and although most vehicles are fairly tight, they still tend to leave small amounts of oil, transmission fluid, and grease behind. Tar from the asphalt that leaches out during warm weather will also be present. While all of this material tends to stay in the cracks of the road (more or less solidified during dry weather), as soon as it starts to rain, this material floats to the surface and mixes with the water. The mixture of lubricants that is then floating on the water becomes extremely slippery and reduces the friction coefficient of the road. It is interesting to note that when a rain first begins after a long, dry spell, accidents increase dramatically during the first half hour. Extremely slick conditions usually last for approximately one-half to three-quarters of an hour after the rain begins and then taper off to a point where the wet street is only twice as slick as it would be if it were dry.

Be especially cautious on hills, since oil buildup is more prevalent there due to the increased engine and drive train strain produced as the vehicle climbs the hill.

Standing water can present several problems for the driver too. A vehicle entering water that is standing on the road will suddenly decelerate since the water acts as a large brake. This resistance can, of course, force the vehicle into a path other than that which is intended by the driver. If both front tires hit a large puddle at the same time, the effect will be that the vehicle will be forced off the crown of the road or the bank of the curve. If the tires on only one side of the vehicle enter deep water, the vehicle will be pulled in that direction, since that side will suddenly have more resistance. Such rapid or uneven deceleration can cause partial loss of control of the vehicle and can also throw EMTs standing or kneeling in the patient compartment off balance, potentially causing further injury to the patient or to the technicians themselves.

Standing water can also affect the brakes. As the water is entered, some of it will find its way into the brake drums, wetting both the drums and the brake shoes. Wet brakes will dramatically extend the distance it takes to slow a vehicle. Even worse, if the brakes become unevenly water-soaked (one side takes on water but the other remains dry) when applied, the brakes will pull violently to the dry side, possibly setting up a skid.

This condition can be avoided by the driver with preplanning. If he knows his coverage area, he will know where the standing water is most likely to collect, and therefore either avoid it or enter it slowly. Once he has left the puddle, he should lightly apply pressure to the brake pedal to see if the brakes work and if they pull evenly. If there is a problem caused by water on the shoes, it can be quickly cleared by driving for a block or two with the left foot slightly depressing the brake pedal. The pressure should be just enough to make the shoes contact the drums or disc. The heat generated will quickly evaporate the water.

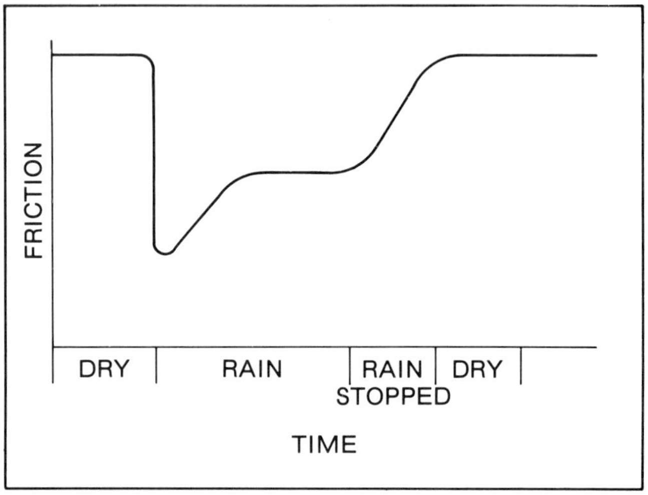

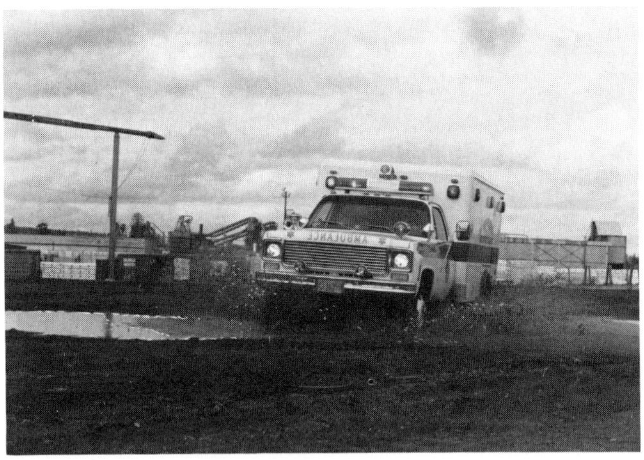

Fig. 11.3a A vehicle entering standing water suddenly decelerates since the water acts as a large brake. This can result in partial loss of control.

Rainy weather can also create visual problems not associated with the windshield. Mirrors cause problems since they are not wiped dry by a blade. Water beading up on the mirrors will distort any image that is seen. For this reason, always double check your mirror before taking any action. Occasionally, wipe the mirrors, and always try to dry them when you must back the vehicle.

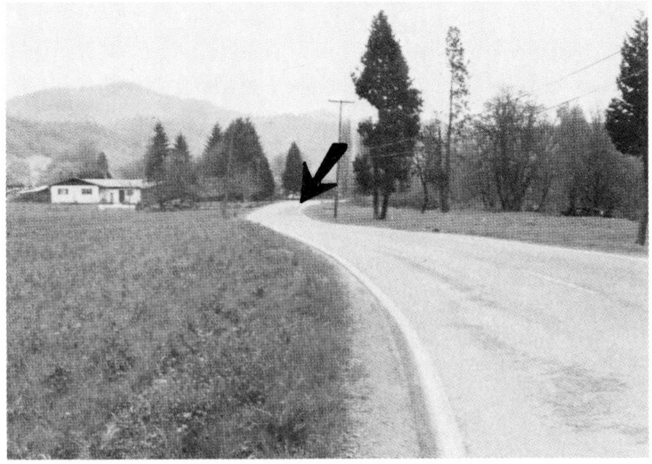

Fig. 11.3b Ambulance drivers should be familiar with hazard locations such as water accumulations in low areas in the area of coverage.

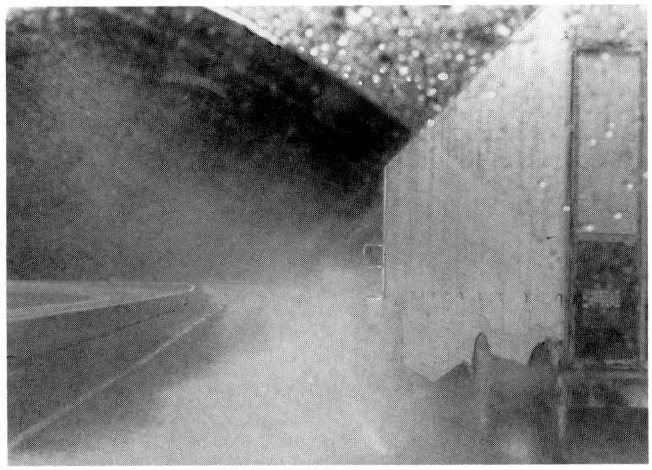

Fig. 11.4a Water spray thrown from truck tires can have a blinding effect. Choose high areas (with little rainwater on the road) for passing trucks.

As areas experience growth and traffic volume increases, streets may be widened or traffic patterns changed on them. Example: A simple two-lane street is transformed into a two-lane street with a center turn lane. When these changes occur, the old lines painted on the street are either burned off or painted over with black paint, and new lines are applied. On a dark, rainy night, the old eradicated lines may be more easily seen in the headlights' path than the newer painted lines that you are supposed to follow. It then becomes difficult for the driver to tell where he is supposed to drive unless he is already familiar with the street, since it will again appear as a simple two-lane street. Any unfamiliar motorist may then find himself driving partially on the turn lane, reducing access for anyone wanting to turn and increasing the potential for a head-on collision. Additionally, at night, lights are reflected from the wet pavement, adversely affecting night vision and distorting the appearance of the road.

Leaves

Certainly if a driver can overlook the effects of rain on streets, he can overlook the hazards associated with streets covered by leaves. Such conditions increase stopping distances since the friction coefficient is greatly reduced. Piles of leaves may also hide toys or other items left behind by playing children. Large piles of dry leaves may actually hide children playing in them. For these reasons, piles of leaves should be avoided and leaf-covered streets should be driven carefully.

Ice

Ice can increase the distance required to stop a vehicle by as much as three times the normal. Once again, if stopping traction is reduced, so too is cornering traction. Many people only think of ice occurring when the thermometer drops below 0° Centigrade (32°F). In reality, the road can have ice on it even when the ambient temperature is above freezing. The reason for this is simply that the ground can be colder than the air. Icy roads that are close to the freezing point are probably the most hazardous to drive of all the adverse conditions the driver can face. At this temperature, ice usually has a fine film of water on top of it caused by either the melting of the ice (by warmer air or from the heat of tires) or new ice creation. This film of water lubricates the already extremely slippery surface, reducing the friction coefficient even further. Under such conditions, it is possible for a standing vehicle to have such poor traction that it will actually slide off the crown of a road. Imagine trying to drive under such conditions. Extreme caution cannot be overemphasized.

Colder ice is actually a little easier to drive upon. When the surface temperature of the ice is well below 0° Centigrade (32°F), it is not as easy for water to form on the surface, and when it does it quickly freezes. Ice, when examined microscopically, is not smooth but rather jagged. Even though the ice is somewhat jagged, the surface can quickly be polished by traffic, once again reducing the already poor friction coefficient.

Have you ever heard the term "black ice"? This term is used to describe patches of ice on an otherwise dry road that often go unnoticed since they tend to blend in with the road itself. It is because these patches of ice occur only intermittently and are not easily seen that they cause so many accidents. Such conditions can easily be forecast by a knowledgeable driver and thus the danger can be reduced. Any time the temperature falls into the thirties or below, black ice should be suspected since it can form at temperatures above 32°F. Be especially watchful on bridges or over culverts, since these areas are prone to have wind blowing under them with a resulting wind chill factor that is below freezing. Additionally, because of their construction, bridges and culverts are also likely to have condensation build up on them, increasing the likelihood of ice forming.

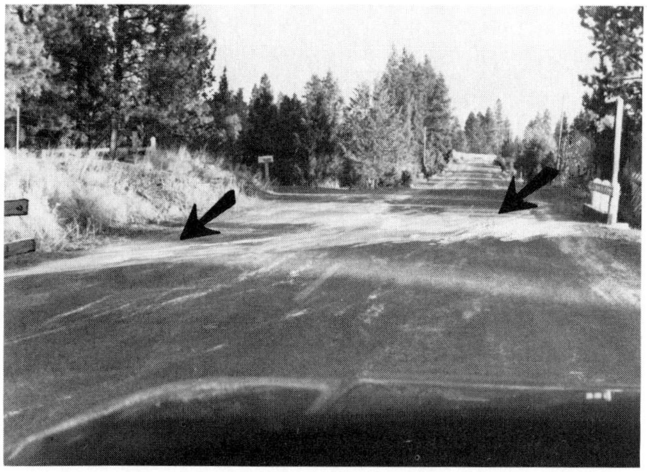

Fig. 11.4b The ice on the bridge is caused by cooler air freezing the road surface from below.

Areas that don't receive the sun during the day should also be areas of concern. Such places include the north side of a hill or mountain, buildings, and even shaded areas formed by roadside trees. Because the sun has an east-to-west arc, the north side of such formations will not receive any sun. Such areas may never be afforded enough heat for the ground to get above the freezing level, even though other areas may become fairly warm and the pavement dry.

Frost forming on the foliage beside the road should also be a clue to the possibility of ice being formed. The frost not only indicates that the ambient temperature is at or near freezing, but that there is some condensation present. That condensation may also contribute to ice being formed upon the road.

Certainly any area where water may be on the road is prone to freezing. The driver needs to be aware that, as temperatures approach freezing, moisture is not easily dissipated. Therefore, it is likely that patches of ice will be present on an otherwise dry road.

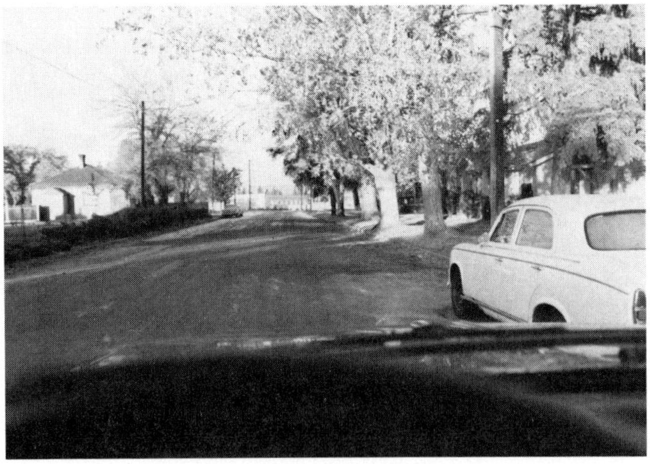

Fig. 11.4c Areas protected by trees or buildings may have a dry road surface while the rest of the road is ice covered, resulting in a very dangerous condition.

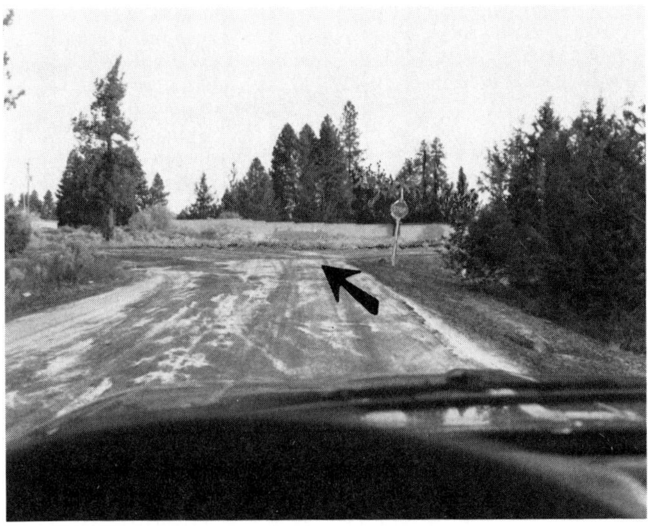

Fig. 11.4d Road surfaces receiving little sun may hide extremely icy patches. Note area to the left of the stop sign shaded by the shrubbery to the right of the road.

Driving On Ice

Icy conditions can cause near panic in some drivers, and certainly a driver should avoid driving in them whenever possible. Unfortunately, people still become sick and injured in such weather. Obviously, the ambulance crew must be able to drive safely and confidently in such conditions.

All movement of the vehicle controls should literally be done in slow motion. The steering wheel is turned very slowly, the accelerator is depressed very slowly, and, when the time comes to brake, the accelerator is released very slowly and the brake depressed the same way. Any abrupt changes can cause a slide. Too much torque applied to the tires will start them spinning. Torque can work in reverse too. By letting off the accelerator too quickly, the tire speed will rapidly slow, once again overcoming the limited traction and causing the vehicle to slide. Turning the steering wheel too fast will cause the front wheels to turn further than the vehicle can handle, given the physical force influencing the vehicle and the limited traction available. Therefore, probably the most important thing the driver can do while driving on ice is to relax. Relaxing while driving on ice is only slightly more difficult to do than relaxing is for the patient with a fractured hip. Such patients are told that by relaxing their muscles they can reduce the pain associated with the fracture. But relaxing can be done.

One trick that will help a driver to relax is to drive without wearing a coat or jacket. Although it may be cold outside and slightly uncomfortable, wearing a coat will have a tendency to bind the arms. Thus, removal will allow more freedom of movement, increasing vehicle control.

The driver must also exercise those good visual habits discussed so much throughout this text. Certainly, he must be prepared to see events developing early on so he may react *slowly* to them. He also must be sure to leave an "out" all around his vehicle. When the road is icy, any vehicle could start sliding without warning. It isn't fun to be beside another vehicle when it suddenly starts to slide, making an accident inescapable. In order to avoid as much as possible those times when two vehicles are close to each other, you should attempt to maintain the same speed as the majority of traffic, neither going faster or slower. When another vehicle must be passed, pick the place carefully so a minimum of traffic will be involved, the shoulders will be wide, and no curves or stops are ahead.

As discussed in an earlier chapter, it is easier to maintain motion than it is to stop and have to develop it again. It is also important to realize that slowing will take longer since resistance (traction) is reduced on ice. So you must look far ahead so the need to slow can be seen early, and slowing done carefully, with the hope that a full stop will not be necessary.

Hills. Icy roads on hills present a special problem because it is so easy to lose traction on them. The trick to driving on an icy hill is to eliminate any wheel spin, since this will rapidly stop forward progress and often cause the vehicle to start sliding backwards. Whenever possible, a safer route should be used to avoid the steeper hills. Additionally, vehicle momentum must be developed before ascent begins. You then must continue up with enough power to maintain traction but not so much that the drive wheels break loose. This is the only way to make it.

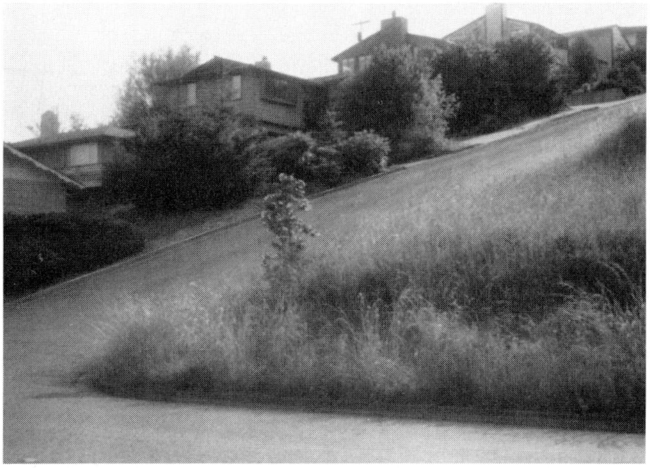

Fig. 11.5 Whenever possible, use an alternative route to avoid steep hills, even if the route is longer.

Increasing Traction

Here are several measures that can be taken to get the most traction possible:

- Driving with a full gas tank increases vehicle weight which aids traction.
- By driving slightly off center of the lane, traction can be increased since the tires are in the sand or salt cast aside by others (quickly thrown out of the tire lanes by the other traffic).
- When pulling away from a stop, the parking (emergency) brake can be set slightly to create an equal drag on both rear wheels so they get equal power. Such a maneuver offsets the normal tendency of a standard rear end to give more power to the right wheel, often causing it to spin. Once this slipping or spin occurs, all power ends up going to that wheel. As you can see, a slight braking effect provided to only the rear wheels (parking brake) can go a long way in diminishing this adverse effect.

During extreme ice conditions, one of two maneuvers can be employed at stop signs or red lights that will assist you in remaining stopped and later leaving that position. While stopped with your right foot on the brake, you should either set the parking brake or place the automatic transmission in neutral. This is because the automatic transmission will continue to apply torque to the rear tires, even when the engine is at an idle. This torque may cause the rear tires to spin slowly on the ice while the front tires are being held by the much stronger front brakes. The result of this slow spin is that the ice under the rear tires becomes so polished that when the time comes to move away, no traction can be obtained. The emergency brake, working only on the rear tires, can prevent this condition from developing.

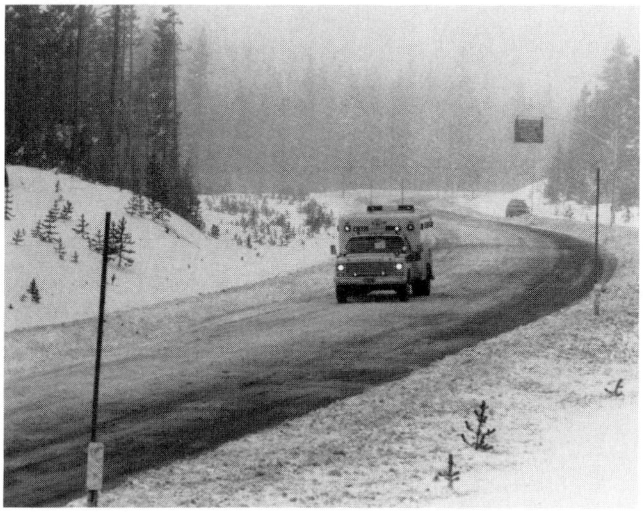

Fig. 11.6 Pumping the brakes is only acceptable on snow-covered or icy roads.

It is a good idea to carry a small pail of sand or road salt in an outside compartment when operating in ice and snow. If you get stuck while stopped on slick but not deep snow, or ice, spreading some of these materials in front of the power tires will help. Commercial cat litter may also help, as some will not only increase the friction coefficient by being abrasive, but the chemicals present will melt and absorb snow and ice.

Traction Devices

Today such devices as studded tires, tire chains and cables, and snow nets are available to help us through snow and ice. Unfortunately, they all have limitations. First, snow tires are of limited value on ice since they are designed to dig down into the snow in order to provide added traction. This action cannot be achieved on ice. (Radial all-season tires are probably the best tire available for ice driving.) Studs embedded in the tire tread increase traction on ice by about ten percent, allowing a vehicle to negotiate conditions that could otherwise be almost impossible. However, the problem with studded tires is that they seem to increase a driver's confidence by about thirty percent. Obviously, this false security can actually lead to accidents. Tire chains and cables also work on ice, but not a lot better than studs. Both chains and cable devices are designed more for snow than for ice. The problem with these devices is that they allow a segment of tire to cross the ground in between each cross link of chain or cable. Each time this occurs, the tire has a chance of slipping since it is going from a condition of more traction to less traction. Once the tire starts slipping, these implements can lose their value unless they are allowed to roll and contact of a cross link is reestablished with the road surface.

Contrary to popular belief, tire chains can be used on radial tires. However, care must be taken to insure that the fasteners that attach to the outside bands have their closure facing out so they don't tear the side wall of the tire. Additionally, if standard chains are used on a radial tire, the rubber tighteners cannot be applied, since they will keep the tire side wall from flexing properly.

A drawback to the use of standard tire chains is that they create extreme noise and vibration. For this reason their use should be avoided whenever possible. Tire cables, on the other hand, don't create as much vibration or noise as standard chains, and are also much easier to apply.

A relatively new device known as a Snow Net is now available for increasing tire traction on snow and ice. According to one manufacturer, they provide easier application and better traction than either standard tire chains or studded snow tires. The manufacturer also states that the snow net significantly reduces the noise and vibration normally associated with tire chains.

These devices, just as studs do, have a tendency to give drivers more confidence than the increased traction they provide dictates. For this reason, care must be exercised in their use. Vehicles equipped with tire chains should not be driven at speeds higher than about thirty miles per hour.

Snow

A fact that many motorists may not realize is that snow often affords more traction than ice, since it can be compacted between the treads as a tire moves over it. It is in such conditions that snow tires excel in providing traction, but as snow is traveled upon, it begins to compact and the surface virtually becomes ice. For this reason, snow should be driven much like ice, since the traction coefficient is roughly the same. Even when the snow is packed, traction can often be improved by driving slightly off-center of the lane to take advantage of the snow that has not been compressed at each side of the tire grooves.

As discussed in the section on ice, the colder the surface of the snow, the better the traction

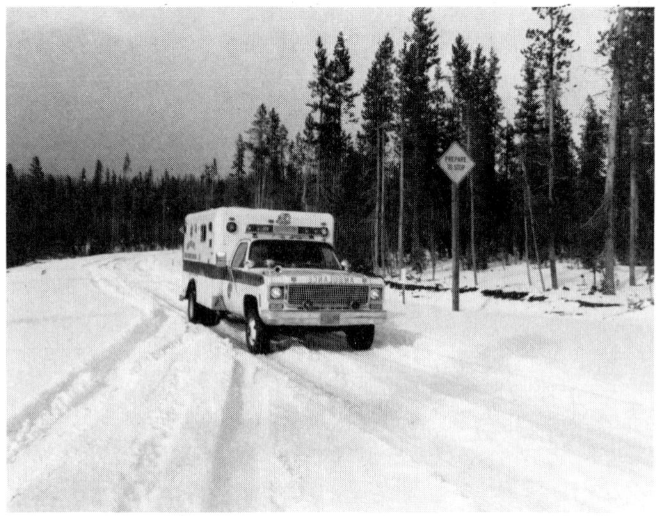

Fig. 11.7 As a snow-covered road begins to compact, the more frequently traveled surface becomes icy. Driving slightly off-center of the compacted area may increase the road's traction.

coefficient. One observation that can help you to judge the slipperiness of the snow is noticing whether snow is sticking to the tires of the vehicle you are following. If the snow is sticking, the leading vehicle's tires will be more white than black. This observation can also be made as the leading vehicle travels on the polished traffic lane and then moves off center into less packed snow.

Another problem associated with snow is that it can quickly clog headlights so they will not cast light as far. Headlights should be routinely checked and cleared at every opportunity to avoid this problem.

Snow can also accumulate on windshield wipers, causing them to lose their wiping ability. The driver may be able to reach out of his window and snap a moving wiper to help relieve the crust while still driving. This act must, of course, be performed with great care since inadvertent turning of the steering wheel is possible.

Emergency lights can also become covered with ice and snow during extreme conditions. When such a condition develops, your emergency lights cannot be seen by anyone in front of your vehicle. Be aware that the siren can also become clogged during a heavy snow storm. The change will be gradual, often going unnoticed by the driver. Ask yourself if the siren is still as loud as usual? If not, your emergency lights may also be so encrusted by snow that they cannot be seen by anyone in front of the vehicle. A misleading observation may be that the light will still be reflecting off of objects to the side of the ambulance. Remember, the snow builds up on the leading edge or front of the lights. An electronic siren may also start to smell like it is burning when the speakers become clogged with snow.

Driving snow can cause extreme problems for the driver. It can mound up on the road, creating small drifts. Small drifts are best negotiated by keeping the wheels straight and hitting the drift squarely. This will cause the snow to fly over the roof of the vehicle, causing a temporary loss of vision.

If a drift is not hit squarely, there is a high potential for a front tire to be grabbed by the drift. This rapid deceleration, coupled with the poor traction coefficient present at the other three wheels, can cause a slide and/or a rapid rollover, caused essentially by the drift tripping the vehicle.

Large drifts should be avoided until they can first be investigated. If you determine that you cannot drive around the drift, and nothing, such as a snow-covered car is inside it, the only way through is once again with momentum, hitting it squarely.

The more common problem associated with drifting snow is the small ridges that build up on the road. These ridges cause the road to become rough. Additionally, they result in a road with a constantly changing friction coefficient. As the tires go over mounds of packed snow and then land on relatively dry pavement, the potential for control loss and slidé increases greatly.

Some services have four-wheel drive ambulances available for use in adverse traction conditions. These vehicles excel in getting where other vehicles cannot, since they can deliver positive traction to all four tires. There are some pitfalls commonly experienced with 4x4s. One problem that people not used to driving four-wheel drive vehicles fail to realize, is that they cannot stop any

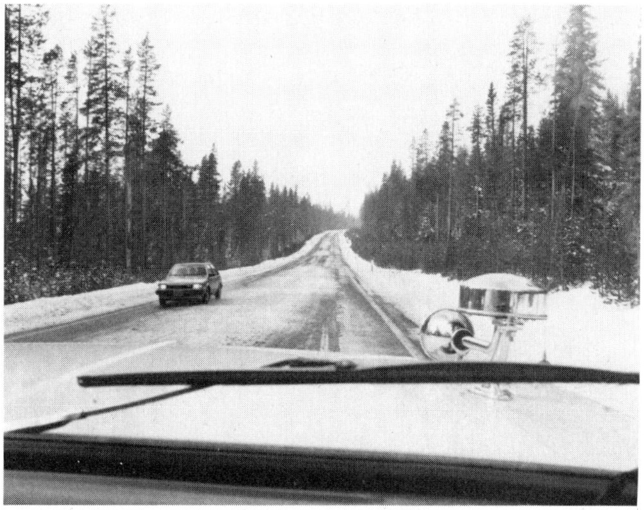

Fig. 11.8 Patches of slush can also cause a vehicle to pull to one side in the same way that brakes would—in much the same way as standing water.

faster than any other vehicle on the road. They will not corner much better than a two-wheel drive vehicle either. Then too, once in a spin, a four-wheel drive vehicle may spin faster and be harder to control than a two-wheel vehicle. Failure to recognize their limitations has caused many accidents for drivers of four-wheel drive vehicles. One word of caution which frequent drivers of 4x4s will give to others: Having a 4x4 only allows you to get deeper in the woods, snow or mud before you become stuck. Keep this in mind when going off the road with a 4x4.

Certainly driving in adverse conditions requires a driver to be at his peak performance. He cannot afford to be driving while fatigued or sick. Under such physical conditions, he should be relieved from driving. The job must be done. The keys to doing it in adverse conditions are proper visual habits and staying relaxed behind the wheel.

12 COLLISION AVOIDANCE

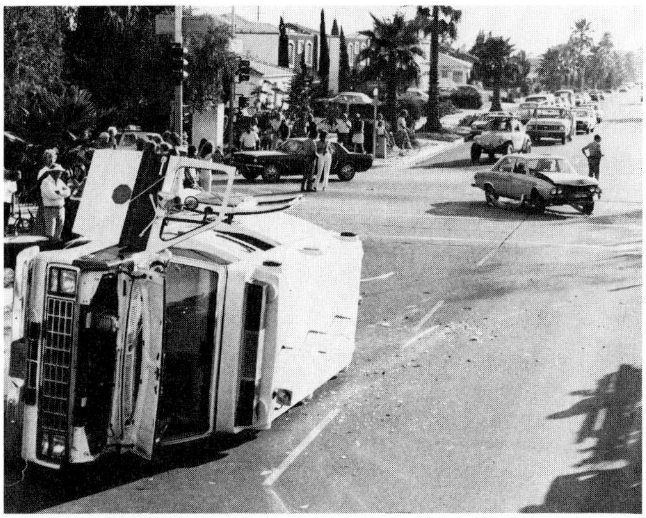

(Photo courtesy of **jems.**)

Statistics point out that one in four drivers will be involved in a major motor vehicle accident sometime in their lives. Ambulance drivers certainly are no more immune from this statistic than other motorists. Although formal driver training on how to handle the vehicle and collision avoidance can go a long way towards preventing accidents, ambulance drivers will still be involved. Collisions can happen to anyone, even those drivers with the best visual habits and safest driving records. Accidents don't have to be the fault of the ambulance driver; sometimes they just cannot be avoided. However, an accident's severity can almost always be lessened if the driver does one thing. He must continue to drive the vehicle!

Unfortunately, when faced with an impending collision, most drivers panic. They might throw their hands in the air and close their eyes, or they might take a death grip on the wheel and anchor the brakes. The point is, these people do nothing to avoid or lessen the severity of the accident. Turning from the path of a head-on collision, going into the ditch, or purposely driving into the shrubbery along the highway can lessen the severity of a collision. A good driver will be able to differentiate between those situations he might be able to squeak out of and those he can't avoid entirely. In either case, he will continue to drive in order to lessen damage and injury.

An old police pursuit driving instructor once told a group of ambulance drivers with whom he was working, "If you're going to go off the road, you'd better go off the road like a gentleman. Drive it all the way." His point was well taken. By continually driving, a simple event such as going off the road can have its impact lessened. By continuing to drive in such a situation, the driver can determine a direction that will avoid trees, poles, and other obstacles in his path. If he is unable to return to the road, he can point the vehicle in such a direction that it will not roll over; thus he can bring the vehicle to a safe stop with less damage or injury. This type of "save" can only be accomplished if the driver keeps on driving!

As Yogi Berra once said about a baseball game, "It ain't over 'till it's over." The same holds true for driving.

Securing Equipment

For passenger safety, vehicles manufactured today must meet rigid criteria for maintaining a safe environment in the occupants' compartment. Ambulances, modified after they leave the chassis factory, often fail to meet such a severe code. Even if they do, the modifications they go through once the EMS agency takes possession often reduce passenger safety in the event of an accident.

At the top of the list of potential safety hazards is the manner in which equipment is stored. Med bags that sit on the floor and monitors only minimally secured on their counters can inflict lethal harm when they start flying around during a collision. Oxygen cylinders mounted to the bulkheads of the ambulance can be easily struck by a technician flying around out of control during a collision. Even safety devices such as fire extinguishers are often mounted where they will be easily struck by one of the occupants.

The cabinetry of the unit, while functional for the purposes of emergency care, may also become hazardous when the vehicle is involved in a collision. A person hitting one of the sharp corners of a cabinet with the forces involved in a collision will easily be injured. In the driver's compartment, the padded dashboard, designed to protect the occupants in a deceleration collision, are often of no safety value because radios and sirens are mounted where they can easily be struck by the head of an occupant.

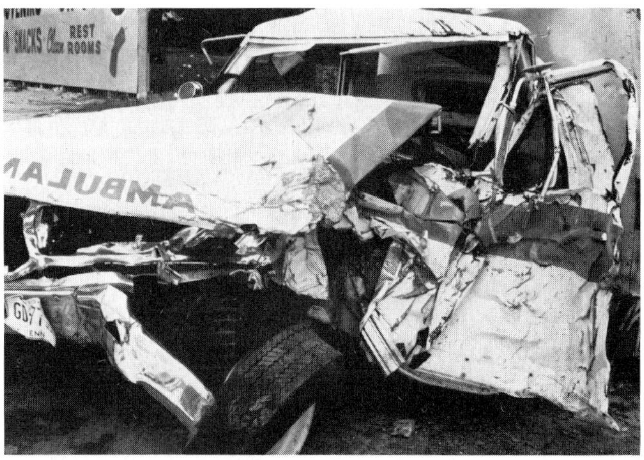

Fig. 12.1 Accidents are not planned, they just happen—no one can predict just how theirs might occur. (Photo courtesy of **jems**.)

It is a good idea for each ambulance crew to go through its unit with an eye for what could happen if the vehicle were involved in a collision. An effort should be made to secure all equipment to keep it from flying about during a collision. Compartment lids should receive special attention since most will open and dump their contents about during a rollover. All equipment should be mounted where it won't be easily struck, e.g., fire extinguishers. All sharp corners should be padded, so that they can afford some protection for the occupants. Whenever possible, the radio equipment should also be mounted where it won't be struck.

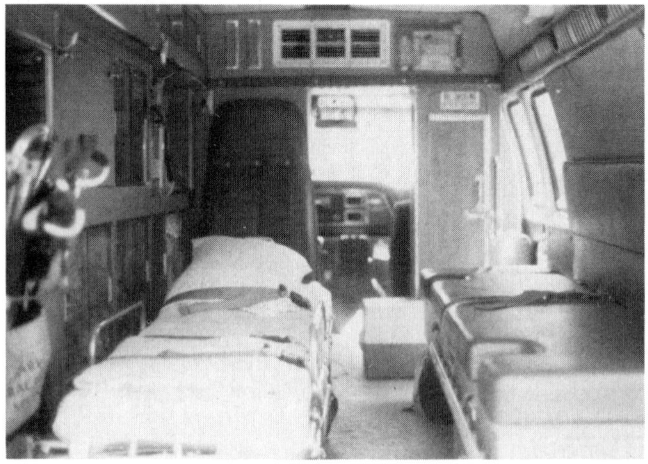

Fig. 12.2 Give special attention to securing compartment lids and the squad bench since most of these open and dump their contents during a roll-over.

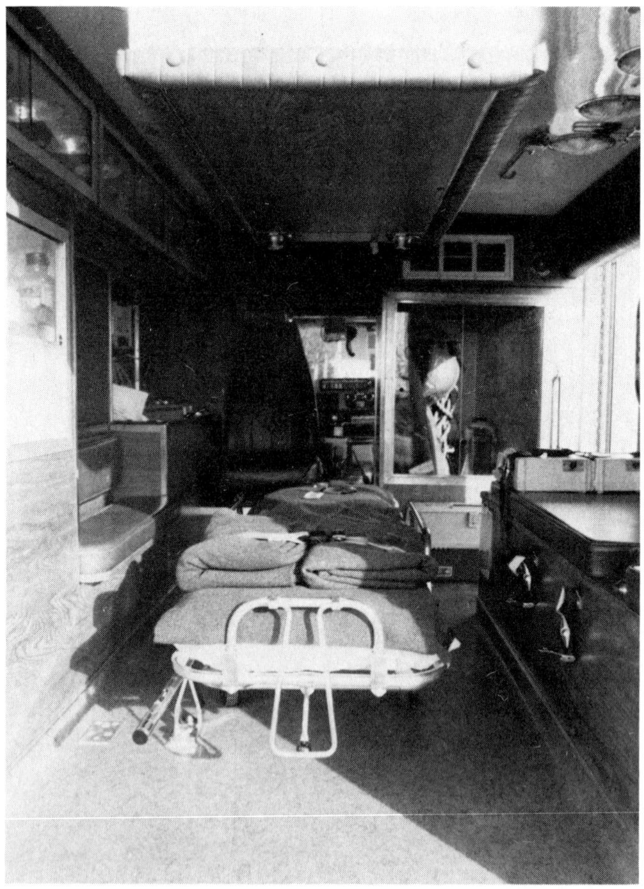

Fig. 12.3 Ambulance crews should go through their unit checking for what could possibly happen in the vehicle in the event of a collision.

The occupants themselves also need to be secured. The driver cannot continue to drive the vehicle if physical forces throw him from his seat because he was not securely belted into it. Even if you disregard the fact that the belt can save a life, keep in mind that it can also prevent an accident from happening in the first place! The other occupants should be secured too. The patient needs to be belted onto the stretcher and the stretcher secured to the chassis. Whenever possible, the technicians in the back should be securely seat-belted. Passengers, such as family members who might be riding along in the ambulance, need to have their seat belts buckled and snugged tight by one of the crew members when they are first placed into the seat. This will insure that belts are on properly and demonstrate concern for all involved in the emergency.

Contingency Plans

Accidents are not planned, they just happen. Certainly no one can predict exactly how an accident they will be involved in will occur. Frankly, most drivers probably avoid such thoughts. While it may seem unpleasant to some, by planning how to avoid accidents, by identifying escape routes and, to some degree, practicing collision avoidance, you can become better prepared to handle the real situation if it should arise. Such planning can actually reduce property loss and severity of injury. The time the accident is developing is really a poor time to start action planning. At that point, you are no longer in control of the situation and have little time to evaluate alternatives to the actual collision.

Get into the practice of looking for escape routes for different types of conflicts while driving. On occasion, take time to look at other vehicles on the road and ask yourself, "What could I do to avoid a collision if the vehicle stopped at the intersection suddenly pulled out in front of me?" Such questioning should incorporate as many different situations as possible, with a wide variety of surrounding conditions.

Example: What would you do if the driver (1) in front of you slammed on his brakes, (2) in front of you braked suddenly in an intersection, (3) beside you slammed on his brakes? Do any other circumstances come to mind? This type of hypothetical exercise should be performed while in traffic, while alone on the highway, on multilane roads, two-lane streets, in short, all different road and traffic configurations. By just looking for escape routes, you can develop habits that may help you instantly identify alternatives which will allow you to avoid a collision or reduce its severity. Of course, you must also practice good visual habits at all times. **S**earch, **I**dentify, **P**redict, **D**ecide, and **E**xecute is the name of the game if you are to avoid collisions.

When a collision is unavoidable, a driver often can choose at what angle he is going to hit. By exercising this choice, damage and injury can be greatly reduced. A head-on collision must be avoided at all costs. Two vehicles approaching one another at 55 mph will collide with an impact force equal to hitting a fixed object at 110 mph! Confronted with such a situation, it is tempting for many drivers to turn into the lane that the oncoming driver has vacated, since it offers a paved driving surface. Although some advanced driving technique instructors suggest this as the best escape route, such a manuever can be extremely risky. The oncoming driver, suddenly recognizing the impending collision, might try to get back into his own lane, thereby completing the collision that all were trying to avoid. Additionally, there may be another oncoming vehicle hidden in the blind spot created behind the offending vehicle. If you drive into the "hole" and are suddenly faced with another oncoming vehicle, it is unlikely you could again avoid a collision. For these reasons, it is recommended that if you are faced with a potential head-on collision you should drive as far to the outside as necessary to avoid the collision, even if it means driving off the road. Only when a clear path can be seen past the oncoming car should driving into the "hole" created by the oncoming car be considered as an escape route.

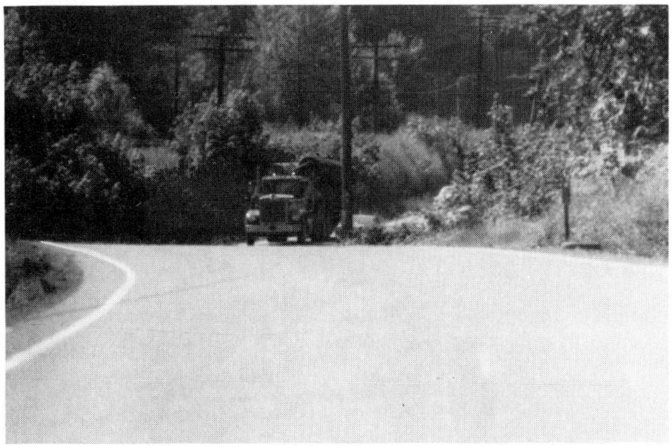

Fig. 12.4 Avoid head-on collisions at all costs. If collision is unavoidable, pick a collision object that is impact absorbing.

Often there are other components which can affect your choice of escape routes. If you have not left yourself an adequate escape route and are forced to collide with an object, try to pick something that is impact-absorbing. Shrubbery will give and break away much easier than a tree. A parked car is preferable to colliding with one that is coming head-on. When possible, avoid concrete bridge abutments, buildings, and large trees which will not absorb impact well and will cause severe damage to the vehicle and possible injury to its occupants. Power poles will also inflict tremendous damage, but if the choice comes down to hitting a wooden power pole or a live tree of the same diameter, the dead wood of the power pole will have less resistance.

If an object, especially a nonimpact-absorbing type, must be hit, damage can be further reduced by trying to sideswipe the object rather than hitting it head-on. However, sideswiping a parked car is preferable to hitting one moving alongside you in another lane since the chance of injury to others is reduced. Once a sideswipe occurs, the driver must be prepared for that action to throw his vehicle back into the path of the more severe head-on collision unless he continues to drive, keeping the wheels turned toward the bank, guard rail, or similar obstacles once contact has been made.

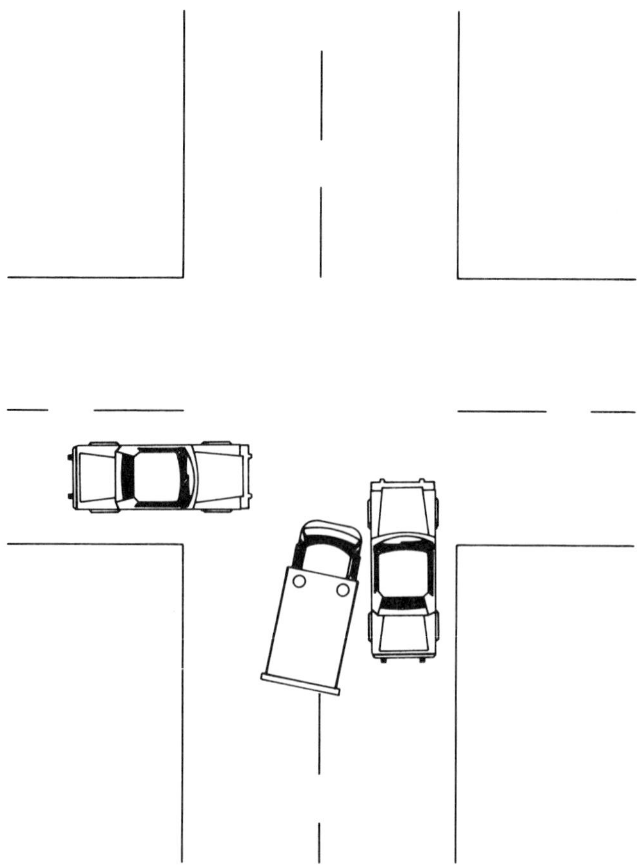

Fig. 12.5 Sideswiping another car, guardrail or other obstacle is preferable to hitting something with full force.

Collision Avoidance

Through proper action, most collisions can be avoided altogether.

There ARE three things a driver can do to avoid a collision: brake, accelerate, or turn to avoid it.

Braking. Of the three alternatives, braking is probably the most commonly employed since it is instinctive. Keep in mind that braking requires a great deal of time and distance to stop an ambulance moving at 30 mph (44 feet per second). By the time the driver recognizes the need to stop and then slows the ambulance to a stop, he will have traveled approximately 125 feet. At 60 mph, he'll be traveling 88 feet per second and require a total distance of approximately 436 feet to recognize the need and get the vehicle stopped. These figures reflect what is required if squeeze braking is done properly on dry, hard pavement. If the brakes are locked up, the distances increase dramatically. If the brake is applied too hard, you must rapidly release the pedal and then instantly reapply it but to a lesser degree. Such a reaction, unless practiced, is nearly impossible. Practice, on the other hand, should only be performed within a properly controlled driving area under the direct supervision of a qualified advanced driving techniques instructor. The important point is that you must have distance available to you for braking. If not, perhaps another alternative will need to be implemented.

Acceleration. The time may come when, after you have already entered an intersection, you observe someone who is going to collide with you and your only choice will be to accelerate, outrunning the collision.

In such situations, all the driver has to do is recognize the problem in time, tromp down on the accelerator, and steer. However, at slow speeds he must, to some degree, temper this action to avoid applying too much torque to the rear tires, causing them to spin. Spinning tires will only make the attempt to outrun the collision take longer. Of course, acceleration is not as viable an alternative for a heavy ambulance as it is for passenger cars.

Steering Out of The Way. There are many situations where steering out of the way is the ONLY alternative to avoiding an accident, but it is seldom thought of since braking is so instinctive. Additionally, most drivers do not realize how far they can "bend" the vehicle from its original path. In order to "bend" the vehicle with the greatest efficiency, that is, to move it laterally the distance needed in the least amount of space, the maneuver has to be executed properly. Most drivers have a fear that in doing so the vehicle will flip over. This is rarely the case, since almost every vehicle will start to slide (losing traction with its rear tires) before it will roll over. Faced with a head-on collision, a glancing blow would certainly be preferable. Collision avoidance training requires a properly set-up course and the direct supervision of a qualified advanced driving techniques instructor. However, a discussion of the techniques involved follows.

For most drivers initially attempting such a maneuver, it would seem logical that it would require heavy braking. As you learned in the chapter dealing with vehicle dynamics, heavy braking is actually detrimental to turning. Conversely, there are some drivers who advocate acceleration as the answer to the problem of collision avoidance. They feel that not only must the vehicle be turned out of the way, but in order to do it more quickly, the vehicle should increase its speed. Once again, if you recall what happens to traction as a vehicle accelerates, you can understand that acceleration is not efficient either.

Almost every potential collision situation requires deceleration, even if nothing more than to buy you more time. In a collision avoidance maneuver where steering is going to be involved, any deceleration is tempered with the understanding of the effects of the resulting loss of traction. Only in rare cases will you want to quickly stab the brake hard, steer, and release the brake to avoid a collision. In most cases, speed should be reduced by the driver removing his foot from the accelerator and then steering. Another key point: the driver will usually steer where he is looking. Instead of looking at the obstacle he is trying to avoid, the driver should be looking at his intended path. During this action, he should look to the far outside of his path. This is because, when turned, the vehicle will track in a tighter radius with the rear tires than with the front. If the driver only looks at or just past the obstacle, it is likely that the front of the ambulance will clear the obstacle while the rear of the vehicle will strike it.

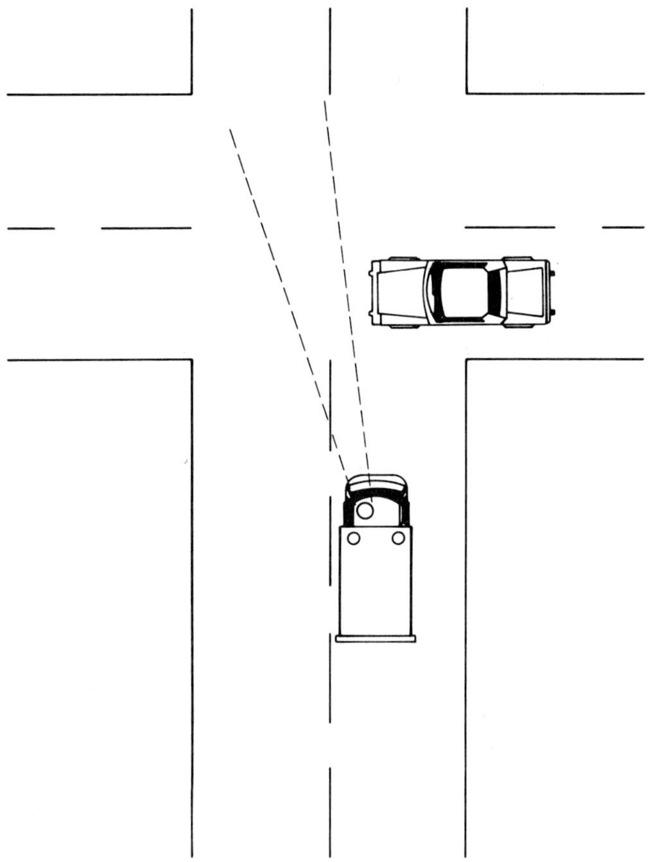

Fig. 12.6 To steer around a potential collision, instead of looking at the obstacle you're trying to avoid, look at your intended path.

A rapid collision avoidance maneuver cannot be done efficiently if the driver has to move his hands on the wheel. For this reason, it is recommended that the hands be properly placed at the nine and three positions before the maneuver is attempted. Another associated with such a maneuver is that most drivers will have a tendency to whip the wheel, turning it faster than the vehicle can respond. This might cause enough overresponse so that the vehicle strikes the obstacle to be avoided. If the obstacle is cleared and the countersteering lags or is excessive, the vehicle can either spin out or fishtail.

Whenever possible, drivers should take collision avoidance instruction so proper techniques can be learned and practiced in a controlled environment.

Off-road Recovery

Collision avoidance may simply mean driving off the road, or the act of driving off the road may in itself comprise the accident. In either case, any time the road is left, you must make every effort to drive off it in a forward direction and return to the road surface. As the road is left, the driver must be prepared to have the vehicle violently pull from the road if the wheels encounter the soft shoulder.

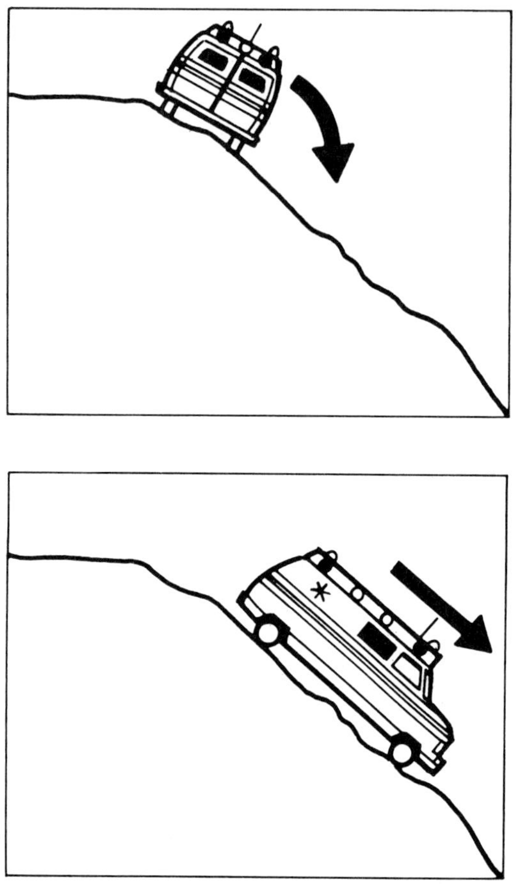

Fig. 12.7 Where road is elevated from the surrounding terrain, if your vehicle leaves the road in a parallel path, a roll-over might occur. Steering straight downhill might avoid this.

The most common reaction of drivers leaving the road surface is to instantly try to get back onto the road. It is this reaction that frequently causes a head-on collision. Typically, a driver will turn his wheels toward the pavement where they will be resisted by the difference in road surface elevation or shoulder surface consistency. This difference may require more steering input. When the vehicle finally does broach the road, it can be violently flung into the oncoming lane which may result in a collision.

To avoid this mishap, a driver leaving the road should immediately release pressure from the accelerator and continue to drive. Rapid deceleration caused by heavy braking can cause certain tires in the softer shoulder to be grabbed and possibly pull the vehicle farther off the road. If no obstacles are in his immediate path, the driver must continue to drive straight ahead until he has established steering control, and slowed the vehicle to a manageable speed for the driving condition. Then he can consider driving back onto the road surface. Before actually attempting to return to the road surface, he must

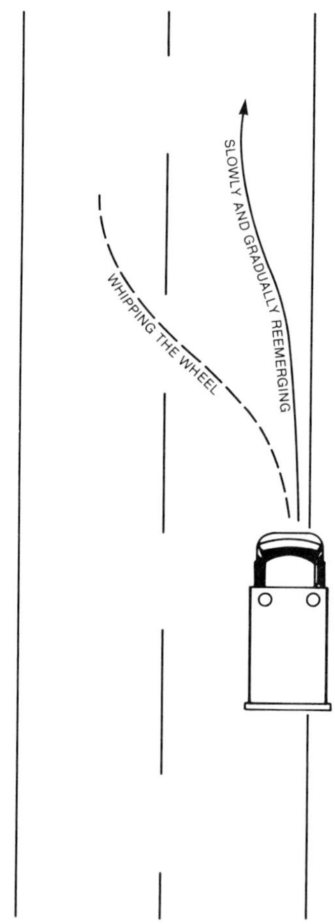

Fig. 12.8 When a vehicle leaves the road bed, avoid the driver's instinct to whip the wheel to get back into your traffic lane and possibly end up in a collision. Just decelerate slowly and continue straight ahead.

select a place where the road and shoulder are at a similar elevation (difference not greater than 4-6 inches). He should also check traffic to the rear and signal his intent to return to the road.

In the event an additional hazard (such as a pole or guard rail) is looming ahead on the shoulder of the road, the driver may have to drive immediately back onto the road, even though he may not yet be fully prepared. This is done by turning (not whipping) the steering wheel toward the road, usually about 90°, and then immediately straightening it as the front tire is felt making contact with the edge of the roadway. The brief period between the steering input and the resulting action should allow the rear tire to also climb onto the road. This rapid maneuver will allow the steering to be corrected before the vehicle is driven into oncoming traffic.

While these procedures may sound easy, their execution is actually difficult. Both should be practiced only under the supervision of a qualified advanced driving techniques instructor.

Vehicle Malfunction

Even the best-maintained ambulance can malfunction. Although statistics place the blame for very few accidents on vehicle maintenance, there are more likely a far greater number caused by partial failure, or at least vehicle inefficiency, than the statistics reflect. Consider the situation where a car is sideswiped by another driver. The driver will probably be cited for failure to maintain control of his vehicle, or possibly failure to maintain his lane. In all likelihood, no investigation will be made that will reveal that the other car was sideswiped because the first driver applied the brakes and his vehicle swerved violently due to a brake system malfunction. While most of these situations can be avoided by proper maintenance, there are occasionally malfunctions that occur to even the best-maintained vehicle.

Tire Blowout. There was a time when one of the chief fears of a motor vehicle driver was a tire blowout. However, tire blowout is not as likely to happen with the tires of today. Still, there is a remote possibility of a tire failure, so you must be prepared for its occurrence.

A blowout, as opposed to a simple flat tire, occurs when the tire is damaged to such an extent that it instantly deflates, often disintegrating in the process. A flat tire loses air over a period of a few seconds or longer. For that reason, the effects of a flat tire on handling are not nearly as dramatic as with a blowout.

During a blowout, occasional adverse handling characteristics can result in a wreck. When the event involves a front tire, the vehicle will have a tendency to pull to the side of the blowout. This will often cause the driver to whip the steering wheel in the opposite direction and overcorrect in the process. On the other hand, a blowout of a rear tire may cause the vehicle to sway back and forth, making it difficult for the driver to keep control through steering. In either situation, you should grasp the wheel firmly and attempt to steer only enough to maintain your lane position. Continuing to look and steer where you want the vehicle to go will help you to maintain your vehicle in the lane.

Another natural tendency for a driver experiencing either a front or rear blowout is to hit the brakes. This reaction can place the driver in serious jeopardy. Heavy braking will increase the negative handling effects of the blowout, causing the vehicle to react even more violently. Even getting off the accelerator too quickly can have this effect. The proper reaction is to ease off the accelerator slowly, monitoring your action's effect on steering as you do so. Once speed has been reduced to the point where steering can be maintained without much difficulty, you can slowly begin braking, still monitoring its effects on steering. Once braking begins, you should signal your intentions and move to a suitable place at the side of the road.

Brake Failure. The most commonly thought of mechanical malfunction is brake failure. Although brake failure does not occur often (especially with today's brakes), it is seen often enough on television and in the movies to cause concern with drivers. If brake failure is encountered, the driver will instinctively try the brake again several times. If pumping the brakes does not work, he must immediately get the transmission shifted into a lower gear so the engine's compression can be used to help slow the vehicle. The parking brake should also be applied since it is engaged mechanically, instead of through the hydraulic system of the conventional brakes. Keep in mind that the parking brake is not nearly as efficient as the fully operational conventional brakes and that its pressure is harder to control. Since the parking brake only activates one shoe on each rear drum, stopping distances will be much longer than normal. Additionally, application of the parking brake may cause the rear wheels to skid, so you must continue to steer.

If speed must be lost faster or if brake failure occurs while going down a hill, the driver must consider sideswiping something in an attempt to slough off speed. Otherwise, he will be out of control if the vehicle is allowed to continue without brakes. Parked cars, guard rail, shrubbery, even a dirt hillside can drain the vehicle of momentum if they are contacted by sideswiping and then the vehicle is steered so contact is maintained with them.

Steering Failure. This is almost always the result of an engine stall on a vehicle equipped with power steering. Steering failure may also result from hydraulic fluid loss from the power steering system. In either case, the vehicle still can be steered. It will just require more physical exertion since the driver must overcome the failure of the hydraulic system.

When steering is applied rapidly in one direction and then the other, the hydraulics may not be able to keep up on a poorly maintained system. This rare occurrence results in a momentary locking of the steering wheel, followed immediately by continued action. The moment when the steering stops may be sufficient to keep the vehicle from completing the maneuver the driver is attempting, causing him to strike the object that he was attempting to avoid. If such a characteristic is encountered, slower steering input may be required until the steering system can be properly serviced.

Although experienced only rarely, in the event of a total steering loss the driver can only slow the vehicle. It is important to avoid using the brake, or at least to apply it slowly, because if one side grabs more than the other it cannot be compensated for by steering and may force the vehicle into oncoming traffic. In almost all steering failures, the driver *will* have control of at least one of the front wheels.

Accelerator Sticking. Such a condition can become extremely frightening. With today's vehicles, the obvious solution (turning off the ignition) cannot be applied since it will also lock the steering wheel, usually in a shallow turn. Even if the ignition switch isn't on the column, turning off the ignition may result in much harder steering if the steering is hydraulically assisted.

If the vehicle has power-assisted brakes, they will also become much harder to use if the ignition is turned off. If the brakes are pumped once or twice, such action will deplete the brake power reservoir, and braking effort will certainly increase.

The best action for most of today's vehicles with stuck accelerators is to shift the transmission into neutral and get the vehicle off the road and stopped as quickly as possible. Understand though that once the resistance of the drive train is released by the transmission the engine will rev up quickly to a very high number of RPMs. If it is not shut off quickly, it will in all likelihood break, causing considerable engine damage. If the engine breaks before the vehicle is fully stopped, the resulting loss of hydraulic assistance will create the problems you're trying to avoid.

Hood Flies Up. While this at first may seem comical, it can be deadly serious, and although it happens infrequently it is almost always preventable. If it should occur, occasionally the driver can find a small gap through which he can look at the base of the hood. If all forward visibility is blocked, he must quickly get his head out the side window and drive the vehicle to the side of the road and stop.

When the Accident Occurs

Accidents usually happen because someone either becomes impatient, travels faster than his senses can respond, misjudges road conditions, experiences a vehicle malfunction, or makes sudden rash movements in an attempt to get around traffic perceived to be moving too slow. Otherwise, accidents are caused simply from the driver's lack of skill and attention. Unfortunately, all of these can affect the driving of an ambulance. The party who is impatient or inattentive might be the ambulance driver. It can also be another driver on the road, who either doesn't realize the ambulance is present or panics when he does recognize the presence of it, responding in less than an ideal manner. Nevertheless, the ambulance driver needs to be aware of such potential situations, mentally anticipating the possible movement of every vehicle on the road. If another motorist makes a mistake and causes an accident because of the mental pressure developed by the presence of the emergency vehicle, it is quite likely the ambulance operator could be found partially to blame. This finding can easily result in action being taken against the ambulance operator in a civil court.

According to the American Ambulance Association's *Loss Control Manual* prepared by Gregg and Associates, the following are the major causes of ambulance accidents while responding to emergency calls:

Following too closely
Failure to sound siren or use the lights properly
Failure to use care in intersections
Driving left of the center line without reasonable notice to other traffic
Driving too fast for conditions
Improper parking or backing
Failure to set the parking brake upon arrival at the scene
Improper passing technique
U-turns
Emergency braking and acceleration

When an accident involves an ambulance, the crew of the ambulance will have certain immediate responsibilities. Their unit should be considered out of service and unable to further respond. Therefore, another ambulance should be dispatched immediately on the original call that the wrecked ambulance was en route toward. The only time the crew should consider leaving the scene prior to a full investigation is when another ambulance cannot respond within a reasonable period of time, their vehicle damage is minimal, and no injuries have occurred. Even under such circumstances, the crew must perform some very important duties before leaving the accident scene.

The first activity a crew must perform following an accident involving their vehicle is to notify the dispatcher, advising him to request the police and to dispatch another ambulance to the original call. Next, the crew must make sure all occupants of their vehicle are safe, and then check all other parties involved. At this time, the crew is in a triage situation and actual care, except for life-threatening conditions, cannot begin until all persons involved in the collision have received a primary survey. If another ambulance is needed at this accident, the dispatcher must be notified immediately, while simultaneous care begins for those injured. While one crew member is caring for the patients, the other has the responsibility of protecting the scene and other traffic by placing warning triangles or flares. This crew member's job will also entail identifying the drivers of any other vehicles involved and obtaining their driver's license numbers from them. In addition, all vehicle registration numbers and license numbers must be obtained. The damage to all vehicles should be quickly assessed.

Even if the ambulance must continue on the original call because of lack of adequate backup, the above information must be obtained. The ambulance driver must then make sure he has adequately explained to the others the reason for his departure. REMEMBER: Do not abandon any injured patients! Understand that any time the ambulance leaves the scene before a complete investigation its crew is setting itself up for trouble. The other parties could easily fabricate an explanation for the incident which is favorable to them if your vehicle has been moved or you are not present to discuss the event with the police.

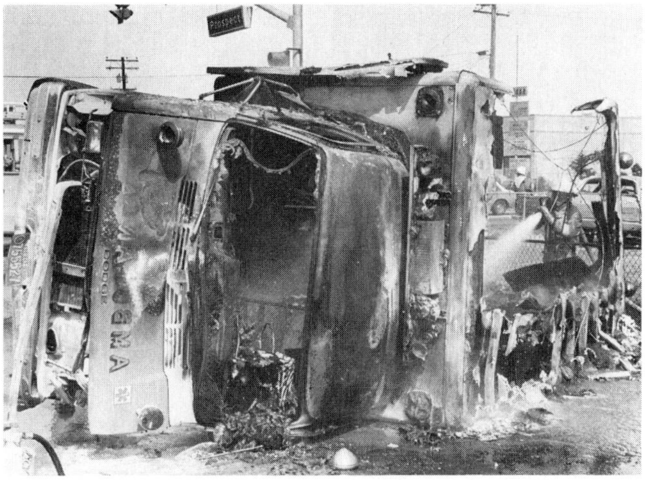

Fig. 12.9a Once involved in an accident, an ambulance may be disabled to a point where it can no longer respond to calls. (Photo courtesy of **jems.**)

Since, in almost all cases, the ambulance will remain on the scene, there is additional information the crew can acquire that will make for better legal preparation. First, no member of the crew should ADMIT FAULT or APOLOGIZE for what happened. Who was at fault will be determined later, with legal counsel, insurance representation, and supervisory participation. Quite possibly, there will be extenuating circumstances that are not clear to the crew at the time of the accident that will have bearing on the determination of who is at fault. Next, as quickly as possible, the crew should identify any witnesses. Ask them simply if they could comment on what they saw. The statements of any witnesses should be carefully written down along with the person's full name, address, and telephone number. The crew should also diagram the scene, indicating to the best of their recollection what occurred, including where the vehicles finally came to rest and how they got there. A further survey of the other vehicles involved should be made to note any prior condition that could have contributed to the collision. Conditions such as a broken headlight that didn't occur in the accident or brake lights that don't work should be noted. The drivers, too, should be cautiously scrutinized. Does the other driver appear to be under the influence of intoxicants? Do his reflexes and mental faculties seem normal? Such observations, entered into an incident report, may become important at a later date. Once the crew has left the scene, they should make further comments in an incident report on everything that could be pertinent to the accident investigation. Such a report must be written as soon as possible after the accident, while the incident is still vivid in each crew member's memory.

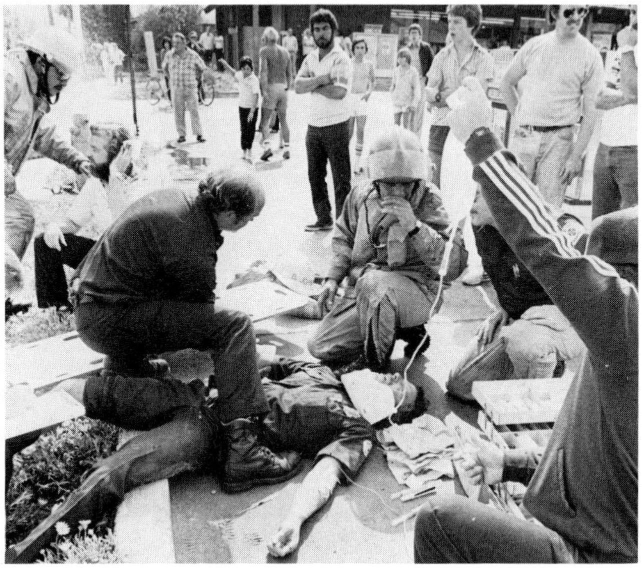

Fig. 12.9b Crew-member being aided following collision which occurred while responding to a call. (Photo courtesy of **jems.**)

Certainly the accident must be investigated by the police. During the on-scene investigation, the ambulance crew should determine which officer is in charge and only address comments to that officer. This will avoid similar questions being answered differently. Conflicting answers can go a long way towards invalidating your testimony should the incident wind up in court. Additionally, do not volunteer information; only answer direct questions.

Discussion of the accident should only take place with the police officer in charge, supervisory personnel investigating the scene, your legal representative, and your agency's insurance representative. Any questions from the press, other investigators, other parties involved, or their representatives should be addressed only by your agency's authorized representatives.

While EMTs see accidents frequently, seldom are they actually involved in them. When they are involved, even in a minor accident, it may produce very traumatic effects. In almost all cases of ambulance accidents, the crew should be relieved of field duty for a minimum of 24 hours with the understanding that a complete incident report will be of first priority, either before relief or upon their return to work. When the crew is relieved of field duty, they need to understand that such relief is not meant as a statement of blame for the collision by supervisors. Rather, it is just an act in both the employing agency's and EMTs' best interests.

Tachograph. Some vehicles are equipped with a tachograph, a recording device attached to the speedometer that records all movement of the vehicle, its speed, time, and other important information such as what emergency equipment was activated. If the ambulance involved in the accident is so equipped, and the police request the graph, the unit should be unlocked only in the presence of the EMS agency supervisory personnel investigating the incident and the police officer in charge of the investigation. The police officer and agency supervisor should sign the graph before it is released to the police as evidence.

In-House Investigation. If an ambulance is involved in a collision, the EMS agency operating the ambulance should immediately respond by sending supervisory personnel to the scene to investigate for the agency. The supervisor should be well versed in all company policy regarding accident investigation. He should be equipped with a camera so that he may record all physical aspects of the scene, including the approach paths of all vehicles, their final resting positions, any damage sustained, and road and weather conditions. This information should then be filed with the incident report provided by the investigating supervisor and each of the crew members.

Review Board. Once all pertinent accident information has been obtained by the agency and the crew involved is able to meet, an in-house review board should be convened to further investigate the incident. In-house reviews are not a duplication of the police investigation which is designed to determine blame. Instead, the review is more of a learning tool to examine what happened and what steps can be taken to prevent such an incident from occurring in the future. The in-house review also must determine if everything was done according to the company's policy and, although legal blame may fall on others, whether the crew's actions contributed to the accident. Such a review may be unpleasant for the crew and all others involved, but it must take place. The crew must not look upon the convening of a board itself as a statement of blame upon the crew, but merely a fact-finding and educational tool intended to reduce future property loss and injury.

Court. While in many accidents the other driver is technically to blame for the collision, if the other parties have a basis to indicate that the ambulance crew contributed to the incident, the case may end up in civil court. For this reason, the crew must be fully prepared for court. The testimony they must give should not vary from the manner they would testify in a medical case, with one big exception. In this case, the crew members will be emotionally involved. As in any court case, it is important for each crew member to prepare himself well in advance by reviewing all documentation available.

During testimony, the crew should only answer the questions they are asked, without elaboration. The crew's response should not vary from what is written in their initial reports. A well-written incident report will contain the answers to any questions that might be asked. If a question is asked which is not adequately covered in the report, the crew member should not attempt to give an answer unless he is positive of the information. Certainly, this is not the time to make suppositions or take guesses. Doing so might easily damage your credibility as a witness and swing the judgment in favor of the other parties.

Review of Common Ambulance Accidents

The following are examples of common ambulance accidents and what a hypothetical in-house review board might determine could have been done differently by the ambulance driver to avoid a collision or reduce property loss and injury.

Example 1

As the ambulance approached the scene, the driver turned off the siren and crossed the center line, driving in the oncoming traffic lane to facilitate getting around the stopped traffic. Vehicle #2 was not signaling for a left turn. However, Driver #2 observed the stopped oncoming traffic and impulsively decided to turn left to avoid the accident scene. The ambulance and the truck (Vehicle #2) collided.

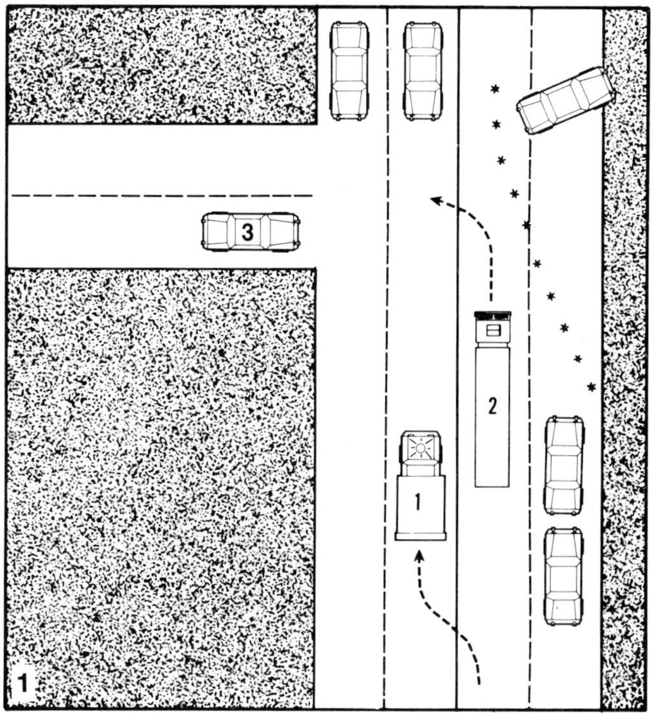

Avoidance

Six measures can be taken by the ambulance driver to avoid or lessen this collision:

1. The EMT driver had turned off his siren because he was approaching the scene and all traffic was stopped. If he had left the siren on, it might have been heard by the driver of the truck.
2. The EMT driver should watch Vehicle #2's driver's head to detect if he is aware of the presence of the ambulance.
3. The EMT driver should watch Vehicle #2's front wheels to see if they are being turned to the left so Vehicle #2 can proceed left.
4. The EMT driver should approach more slowly, allowing himself more reaction time.
5. The ambulance driver can pull into the oncoming traffic lane sooner, giving the truck driver more time to observe him.
6. The ambulance driver can give wider berth to the truck to give himself more reaction time. However, in a situation such as this, he must be careful not to go too far left, in case the car (Vehicle #3) on the side street should decide to turn without first looking.

Example 2

On a cold, sunny morning, the EMT unit is responding in an emergency mode on a dry road.

The temperature is 35°F. While rounding a shaded corner, the unit hits some ice and spins out.

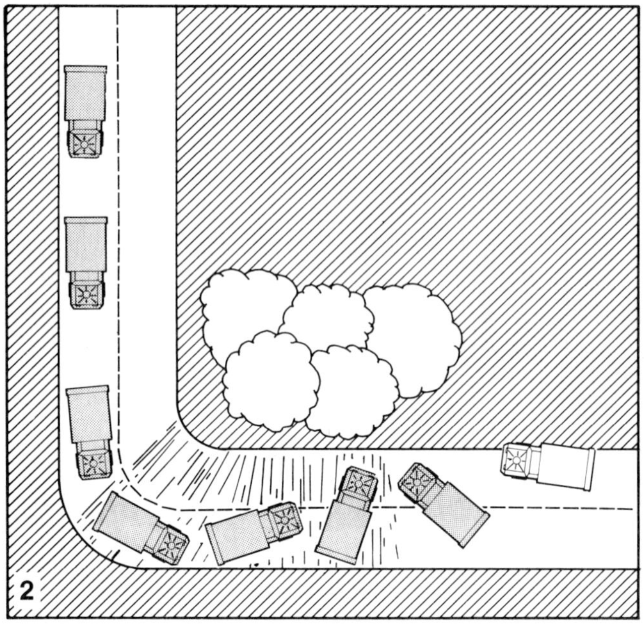

Avoidance

The paramedic driver should consider the outside temperature and anticipate the road surface to be a few degrees colder in the shade. Additionally, he should realize the moisture from the previous night may not have evaporated in the shade.

Example 3

On a day when the temperature was right at freezing and the road wet, the crew encountered several icy spots, but none within the last few minutes. Upon entering a sweeping high-speed curve, the ambulance lost traction and spun.

Avoidance

The EMT driver should anticipate ice and drive slower.

Example 4

The ambulance is responding in an emergency mode. Noting that the vehicle ahead was signaling for a left turn, the EMT driver passed on the right. When the driver of Vehicle #2 heard the siren, he suddenly headed for the right shoulder, hitting the ambulance.

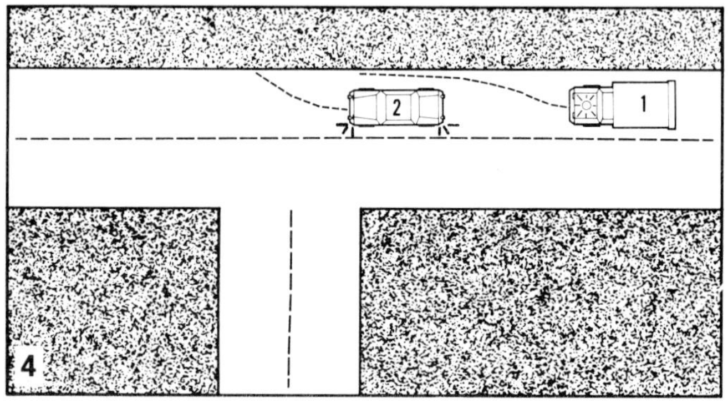

Avoidance

The ambulance driver should not attempt to pass a motorist signaling his intent to turn. The ambulance driver should let Driver #2 make his turn and then proceed.

Example 5

While driving in an emergency mode down a highway, the ambulance driver attempted to pass the vehicle ahead, which was stopped to

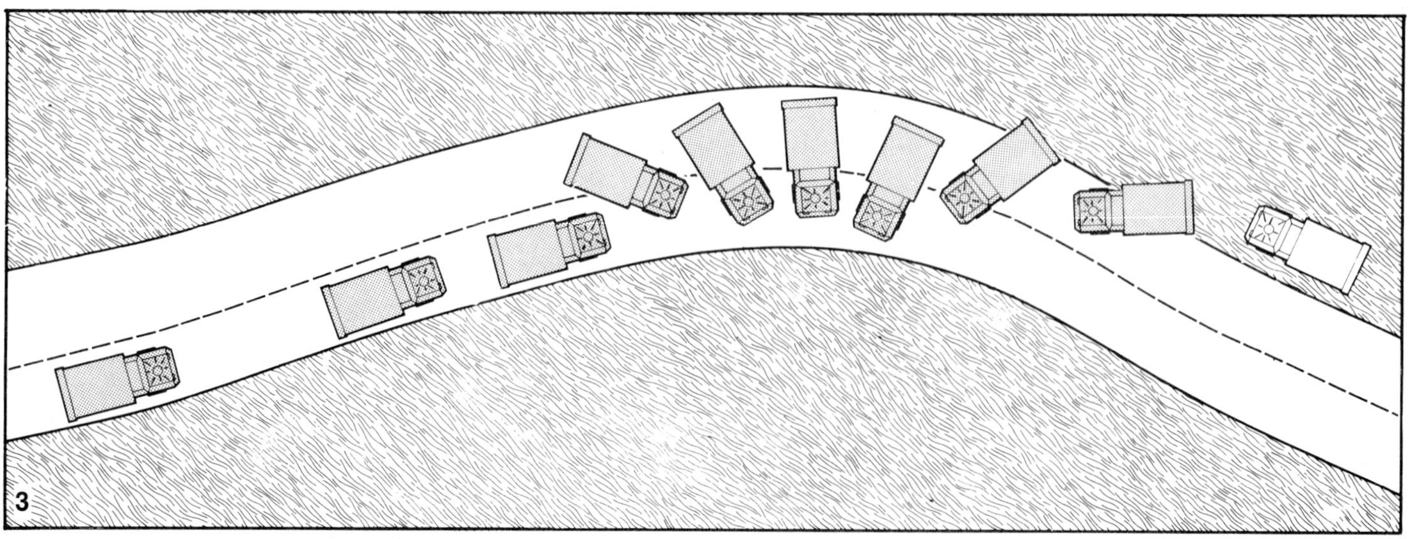

make a left-hand turn. The ambulance passed on the left and was hit when the vehicle (#2) ahead turned into its path.

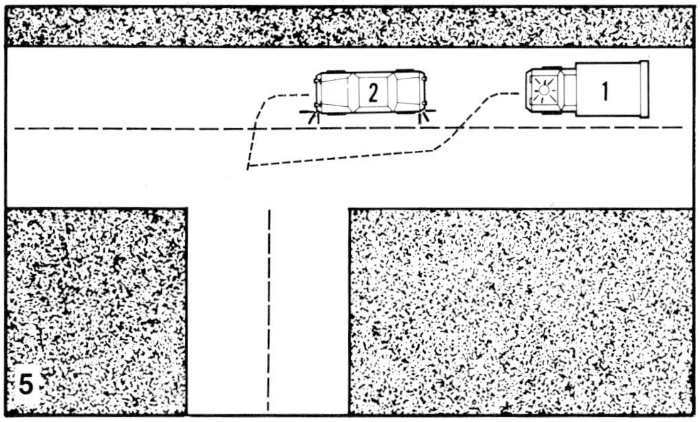

Avoidance

The ambulance driver should not attempt to pass a vehicle whose driver is indicating his intention to turn left. Many ambulance accidents are caused by this one error. Let the motorist ahead of you complete his turn so you can eliminate possible collision with the lead vehicle.

Example 6

While traveling in an emergency mode on a rural road, the ambulance driver observed an approaching vehicle (#2) pull to the shoulder of the road in an attempt to yield. The vehicle (#3) following the approaching car (#2) became impatient at the slowdown and apparent uncertainty of Driver #2 and pulled into the oncoming lane of traffic to pass. Driver #3 apparently did not look ahead to see if any traffic was approaching. A head-on collision was the result of this act with damage primarily to the left front of both Vehicles #1 and #3. According to witnesses, both vehicles were traveling within the posted speed limit and the driver of the ambulance attempted to evade.

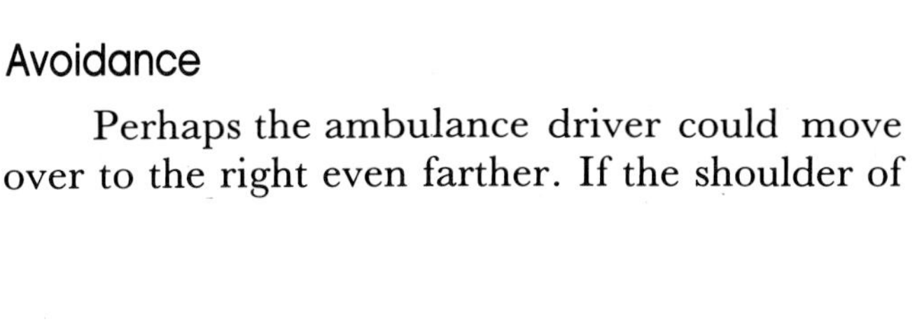

Avoidance

Perhaps the ambulance driver could move over to the right even farther. If the shoulder of the road dropped off significantly, further maneuvering to the right would entail going off the shoulder and, in all likelihood, rolling the ambulance. Additionally, if the ambulance driver sees the potential for such a situation developing early, he may be able to slow before impact.

Example 7

An ambulance on an emergency run is climbing a steep, ice-covered hill. Just prior to reaching the crest of the hill, the engine of the vehicle dies. The vehicle loses traction and slides down the hill backward.

Avoidance

The vehicle should be checked out by a competent mechanic and placed in top condition. Such an incident might be avoided if the driver takes another street which is less steep.

Example 8

While returning to quarters in a nonemergency mode, the ambulance traveling in the center lane has a vehicle pull from the far right lane crossing in front of the ambulance while attempting to get into the left lane. The traffic in the left lane is stopped. Because of the stopped traffic, the offending vehicle (#2) is forced to stop abruptly across the center lane. The ambulance driver, faced with hitting a stopped vehicle in the

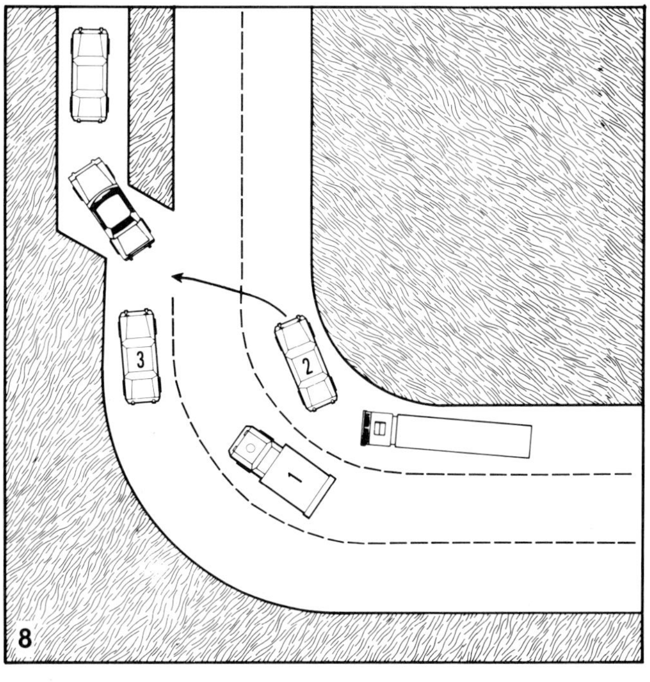

side, or sideswiping another vehicle (#3) stopped in the left lane, may decide to sideswipe Vehicle #3 in an attempt to minimize damage and injuries.

Avoidance

Such a maneuver undoubtedly will save much damage and probably injury. With proper visual habits, the ambulance driver may see the situation developing sooner and therefore have more options available to help avoid a collision.

As you can see from the many examples listed above, there are ways of preplanning escape routes that can help you to either avoid collisions or reduce property loss and injury. Having an accident is not an enjoyable experience. Certainly anything you can do to lessen its severity is good for all parties, no matter who is at fault.

13 EXERCISES YOU CAN DO

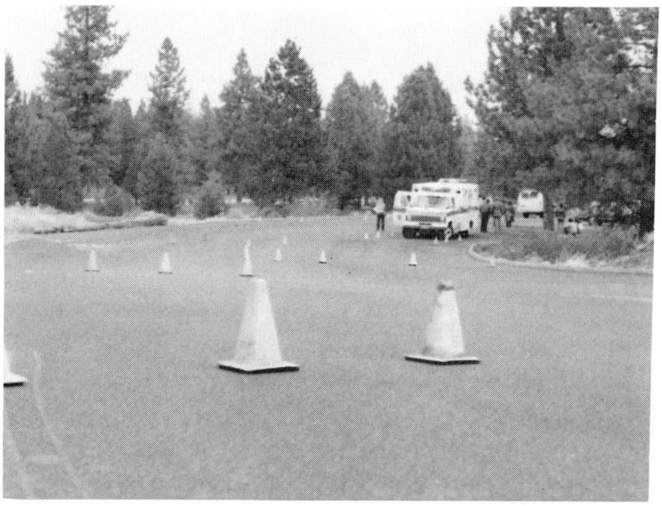

As serious a task as driving is, there is no reason it can't also be fun. In fact, driving can be made safer and more interesting with the employment of some simple games and exercises.

In order for you to gain the most impact from these exercises, you must enter into them with the understanding that even the most experienced driver can benefit from them. It is already a given fact that the ambulance driver has certain abilities, so participation in such exercises need not threaten. Instead of testing ability, these exercises are designed to enhance your current ability.

There are several exercises available to develop almost any driving skill. Many of these are complex and require the involvement of a qualified advanced driving techniques instructor in order that you may properly learn under safe conditions. These more advanced or dangerous exercises have not been included in this text. The exercises that have been included are by no means the only ones that can be performed. They are presented simply as one method of developing each driving skill. As these exercises become familiar to the driver, they can be modified and others developed to further enhance each ability. It can also be fun to develop new exercises. When inventing new exercises, keep in mind the goals that you are trying to achieve with each exercise. Do not make them so difficult that they become discouraging, or waste the driver's time with pointless exercises.

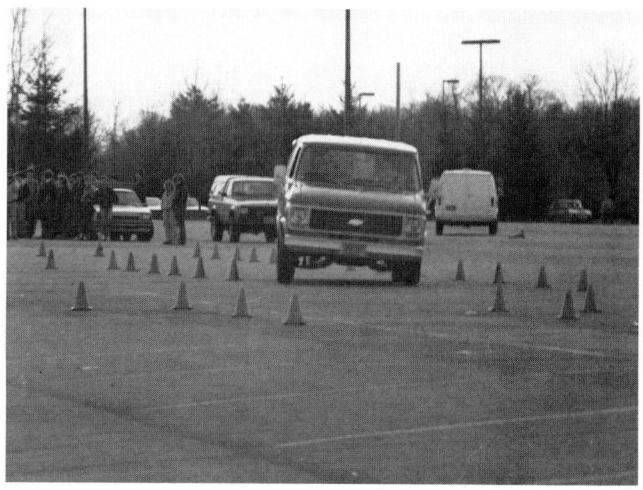

Fig. 13.1 Many complex driving exercises require the involvement of a qualified Advanced Driving Techniques instructor to be done under safe conditions.

Fitting the Traffic

Probably one of the most important driving skills that you can improve is called "fitting the traffic." It is with this exercise that we will begin this chapter. Fitting the traffic is simply the driver ability to blend easily into the traffic flow, making minute adjustments in speed early enough to avoid sudden stops or tight situations. Obviously such driving requires the use of excellent visual skills so the driver can quickly see those things happening around him that might affect his driving. Early recognition of problems will help you to react to them quickly and in a proper manner. Driving to fit traffic conditions is important for a smooth ride and your safety. It is also important in reducing strain on the vehicle and, therefore, costly maintenance.

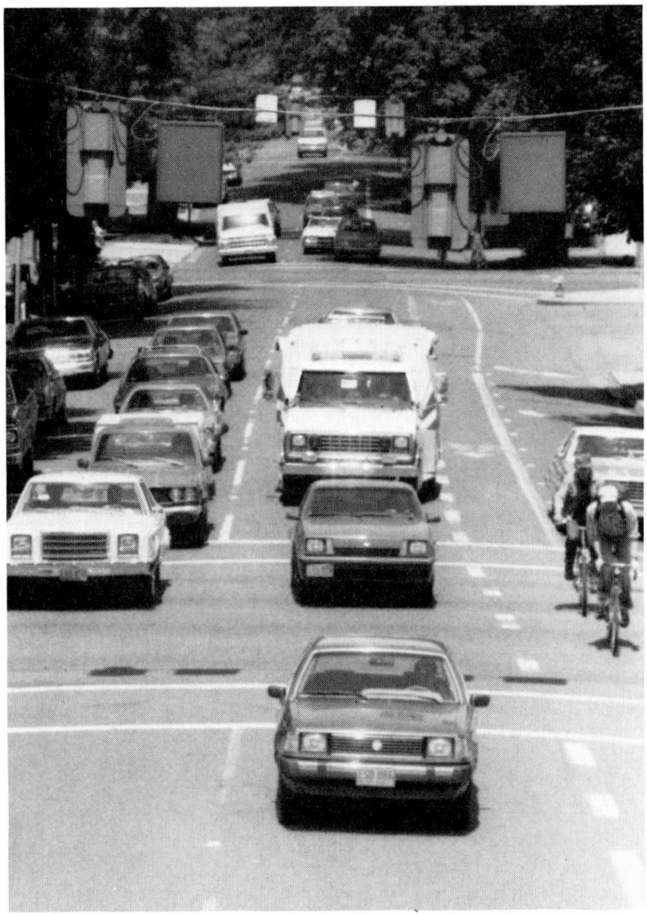

Fig. 13.2 Fitting the traffic is an important driving skill which can be improved by using commentary driving exercises.

Commentary Driving. Proper visual habits can be difficult to develop. Knowing those habits that must be developed is only the beginning and does not mean they will get developed. Here is a simple exercise that will help develop proper visual habits.

While driving, start vocalizing (talking out loud) about anything you see that might in any way affect your driving. By vocalizing out loud, you force yourself to look around more than you might otherwise. Typically, a driver starting to do this exercise in moderate traffic will find himself commenting on only a few things around him and then pausing until something else appears. As commentary driving is practiced, the driver soon finds he does not have enough time to comment on everything that IS happening around him. This is because he starts noticing conditions that were previously unrecognized. Soon, you will start to realize there are more conditions present that can affect your driving. Commentary driving can and should be done on the open road under a variety of driving conditions, including heavy urban traffic, lighter traffic on rural roads, and on the expressway. The key to this exercise is not to stop talking.

If nothing seems obvious or worthy of comment, look harder. Comments should not only include such things as the traffic before you, but also what is happening behind you and to the sides, the width of the road, what the shoulders are like, weather conditions, the speed you are traveling, and how you intend to deal with upcoming events. Pertinent negatives such as the fact that the intersection ahead appears free of traffic, or that the vehicle parked alongside the road does not have a driver in it should also receive comment.

A typical episode of commentary driving might sound something like this: "I'm on a two-lane road, curbed with wide paving, in moderate traffic. This is a residential area, so I'm watching for children and cars coming out of driveways. I'm following 3-1/2 seconds behind the vehicle in front. The vehicle behind appears well back. Traffic is approaching in the oncoming lane. It appears to be maintaining its lane. My speed is 30 mph. I am approaching an intersection. I have the right of way. I will slow my speed slightly, anyway. The car ahead is now signaling a right-hand turn. I will slow additionally in anticipation of his slowing to turn. Checking my mirrors, the car is still well behind. Slowing, since I'm approaching the intersection. I'm watching the other traffic to make sure no one enters the intersection, or turns. It appears all clear. The car in front is making his turn. I'm proceeding on through. There is a car parked ahead, it has a driver in it. I don't see any exhaust. Will slow and give it wide berth. The car behind is still well back. I'm past the parked car. There is a slow moving car approaching in the oncoming lane. Will keep an eye on it. Checking my instruments. All look good. Now there is a car in front of me. The approaching car is now going past. Driver appears to be looking for an address; is not attentive to driving. I'm going to count distance between me and car in front, . . . one thousand one, one thousand two, one thousand . . . I'm traveling about two and a half seconds behind. Will maintain this distance."

Reading the previous example makes it easy to see that events happen very quickly, even in light or moderate traffic. In fact, you will not have time to comment on everything and will find yourself talking faster and becoming frustrated when you can't remark on everything you observe. This indicates that your seeing habits are beginning to properly develop.

Because commentary driving is very demanding of the driver, it should only be done for a short duration (five to ten minutes at a time). When a driver first performs commentary driving, it should be done in light to moderate traffic.

One episode of commentary driving will not be enough to sharpen your skills. You should practice it four or five times a week until you feel you have firmly established the needed habits. Then sit back and drive. Keep in mind that those good habits will deteriorate after a period of time; so every few weeks, break out the commentary driving, dust it off and again go through a few episodes. After a while, good visual habits will become firmly ingrained and commentary driving will be less frequently needed. However, you should never abandon commentary driving. It should be with you for the rest of your driving career. Occasionally, you might be driving down the road and discover you have had to stop rather abruptly, or that a car passed that you didn't realize was behind you. When something like that occurs, it's time to once again break out the commentary driving. It may take only one or two episodes to sharpen your visual habits. In addition, whenever a driver becomes tense while driving, it is often the result of a breakdown of those visual skills. Employing commentary driving at such times can open up your field of vision and relieve the tension.

Driving Without Brakes. Most drivers rely on their brakes far more than necessary. It seems as though a foot on the pedal provides a certain security for the driver. When that foot isn't using the accelerator, it is immediately placed on the brake pedal. As you know, this is not necessary. Incorporating proper visual habits will allow plenty of time for slowing so it doesn't have to be done rapidly. Instead, slowing can take time and distance. In many situations, the use of the brake is not at all needed if the driver only perceives the need to slow early enough and gets off the accelerator.

The following exercise or "game" has been developed to help you look ahead, smoothing the ride and thus reducing vehicle wear and maintenance. This exercise can and should be performed on the open road, preferably in moderate to heavy traffic. In addition, the exercise should be done over a familiar route that is frequently driven, e.g., from the hospital to the base. The driver can compete with himself or with his partner. The object of the game is simply to count every time the brake pedal is depressed, even a small amount. In a short period of time, the driver will begin to anticipate traffic, and let up lightly on the accelerator so he won't have to use the brake. Don't be consumed by the desire to win and take unnecessary chances.

Smoothing It Out

Even drivers with good visual habits sometimes do not provide a good smooth ride. They may enter corners wrong, improperly squeeze the pedals, or disregard the early indications to start slowing. As you know, smooth ride is important for vehicle maintenance and patient comfort. A couple of the following tricks will quickly add smoothness to almost any driver's ability.

Driving With a Glass of Water. Placing a small glass filled with water in the driver's compartment will quickly develop a smooth ride. This exercise should be performed on the road in moderate traffic, and only after some practice in heavy traffic. If the floor of the vehicle is carpeted, the cup should be placed on a board for a more stable footing. It is imperative that spilled water not come in contact with any electrical components or wiring. The cup is filled to the rim with water and driving begins. Since it is harder to spill the water than it might seem, care should be taken to make sure the cup is as full as possible. Because the cup is out of the driver's normal field of vision, someone else should monitor the results, letting the driver know whenever water sloshes over the rim. Usually, only small drops of water will be spilled, but the observer should be ready with a towel in case a large spill occurs.

Driving With Eggs. This exercise should be done in a parking lot that is not in use or in an area where traffic is not a consideration. This environment will allow the driver to concentrate more fully on braking and acceleration. The object of this exercise is to help develop smooth braking and acceleration skills. This particular exercise is of great benefit for drivers who habitually drive in a rough manner.

Begin the exercise by checking the pedals to see if they can be used without a lot of force. A few vehicles have such strong return springs on the brake pedal that this exercise won't work. Next, tape an unboiled egg to each pedal and have the driver remove his shoe. The shoe is removed to give the driver a better feel of the pedal, the egg, and the force that is used. It also reduces the likelihood of the egg breaking. In addition, the raw egg adds incentive for the driver to get it right, soon!

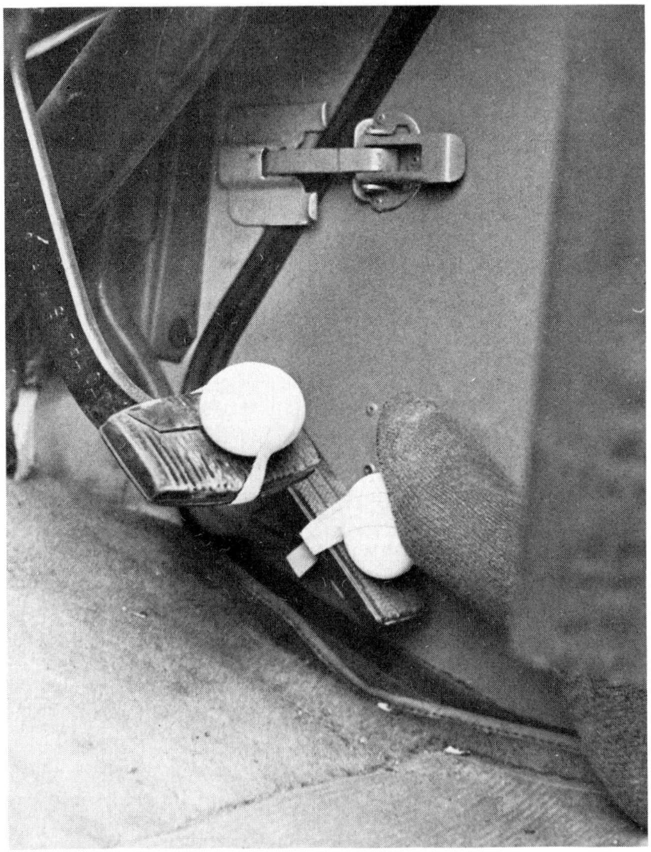

Fig. 13.3 By driving in a controlled area with eggs taped to the pedals, you'll soon develop smooth braking and acceleration skills. (Photo courtesy of jems.)

During the driving exercise, the driver must learn to accelerate quickly to different speeds and then brake, bringing the vehicle to a complete stop in as short a space as possible. Soon he will develop the proper feel for squeezing the pedals. A bonus of the results from this skill improvement will be improved gas mileage.

Backing

Backing is an especially tricky skill since it involves limited vision which is further distorted by the use of mirrors. Additionally, the driver may be unaccustomed to the maneuvering that occurs when the steering wheels are at the rear of the vehicle. In all there are five components which need to be developed in backing exercises. They are: (1) comfort with the use of mirrors and their distortion; (2) improving depth perception in the mirrors; (3) the ability to switch between mirrors as well as observing the front of the vehicle; (4) a feel for the tracking of the tires and therefore vehicle placement, and (5) awareness of where the rear tires are in relation to what is seen in the mirrors at the back of the vehicle.

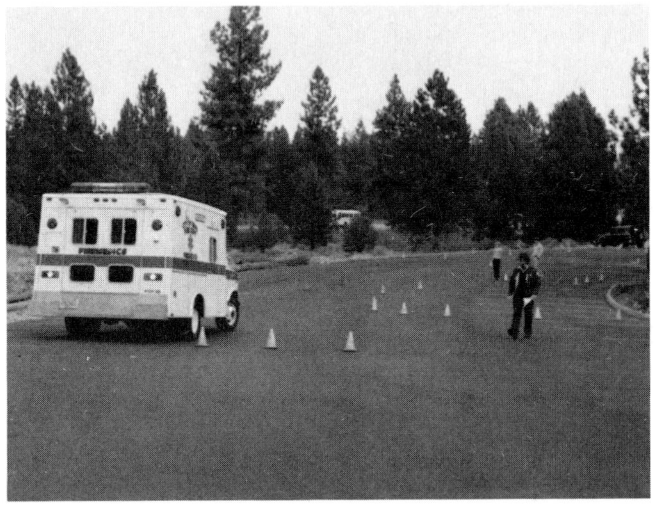

Fig. 13.4 Backing, an especially tricky skill can be developed through exercises set up in any area free of traffic.

By developing each of these components, a driver will be able to back comfortably and safely when the need arises. Keep in mind that backing should never be performed when it can be avoided, and that a spotter is needed when backing the ambulance in real situations.

The following exercises should be set up in an unused parking lot or other area free of traffic. Each exercise should be set up one after the other, so the drivers can quickly go between them, exercising all aspects of backing. You should not be concerned with speed as much as you should about maneuvering safely. Remember, each obstacle hit represents potential damage in a real situation. Additionally, it is not as big of a concern if the driver occasionally has to pull forward to reposition his vehicle instead of making one continuous movement and hitting cones. In due time, you will learn vehicle positioning so you won't have to reposition as often. Again, the emphasis should be on completing the course safely.

For these exercises it is best to use traffic cones twelve, eighteen, and twenty-four inches in height. The shorter cones are used to mark out the routes while the tall cones are used at corners to indicate critical pivot points. This is important since a pattern of cones seen in a rearview mirror can be very confusing. If cones are not available, cardboard boxes or other items that won't damage a vehicle or its paint, may be used. The measurements given on the following diagrams are for a van ambulance (Type II). The longer Type I and III vehicles may require the course to be enlarged to facilitate their turning radius.

Narrowing Channel

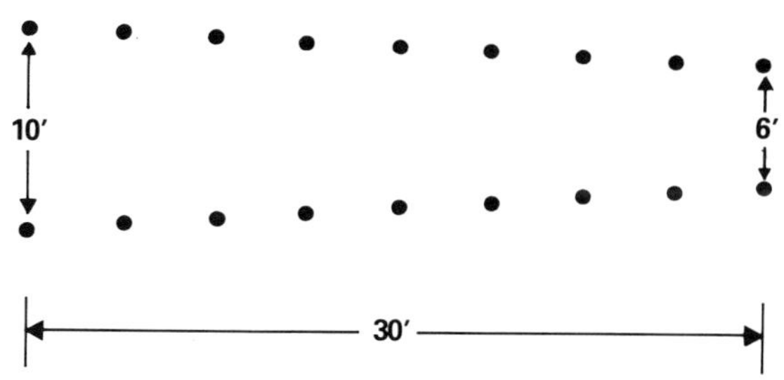

OBJECTIVES:

1. To help the driver recognize width using his mirrors.
2. To help the driver learn how to center the vehicle.

SETUP

Two rows of tall cones, 30 feet long, opening width 10 feet, end width 6 feet. Driver backs in as far as possible without hitting cones.

Equipment required: 18 cones on 3-foot centers.

Serpentine

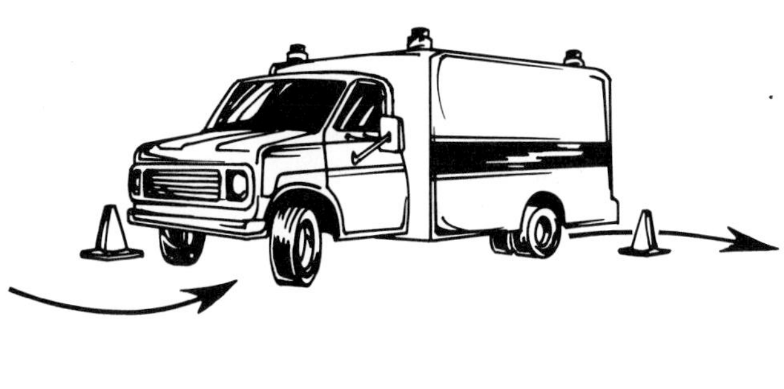

OJECTIVES:

1. To help the driver recognize the tires as the pivot point and not the rear bumper.
2. To help the driver alternate mirrors use and to become familiar with them.

SETUP

One row of six tall cones set at 50-foot centers in a straight line.

Equipment required: 6 cones.

Backing Along Curb

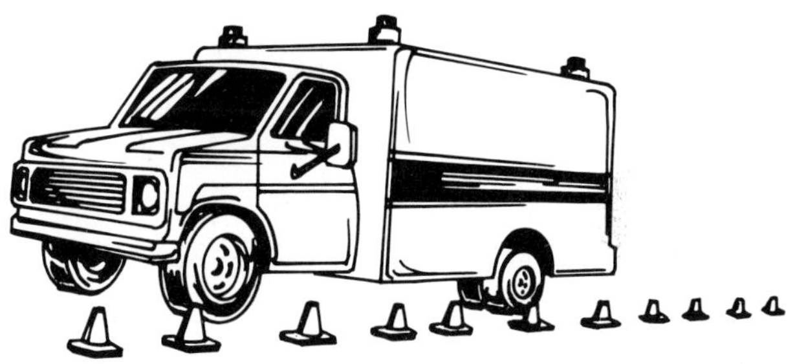

OBJECTIVES:

1. To be able to back straight following a low curb.
2. To stay as close to the curb as reasonable to avoid obstructing traffic.
3. To back using mirrors.

SETUP

One row of low cones set in a straight line for 40 feet.

Equipment required: 11 cones on 5-foot centers.

Backing Under Height

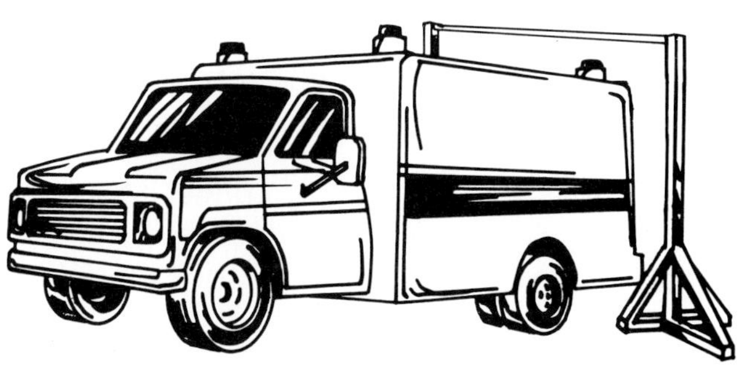

OBJECTIVES:

1. To gain depth perception while using mirrors.
2. To gain height perception while using mirrors.

SETUP

Two standards with variable height and a 10-foot horizontal wand. The driver must back as close as possible to the wand.

Equipment required: 8 cones, 2 standards, and 1 wand.

Backing to Wall

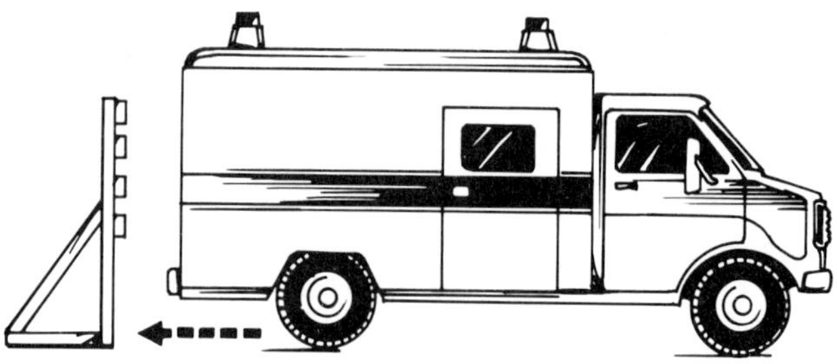

OBJECTIVES:

To gain depth perception while backing with mirrors.

SETUP

Set up a fence barrier. The driver is to back as close to the wall as possible without hitting it.

Driveways

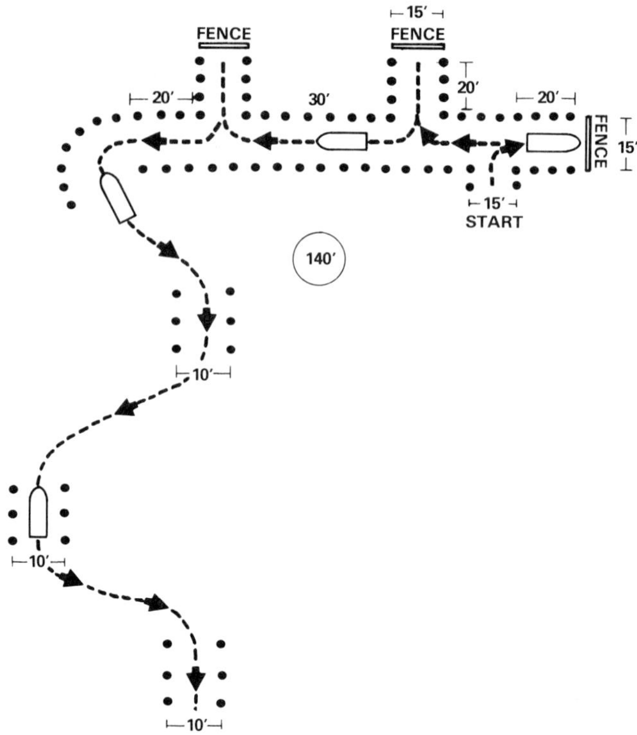

OBJECTIVES:

1. To bring together all of the exercises into a sustained backing exercise.
2. To help the driver understand the principle that turning while backing offsets the front laterally.

SETUP

Set up a system of cones in the following pattern.

Equipment required: 30 cones, 3 fence barriers.

Know Your Vehicle

It is important for every driver to know where his vehicle is in relation to everything else around it, and how the vehicle handles. You can develop a feeling for these relationships through the following exercises.

Serpentine. This course is laid out just like the backing exercise. Driving through a serpentine teaches you the amount of steering available to you and familiarizes you with utilizing the vehicle body motion. It will also make you aware of the physical limitations of the vehicle as well as your own limitations. Serpentine driving will help develop coordination between hand and foot controls, and the placement of the vehicle in relationship to objects around it.

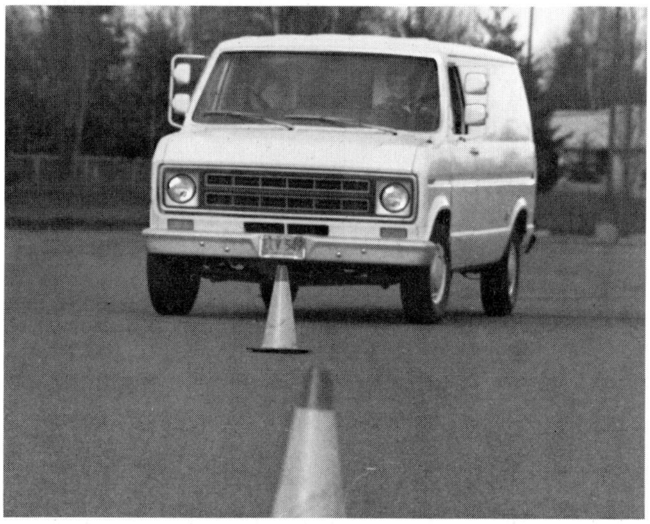

Fig. 13.5 The serpentine is designed to familiarize drivers with using vehicle body motion.

In order to perform this exercise properly, you should approach the first cone as closely as possible and keep your hands at the nine and three positions on the wheel. Use a smooth, rhythmic motion, first turning the wheel one way and then the other, passing each cone as close as possible and pivoting the rear tire around it. This is a deceptively complex exercise when done properly. Any mistake made will be magnified as each cone is passed. A mistake at the beginning will make it extremely difficult to properly negotiate the last cone. The keys to this exercise are: First, do not let your arms rest. The initial turn of the wheel is approximately 90°, the rest will be about 180°. As soon as the turn out is completed with your arms, you must immediately begin the turn back in the opposite direction. The second key is to maintain a constant speed. This means that you leave the exercise at the same speed you entered. It's not easy, but by doing so, the constant wheel turning becomes easier since the same amount of time elapses between each cone. Since this exercise is intended to develop coordination and proximity judgment, it should only be performed at speeds between 20 and 25 mph. Performing this exercise at speeds in excess of 25 mph will be of no value and may only serve to frustrate the driver and create improper habits.

The Esses

As you know, the rear wheels track closer in a curve than the front. The amount of difference varies according to the acuteness of the turn and the wheel base of the vehicle. In this exercise, the driver travels through a long pattern of cones laid out in a winding pattern. The exercise will demonstrate that if you do not stay to the outside of the curves you will undoubtedly strike cones with the inside rear tire. Once this simple skill has been mastered, the course can be made more difficult by causing it to progressively narrow. It might be a couple of feet wider than the vehicle at the beginning and then narrowed to only two inches of excess clearance at the end. Difficulty can also be increased by increasing the severity of curve. When this is done, the course may have to be adjusted several times to obtain the desired effect, since increasing the amount of curve also increases the tracking ratio of the tires.

Additionally, this exercise can be used to strengthen backing technique. It should be performed at a constant speed, utilizing the nine and three hand position.

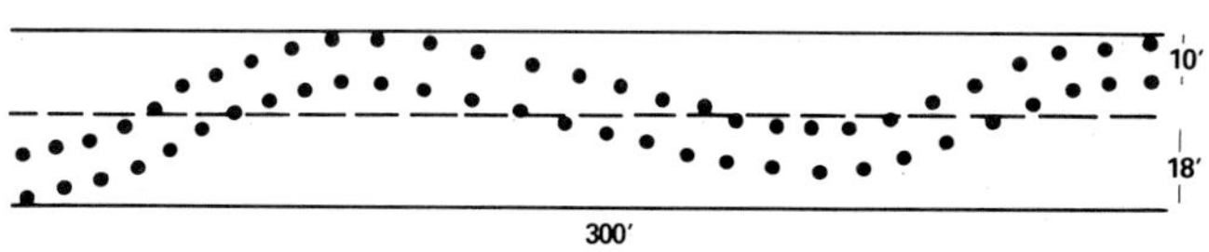

PATIENT RIDE

Equipment required: 150 cones placed every four feet.

Patient Ride

At least every six months every ambulance driver should take the opportunity to ride on the stretcher while someone else drives over a variety of road conditions. This will help you to develop an appreciation of what the patient experiences.

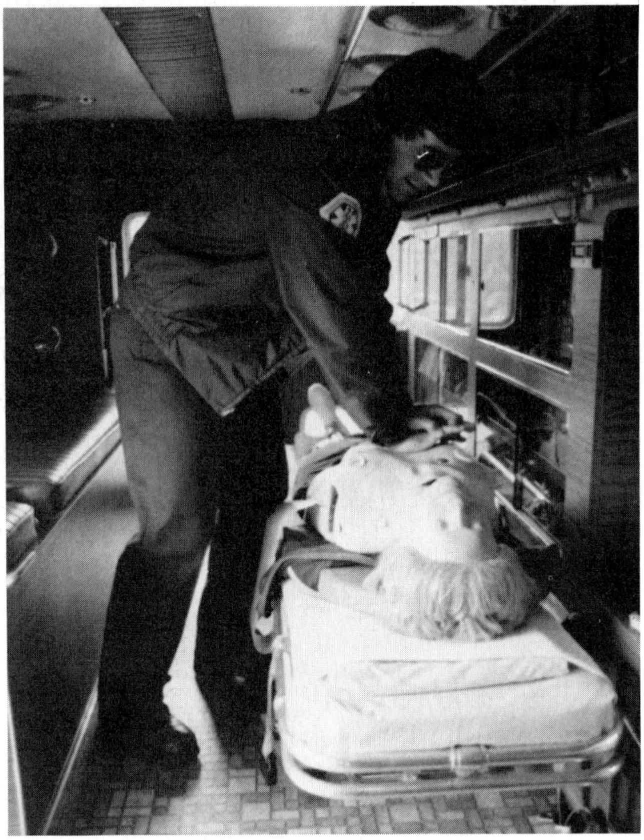

Fig. 13.6 You can develop a better understanding of the need for a smooth patient ride by evaluating your CPR skills on a recording mannikin while traveling in an ambulance in a prescribed course.

If this knowledge is routinely reinforced, the experience will not be forgotten.

Ambulance Rodeo

Many of the exercises listed in this chapter can be combined to create a game that is fun, as well as beneficial to all participants. An ambulance rodeo, as the game is often called, has the ambulance driven through a given course while several judges observe for errors in judgment or skill. The judges will not only observe for the obvious, such as cones being hit, but also such things as proper signaling and mirror usage. To add an additional degree of difficulty, CPR is performed on a recording-type resuscitation manikin while the course is negotiated. The recording strip is then scored and the judges submit their sheets to determine the contest winners.

As you can see, there is more to properly driving an ambulance than just steering and braking. Your vehicle must receive a thorough inspection at the beginning of each shift to ensure its preparedness and safety. You must be able to perform both fundamental and advanced driving techniques while maintaining proper attitudes and habits. You have learned the importance of route planning, as well as some of the skills required to operate your vehicle safely in a variety of traffic and weather conditions. Through the application of some of the exercises in this chapter, you will "fine tune" your skills and certainly become more proficient.

It is the combined hope of the authors that this text will help you to drive more safely and confidently for both the patient and yourself.

A-INFECTION CONTROL IN THE AMBULANCE

The first chapter of this book discussed the external and mechanical maintenance of your vehicle. This appendix will address the maintenance required for the interior of the vehicle—the patient care environment.

Describing the interior of the ambulance as a patient care environment should not surprise you. Today, intensive care is rendered in the vehicle, care which was previously rendered only in the hospital setting. Today's ambulance serves as a mobile hospital. This environment, as in the hospital, can harbor organisms which can pose hazards to your patient and you, the care provider.

When patient care is rendered, microorganisms (bacteria and viruses) are exchanged between the patient and the environment.[1] In most instances, this exchange is made by the individual providing the care. The care provider is touching equipment and then touching the patient. The result can be acquisition of an infection by the patient or the care provider. Your risk from the environment comes from your touching surfaces and equipment and then engaging in hand-to-nose or hand-to-mouth activities. Many bacteria and viruses can survive on surfaces for long periods of time. For example, the Hepatitis-B virus has been shown to survive on a surface six weeks or longer without the visible presence of dried blood.[2] This is but one example of the possible risks that exist.

Let's examine the areas which can present a risk and what can be done to reduce the risk.

First, identify the areas which present a risk; attention should be given to items which are in direct contact with patient's blood or body fluids. These items include: bag-valve-masks, antishock pants, suction tubing, and airways. Concentrate on cleaning high patient contact items. The areas in the ambulance which present a possible risk are: stretchers, the monitor-defibrillator, and portable suction equipment (walls and floors do not present a hazard unless visibly soiled by blood or body fluids).[3,4]

Second, risks can be reduced most simply by cleaning. The published recommendations by the CDC (Centers for Disease Control) state that any EPA-approved disinfectant-detergent which is viricidal and germicidal may be used for cleaning.[5] There are many products on the market that meet this criteria. Evaluate which product meets your specific needs while considering cost, effectiveness, and the safety of the solution on the interior surfaces of the vehicle (whether the solution would damage a surface). Example: Bleach will cloud plexiglas and cause corrosion of metals.

The recommended procedures for cleaning follow:

Cleaning of Blood. This should be your first priority. Use a solution of one part bleach to 10 parts water. The individual responsible for cleaning the ambulance should wear disposable gloves and clean all blood-covered areas with the bleach solution.

Routine Cleaning. Cleaning should be carried out on all surfaces daily. A "pistol-grip" hand spray bottle should be used to apply the cleaning solution. The spray application insures that a concentration of solution reaches the surface to be cleaned.

Disposables. Any item labeled "one-time use" or "disposable" must be discarded after use. (A federal regulation against their reuse exists.) Disposables usually include items such as airways, suction catheters, and O_2 delivery devices.

Bag-valve-masks. Disassemble and sterilize after each use. A cold liquid sterilization solution can be used. Air dry, reassemble, and check for proper operation.

Suction Equipment. Disposable equipment should be bagged and set aside for incineration. Nondisposable sets should be carefully cleaned. Bottled contents should be emptied in such a manner that would reduce splashing. Collection bottles should be washed with an appropriate cleaning solution and allowed to air dry. All nondisposable tubing should be cleaned in a similar manner.

Pneumatic Counter-pressure Devices (MAST). PCPDs should be cleaned to remove any blood or secretions. The method of cleaning depends on whether the bladders are removable or nonremovable. If covered with large amounts of blood, the recommended cleaning method is gas sterilization. A cold liquid sterilization solution is acceptable,but this procedure is difficult for EMS personnel to monitor at the base station. The reason this procedure is difficult is threefold. First, the "in date" solution must be properly mixed. Second, the PCPD (bag-valve-mask, etc.) must be soaked for at least 20 minutes. And finally, the device must be allowed to *completely* air dry. A PCPD or bag-valve-mask damp with cold liquid sterilization solution is quite likely to cause burns to skin it may contact. Whenever possible, PCPD sterilization procedures should be performed by the hospital.

Airing Vehicle. Airing the vehicle following the transportation of a patient with a possible or confirmed communicable disease is not necessary. Simply clean all contact areas with the designated cleaning agent.[6,7]

As is usually the case when new procedures are introduced, these cleaning measures may appear to be time-consuming. These recommendations have been scientifically studied and are in operation in all aspects of the hospital setting. The measures are practical; they reduce the risk of infection for you and your patients.

Contributed by:

Katherine H. West, R.N., B.S.N.
Consultant for Infection Control Aspects of Emergency Medical Care
Springfield, Virginia

References

1. "Guideline for hospital environmental control," *Guideline for Prevention and Control of Nosocomial Infection,* Centers for Disease Control, Atlanta, Georgia, 1981.
2. Francis DP, Favero MS and Maynard JE: "Transmission of Hepatitis B virus," *Seminars in Liver Disease,* Vol. 1 (1), 1981, 90–95.
3. West KH, "Infection Control," *Emergency Medical Services,* Vol. 12 (1), 1983, 53–54.
4. "Environmental Guidelines: Disinfecting, Sterilizing, and Housekeeping," *Conversations in Infection Control,* Stuart Pharmaceuticals, Vol. 13, September, 1982, 1–12.
5. "Cleaning, Disinfection, Sterilization," *Guidelines for Prevention and Control of Nosocomial Infection,* CDC, Atlanta, Georgia, 1981.
6. "Guideline for Prevention of Nosocomial Pneumonia," *Guideline for Prevention and Control of Nosocomial Infection,* CDC, Atlanta, Georgia, 1981.
7. West, KH: *Infection Control Recommendations for Rescue Vehicles,* 1982, available from author.

Appendix B: Daily Patient Care Equipment Checklist

PATIENT CARE EQUIPMENT:

Oxygen (medical)
- Portable – 2 hr supply @ 10 liters per min.
- Installed – 2000 liters
- (If there is only one, it must be portable)

Oxygen Masks With Tubing
- Adult – 3
- Pediatric – 3

Oxygen Nasal Cannulas
- Adult 3

Bag Mask Ventilation Device
- One device with transparent and pre-inflated mask for adults and children.
- One device with transparent and pre-inflated mask for pediatric/infant.

Airways (plastic or rubber)
- Infant – 2
- Child – 2
- Small Adult – 2
- Medium Adult – 2
- Large Adult – 2
- Extra Large Adult – 2

Suction
- Portable (battery, oxygen powered or manual)
- Installed (independent of oxygen supply)
- (if there is only one, it must be portable)
- Assorted Suction Catheters

Litters
- Wheeled Cot With Mattress – 1
- Folding, Number Based on Litter Carrying Capacity of Vehicle

Traction Splint
- Adult – 1
- Child – 1
- Or Combination – 1

Splints
- Lower Extremity – 3
- Upper Extremity – 3

Extrication Collars
- Small – 1
- Medium – 2
- Large – 2
- Extra Large – 1

Scoop Stretcher (folding or nonfolding)

Dressings
- Elastic Gauze – 24 (minimum of 12, must be sterile)
- 4″×4″ Sterile Gauze Sponges – 36
- 4″×4″ Sterile Non-Porous Dressing – 4
- 8″×30″ Sterile Bulk Dressing – 4
- Tape, 1″ Roll – 3
- Disposable Gloves – 3 pairs
- Clean and/or Sterile Burn Sheets – 60″×90″ – 2
- Rigid Eye Shields – 2

Obstetrical Kits – Disposable – 1

Anti-Shock Trousers – 1, (Must have no less than three inflatable sections.)

MISCELLANEOUS EQUIPMENT:

Emesis Basins – 2

Stethoscope – 1

Sphygmomanometer
- Adult – 1
- Pediatric – 1

Sand Bags – 4

Bite Sticks – 2

Linen Supplies
- Pillow with Plastic Cover – 1
- Cot Sheets – 6
- Blankets – one each stretcher

SECURITY AND RESCUE EQUIPMENT:

Fire Extinguisher (2A-10BC Type) 5 lb – 2

Road Flares, 30 min. – 6

Flashlight – 2

Gauntlets – 2 pairs

Crowbar, 24″ – 1

Wrecking Bar, 51″ – 1

*K-Bar-T may be substituted for crowbar and wrecking bar

COMMUNICATION EQUIPMENT:

VHF or UHF Radio, to allow voice contact between ambulance and hospital and/or medical control)

Patient Care Report Forms

ADVANCED LIFE SUPPORT:

Have all above equipment, plus:

Portable Monitor/Defibrillator Operate independent of an electrical outlet, provide continuous monitoring by oscilloscope, provide a paper tape write-out

Contact Gel – 1 tube and/or

Defibrillator pads – 3

Monitoring Electrodes – 12

Patient Cable – 1

EKG Paper – 3 rolls

Airway Care
- Laryngoscope Handle – 1

Laryngoscope Blades
Adult – 1
Infant – 1
Intubation Tubes
Number and size to be indicated in medical advisor's standing orders
Sterile Intravenous Agents & Medications—number and type authorized by medical advisor
Copy of Standing Orders

Appendix C: Emergency Medical Service Ten-Codes

EXAMPLE LIST OF TEN-CODES*

10–1	Signal Weak
10–2	Signal Good
10–3	Stop Transmitting
10–4	Affirmative (OK)
10–5	Relay (To)
10–6	Busy
10–7	Out of Service
10–8	In Service
10–9	Say Again (Repeat)
10–10	Negative
10–11	___ On Duty
10–12	Stand By (Stop)
10–13	Existing Conditions
10–14	Message/Information
10–15	Message Delivered
10–16	Reply to Message
10–17	Enroute
10–18	Urgent (Quickly)
10–19	(In) Contact
10–20	Location
10–21	Call (________) by Phone
10–22	Disregard
10–23	Arrived at Scene
10–24	Assignment Completed
10–25	Report to (meet)
10–26	Estimated Arrival Time
10–27	License/Permit Information
10–28	Ownership Information
10–29	Records Check
10–30	Danger/Caution
10–31	Pick-Up
10–32	___ Units Needed (Specify)
10–33	Help Me Quick (Emergency)
10–34	Time
10–35	–Reserved–
10–36	–Reserved–
10–37	–Reserved–
10–38	–Reserved–
10–39	–Reserved–

*Reserved codes could be adopted to communicate
public in the area, attempted suicide, suspicion of intoxicants, and behavioral problems.

Appendix D: Phonetic Alphabet

A	Adam
B	Boy
C	Charlie
D	David
E	Edward
F	Frank
G	George
H	Henry
I	Ida
J	John
K	King
L	Lincoln
M	May
N	Nora
O	Ocean
P	Paul
Q	Queen
R	Robert
S	Sam
T	Tom
U	Union
V	Victor
W	William
X	X-Ray
Y	Young
Z	Zebra

Appendix E: Inventory—Trauma Crash Bag

TOP TRAY

2 – 14G Bard I Cath } 8″ cath
1 – 18.5 Bard I Cath } 8″ cath
2 – 14G Bard a Cath
2 – 16G Angio
2 – 18.5 Bard a Cath
2 – 21G Jelco
1 – 19G butterfly
? – opsite
1 – 1″ tape roll
1 – ½″ tape roll
1 – disposable razor
1 – note pad
1 – tourniquet

MIDDLE TRAY

8 – Kling
15 – 2″ × 2″ gauze sponges
2 – ice pak
15 – alcohol swipes
10 – Neosporin
15 – Bandaids
1 – oval eye pad

BOTTOM TRAY

1 – ring cutter
1 – window knife
1 – window punch
4 – triangular bandages
15 – towelettes
5 – oral airways
1 – bite stick
1 – scissors

BOTTOM AREA

2 – Adaptic
1 – Vaseline gauze
6 – 3″ × 3″ gauze sponges
12 – 4″ × 4″ gauze sponges (sterile)
1 – 7″ × 8″ abdominal pad
1 – trauma dressing
2 – Kerlix
stack of open 4″ × 4″ gauze sponges (non-sterile)
1 – arm splint
1 – BP cuff
1 – stethoscope
2 – ringers.
2 – macro I.V. sets
1 – I.V. kit

Appendix F: Inventory—Cardiac Crash Bag

TOP TRAY

laryngoscope w/3 blades
6 – oral airways
1 – 12cc syringe w/one-way valve
1 – 90° elbow
1 – scissors
2 – lasix
3 – lidocaine
3 – atropine
3 – epi (1:10,000)

MIDDLE TRAY

2 – 18G Bard I Cath } 8″ cath
2 – 16G Bard I Cath }
2 – 14G Bard a Cath
2 – 16 Angio
2 – 18G Bard a Cath
2 – 22G Jelco
1 – 19G butterfly
1 – 21G butterfly
1 – tourniquet
? – opsite
1 – 1″ wide tape
1 – ½″ wide tape
1 – disposable razor
1 – note pad
6 – electrodes

BOTTOM AREA

1 – BP cuff
1 – stethoscope
1 – I.V. kit
1 – bag, valve device
2 – face masks
5 – E.T. tubes (9.0, 8.0, 7.0, 5.0, 3.5)
2 – stylettes (lg & sm)
1 – Magill forceps
3 – bicarbs
2 – D5O
2 – D5W
1 – D5W w/0.4% lidocaine
3 – microdrip admin. sets
1 – arm splint
1 – Kerlix
2 – 3″ × 8″ adapties

BOTTOM TRAY

2 – 3″ Kling
1 – 30 ml ipecac syrup
1 – activated charcoal
1 – contact lens holder & solution
10 – 2″ gauze sponges
15 – Bandaids
10 – Neosporin
15 – alcohol swipes
1 – 2½cc syringe
1 – 3cc syringe
1 – 6cc syringe
1 – 12cc syringe
1 – tubex syringe
5 – narcan
3 – epi (1:1,000)
2 – m.s.
5 – monoject 21G
5 – monoject 19G
2 – red top holders
3 – red tops

Appendix G: Daily Emergency Vehicle Inspection Checklist

Name: ______________________ Date: ____________ Time: ______

Vehicle Identification No.: ______________________ Location: ______________

		OK	FIX		OK	FIX
APPROACH VEHICLE	Vehicle Attitude	☐	☐	Body Damage	☐	☐
	Remarks: ______________________					
UNDER HOOD	Hoses	☐	☐	Belts	☐	☐
				Oil	☐	☐
Fluids:	*Radiator	☐	☐	Steering Fluid	☐	☐
	Windshield Washer	☐	☐	Brake Fluid	☐	☐
	Battery	☐	☐	Transmission Fluid	☐	☐
	Remarks: ______________________					
IN VEHICLE	Cleanliness	☐	☐	Oil Pressure	☐	☐
	Seat Adjustment	☐	☐	Brake Action	☐	☐
	Seat Belt	☐	☐	Air Pressure	☐	☐
	Outer Mirrors	☐	☐	Turn Signals	☐	☐
	Interior Lights	☐	☐	Communications	☐	☐
	Fuel Gauge	☐	☐	Siren/Audibles/Horn	☐	☐
	Alternator	☐	☐	PA System	☐	☐
	Temperature	☐	☐	Fire Extinguisher	☐	☐
	Windshield Wipers	☐	☐	Parking Brake	☐	☐
	Inner Mirrors	☐	☐			
	Remarks: ______________________					
WALK AROUND VEHICLE	Headlights	☐	☐	Emergency Lights	☐	☐
	Running Lights	☐	☐	Flood	☐	☐
	Brake Lights	☐	☐	Body	☐	☐
	Four-Way Flasher	☐	☐	Wheels	☐	☐
	Tires	☐	☐	Windshield	☐	☐
	Doors	☐	☐	Turn Signals	☐	☐
	Remarks: ______________________					
DYNAMIC VEHICLE INSPECTION	Steering/Smoothness	☐	☐	Brakes	☐	☐
	Unusual Noises	☐	☐	Suspension	☐	☐
	Remarks: ______________________					

*Radiator must be cool to avoid injury and to make accurate inspection.

BIBLIOGRAPHY

American Academy of Orthopaedic Surgeons. *Emergency Care and Transportation of the Sick and Injured*. 3rd Ed. Chicago, IL: American Academy of Orthopaedic Surgeons, 1981.

Caroline, Nancy L., M.D. *Emergency Care in the Streets*. 2nd Ed.Boston, MA: Little, Brown and Company, 1983.

Clark, J. M. *Emergency and High Speed Driving Techniques*. Texas: Gulf Publishing Company, 1976.

Drake, G. N. *Let's Drive to Survive! A Guide to Cost-effective Advanced Driver Training*. Massachusetts: Phoenix Books, 1981.

Gregg and Associates. *American Ambulance Association Loss ControlManual*. Phoenix, Arizona, 1982.

Grant, H. *Vehicle Rescue*. Maryland: Robert J. Brady Publishing Co., 1975.

Grant, H., Murray, R. H., Jr., Bergeron, David J. *Emergency Care*. 3rd Ed. Maryland: Robert J. Brady Company, 1982.

Hanna, J. A. *Ambulance and EMS Driving*. Virginia: Reston Publishing Company, 1983.

Misener, W. R. *Defensive Pursuit Driving*. Mid-State Technical Institute.

National Safety Council. *Student Workbook and Defensive Drivers Manual*. 7th Ed. National Safety Council: 1975.

Schults, D. P., Dobey, R. G. *Advanced Driving Techniques, Operational Handbook*. Minnesota: St. Cloud State University, 1980.

Traffic Safety Institute College of Law Enforcement, Eastern KentuckyUniversity. *Advanced Driving for Law Enforcement Personnel*. Kentucky: Eastern Kentucky University, 1976.

U.S. Department of Transportation. *National Highway Traffic Safety Administration: Training Program for Operation of Emergency Vehicles*. Washington, DC: U.S. Government Printing Office, 1978.

West, Katherine H., R.N. B.S.N. *Infection Control Recommendationsfor Rescue Vehicles*. Alexandria, Virginia: 1982.

Index

NOTES

NOTES

NOTES

NOTES